Textbook of MICROBIOLOGY for Nursing Students

SECOND EDITION

RR Rao MD MAMS (FICpath)
Professor and Head
Department of Microbiology
Kamineni Academy of Medical Sciences
Hyderabad, Andhra Pradesh, India

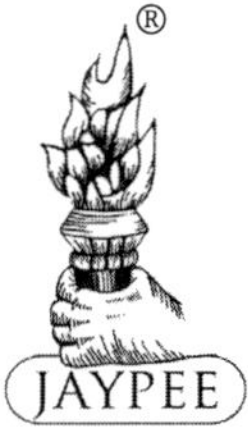

JAYPEE BROTHERS MEDICAL PUBLISHERS (P) LTD

New Delhi • London • Philadelphia • Panama

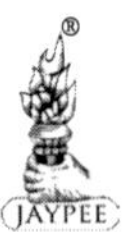

Jaypee Brothers Medical Publishers (P) Ltd

Headquarters

Jaypee Brothers Medical Publishers (P) Ltd
4838/24, Ansari Road, Daryaganj
New Delhi 110 002, India
Phone: +91-11-43574357
Fax: +91-11-43574314
Email: jaypee@jaypeebrothers.com

Overseas Offices

J.P. Medical Ltd
83, Victoria Street, London
SW1H 0HW (UK)
Phone: +44-2031708910
Fax: +02-03-0086180
Email: info@jpmedpub.com

Jaypee-Highlights Medical Publishers Inc
City of Knowledge, Bld. 237, Clayton
Panama City, Panama
Phone: + 507-301-0496
Fax: + 507-301-0499
Email: cservice@jphmedical.com

Jaypee Medical Inc
The Bourse
111 South Independence Mall East
Suite 835, Philadelphia, PA 19106, USA
Phone: + 267-519-9789
Email: joe.rusko@jaypeebrothers.com

Jaypee Brothers Medical Publishers (P) Ltd
17/1-B Babar Road, Block-B, Shaymali
Mohammadpur, Dhaka-1207
Bangladesh
Mobile: +08801912003485
Email: jaypeedhaka@gmail.com

Jaypee Brothers Medical Publishers (P) Ltd
Shorakhute, Kathmandu
Nepal
Phone: +00977-9841528578
Email: jaypee.nepal@gmail.com

Website: www.jaypeebrothers.com
Website: www.jaypeedigital.com

Inquiries for bulk sales may be solicited at: jaypee@jaypeebrothers.com

Textbook of Microbiology for Nursing Students
First Edition: 2005
Reprint: 2007
Second Edition: ***2014,*** Reprint: 2023

ISBN 978-93-5090-977-5

Printed in India

Dedicated to

My Grandfather

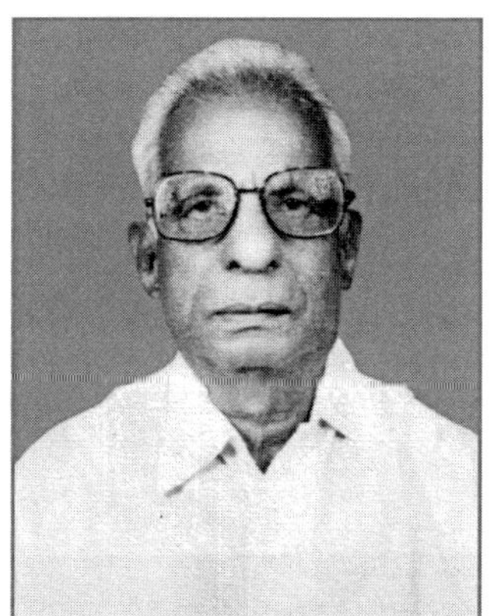

(1914–2004)

Late Sri B Harisarvothama Rao

Preface to the Second Edition

During the last 5 to 10 years, the importance of microbiology has been well recognized by all categories of healthcare personnel. With many hospitals undergoing for accreditation by the National Board of Hospitals (NABH), more stress is on infection control. At present, many known pathogens causing infections in humans both in the hospital and at the level of community are showing increasing resistance to various antibiotics including the Penicillins and Cephalosporins. Apart from increasing resistance, new organisms are emerging as pathogens, which were earlier considered as commensals or harmless microorganisms. Therefore, it is becoming more important to take adequate steps to prevent or control the infection rather than treating it after getting established. Infection control committee is playing an important role in many hospitals. Keeping in view of these changing trends and also taking into the consideration of experts' constructive comments on the first edition of this book, it has been decided to revise the *Textbook of Microbiology for Nursing Students* by expanding its frontiers by including more information to the existing one. Accordingly, several topics have been expanded or introduced freshly. In addition to the chapters like 'Hand Hygine' and 'Biological Waste Management', a new chapter on 'Infection Control Guidelines' has been included.

I am glad that the students of nursing profession as well as faculty from all over the country welcomed the first edition of this book and appreciated the simplified principles of microbiology. I am of the opinion that with the same zeal, they would also welcome this revised second edition and expand their knowledge of microbiology.

I thank all those experts who spared the time to review the first edition of this book and provided valuable comments. As far as possible, their suggestions have been implemented in this second edition. I hope, the students of nursing profession will be comfortable in reading the second edition and practice the implementation of principles of microbiology in preventing the infection and/or in controlling it.

RR Rao

Preface to the First Edition

Microbiology is relatively a new specialty of medicine. But, during the last 50 years or so, it grew tremendously and made a strong impact on not only among the medical professionals but also on the public health. The importance of infectious diseases has been widely recognized and a number of textbooks written by distinguished authors are available that provide vast information, which is being updated continuously. Considerable importance has been given to microbiology in the curriculum of medical and paramedical courses to understand, to diagnose, to treat, and to control a variety of infectious diseases both communicable and non-communicable. However, a student nurse entering the nursing profession is in dilemma that how much information is needed for her/him to remember and practice microbiology in routine. Moreover, a first year nursing student is supposed to undergo training in as many as ten subjects related to nursing along with microbiology. To lessen the burden on the students and to emphasize on only the most practicable fundamentals of microbiology, an attempt has been made in this book to abridge the available information, stressing more importance on proper collection and transportation of microbiological specimens, adequate knowledge on disinfection and sterilization procedure, management of biological waste, and last but not least, the role of "Hand Hygiene". Detailed descriptions of morphological, cultural and biochemical characters of various microorganisms and their complex antigenic structures are simplified, as they are not necessary for a student of nursing. Instead, adequate importance has been placed on the clinical signs and symptoms of various infectious diseases for their early recognition, so that nursing staff are geared up to apply appropriate preventive measures to curtail the spread of the infection, either in the hospitals or in the community. This textbook has been divided into different sections without discontinuity, in order to make the student feel comfortable and develop interest to read and remember the contents of the respective sections. Detailed discussions on some topics have been avoided keeping in view of their rare occurrence in day-to-day practice. An attempt has been made to provide more illustrations to create a visual impact that creates a long-lasting memory.

I take this opportunity to express my sincere gratitude to my professor and mentor Dr CS Bhaskaran who always encouraged me in all my attempts. I also express my respects to my teachers like Prof Dr KC Agarwal, Prof Dr RC Mahajan, Prof Dr NK Ganguly, Prof Dr SN Saxena, under whom, I had the opportunity to work and improve my skills and knowledge in this specialty.

RR Rao

Contents

Section 1: General Microbiology

Section 2: Immunology

Section 3: Study of Infectious Diseases

PLATE 1

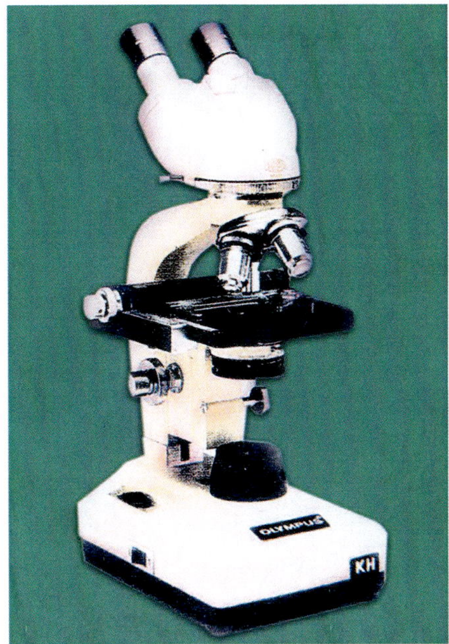

Fig. 1.1: Binocular compound microscope

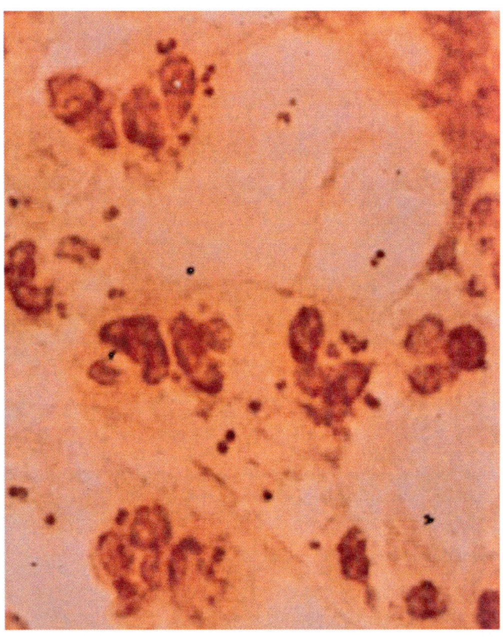

Fig. 3.1: Gram-negative intracellular cocci (meningococci) (×100)

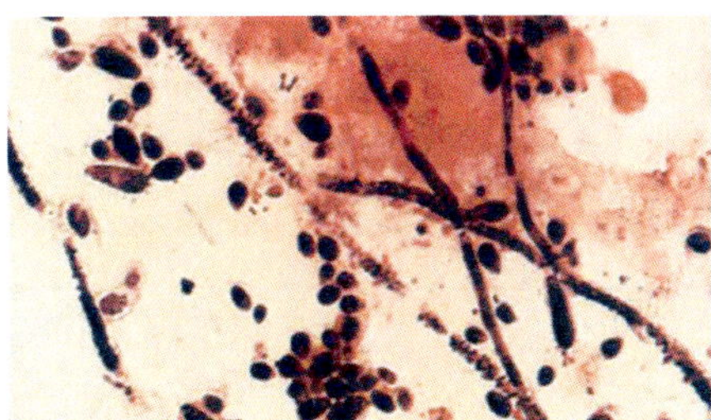

Fig. 3.4: Yeast-like budding cells along with pseudomycelia *Candida albicans* (×100)

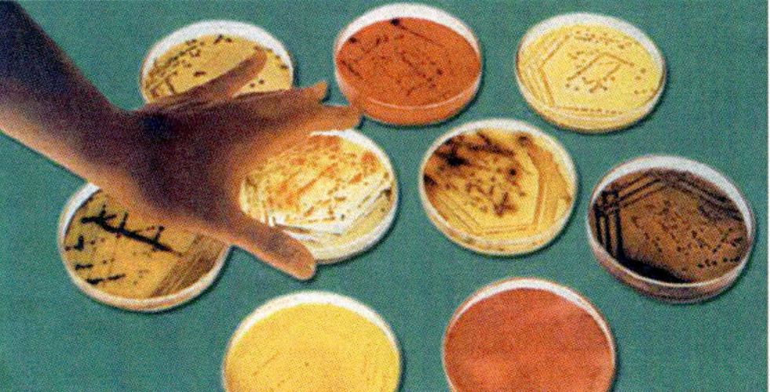

Fig. 6.1: Various types of nutrient media which support the growth of bacteria

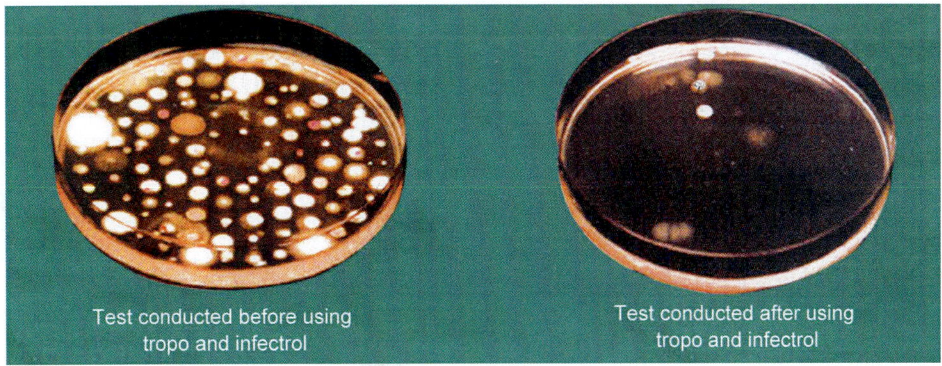

Fig. 7.1: Nutrient agar plates showing the effect of disinfection. Note the number of colonies have reduced after disinfection (right side)

PLATE 2

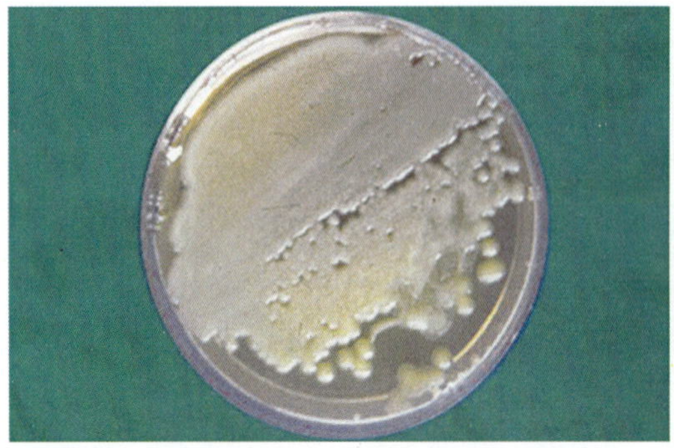

CL 1: Agar plate showing mucoid colonies of *Klebsiella pneumoniae*

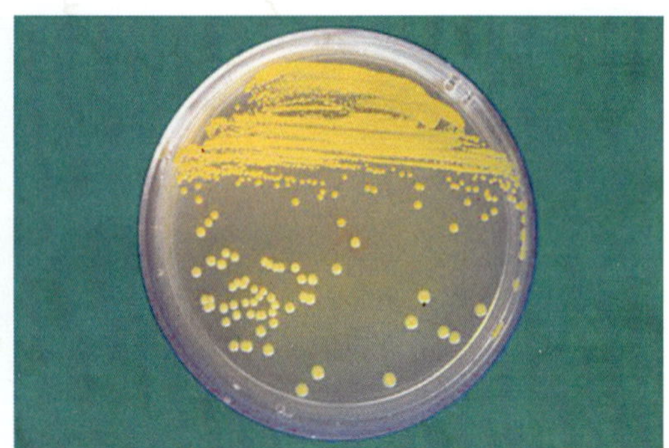

CL 2: Agar plate showing discrete colonies

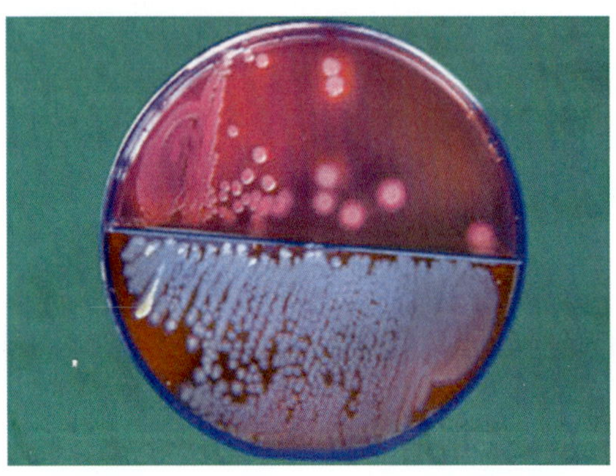

CL 3: Colonies of blood agar and MacConkey/ CLED agar

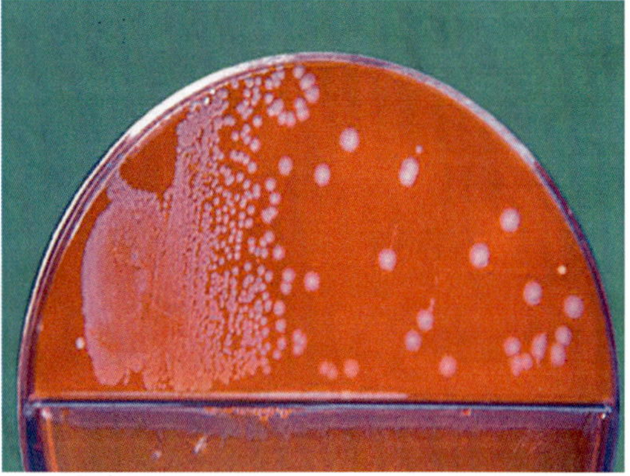

CL 4: Blood agar showing colonies of staphylococci

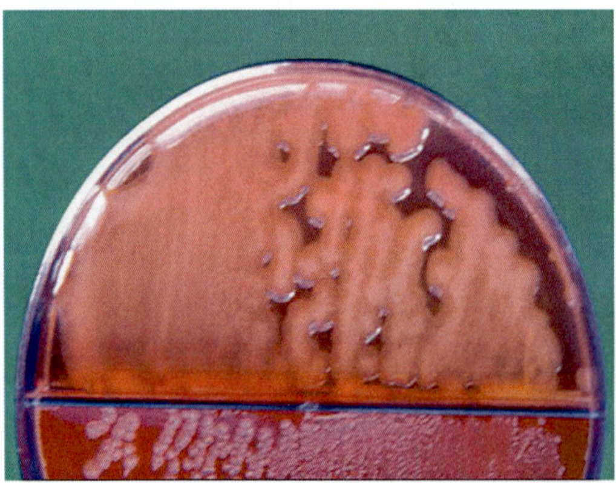

CL 5: MacConkey agar showing pink colored mucoid colonies of *Klebsiella pneumoniae*

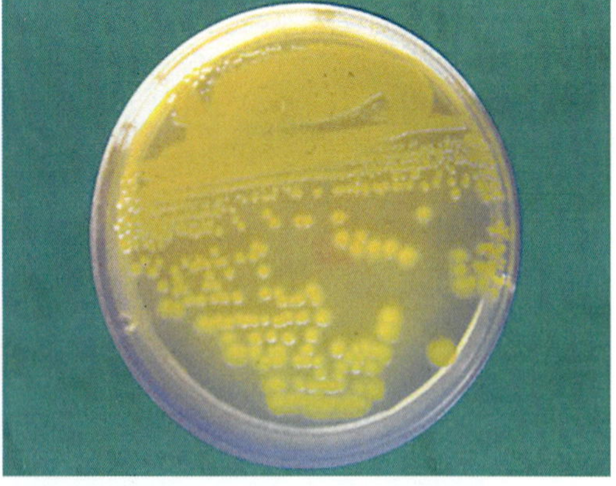

CL 6: CLED agar plate showing yellowish colored colonies due to lactose fermentation

Fig. 6.3: Enteric media (CL 1 to 6)

PLATE 3

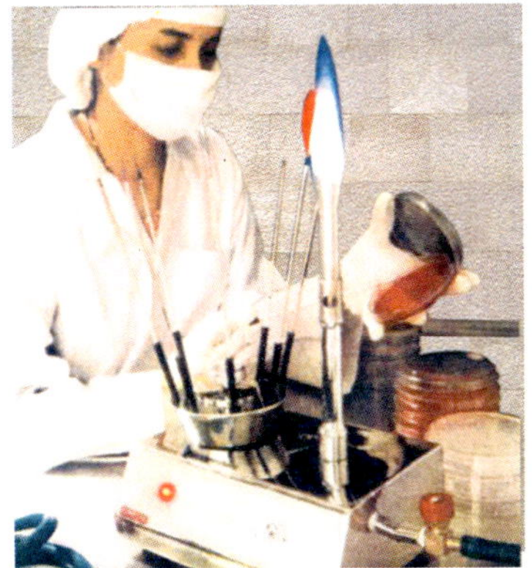

Fig. 6.2: Inoculation of specimen on culture media

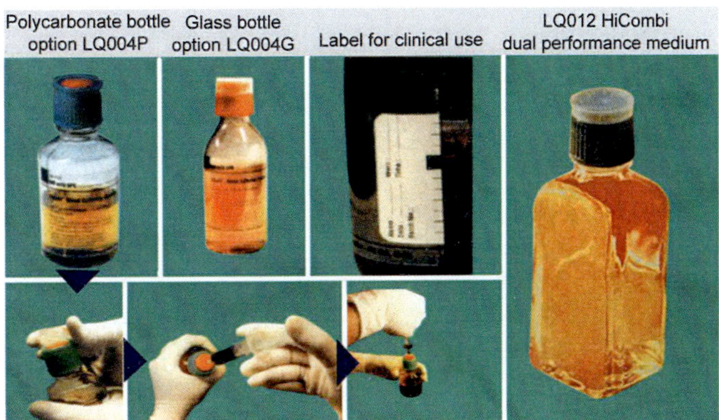

Fig. 8.1: Blood culture bottle and collection of blood for culture under aseptic conditions. LQ—Liquid medium store between 2–8°C, SPS—Sodium polyanethol sulfonate (liquid)

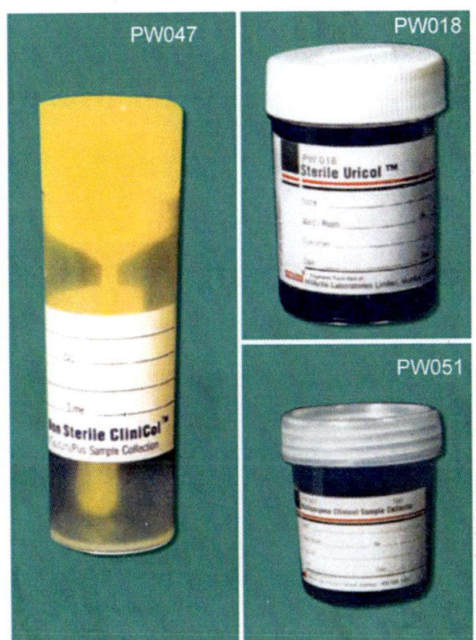

Fig. 8.3: Specimen collectors for urine, feces, and sputum

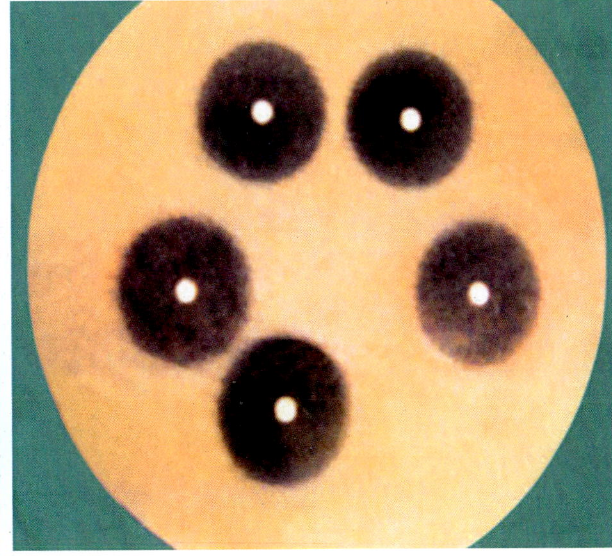

Fig. 8.4: Antibiotic sensitivity testing. Note the clear zone around the antibiotic disk indicating that the organism is sensitive to that antibiotic

PLATE 4

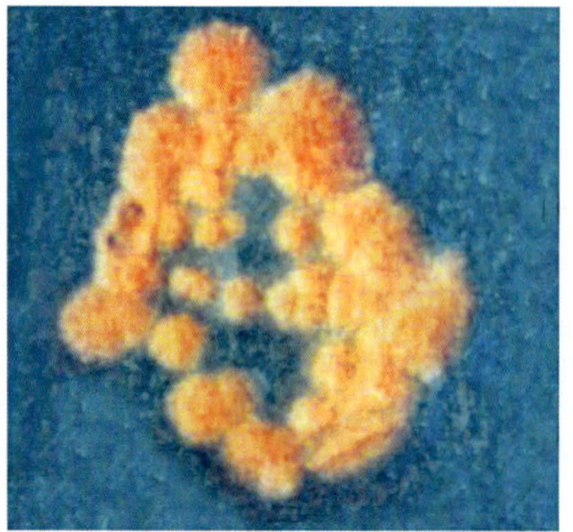

Fig. 17.1: Growth of *M. tuberculosis* on LJ medium. Note the color and shape of the colony

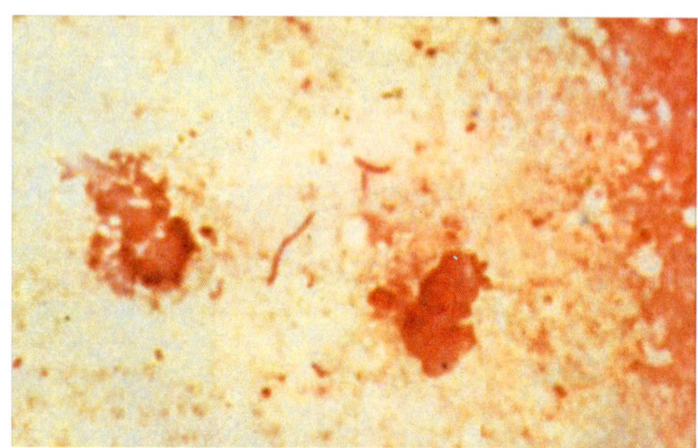

Fig. 17.2: Gram-stained film of the CSF from a patient of *Haemophilus influenzae* meningitis

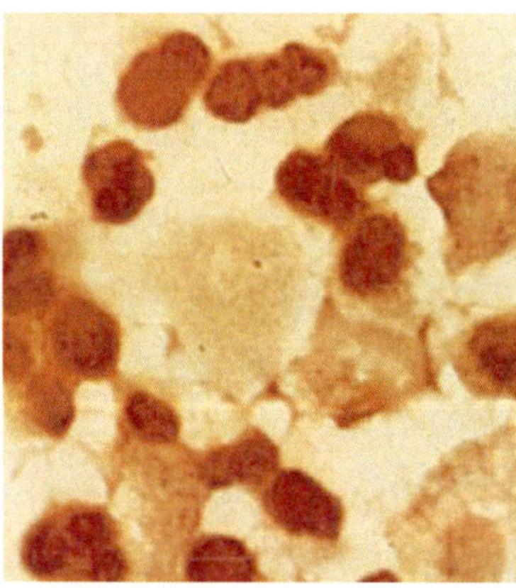

Fig. 17.3: Gram-stained film showing Gram-negative diplococci within the cells (meningococci) (×100)

Fig. 17.4: Rose spots in a patient with typhoid fever

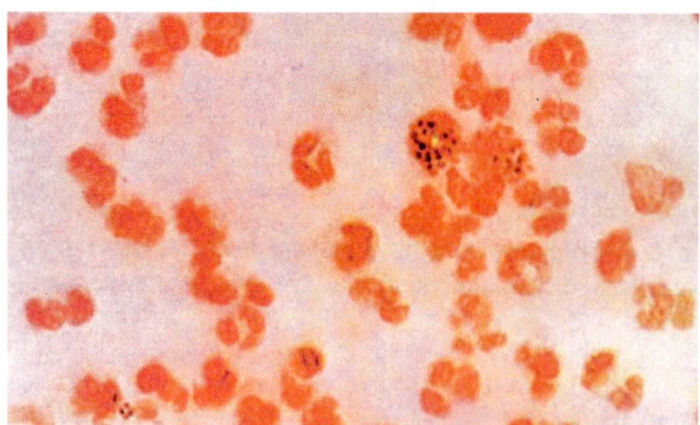

Fig. 17.5: Intracellular gram-negative cocci in pairs. Gonococci (×100)

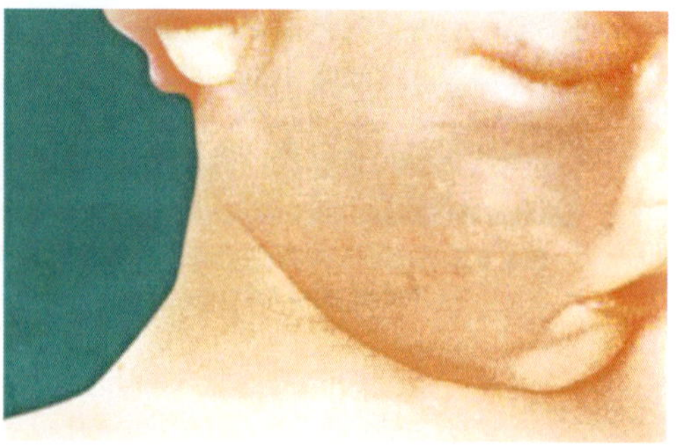

Fig. 17.7: Staphylococcal infection

PLATE 5

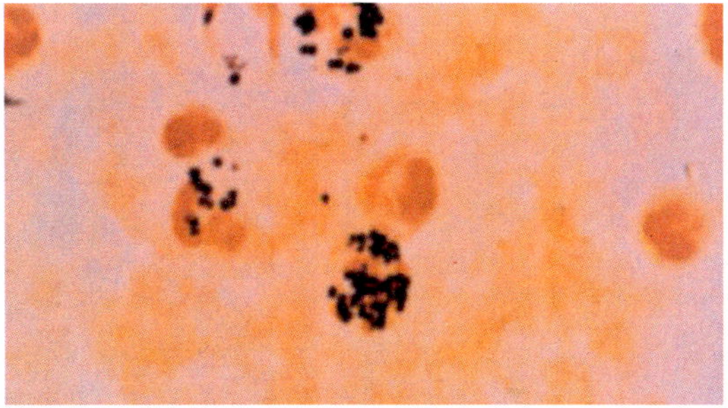

Fig. 17.8: Gram-positive cocci in clusters. Note many of them are intracellular staphylococci (×100)

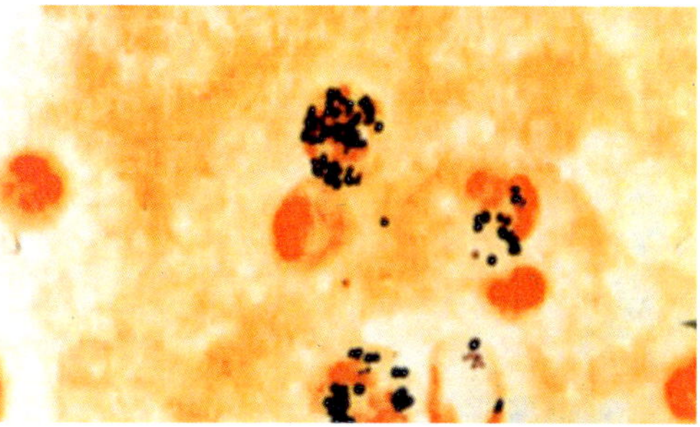

Fig. 17.9: Gram-positive cocci in clusters along with pus cells. Staphylococci (×100)

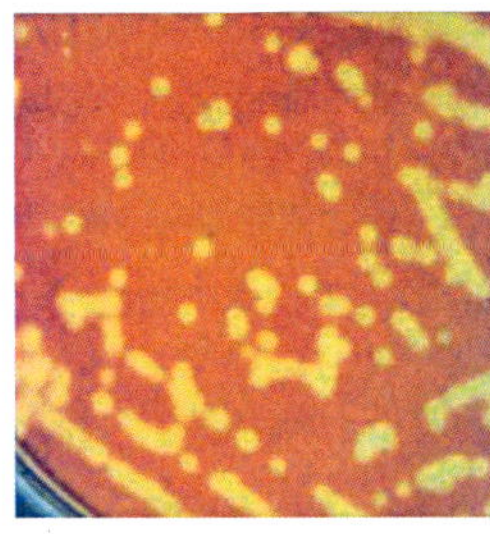

Fig. 17.10: Colonies of β-hemolytic streptococci. Note the clear zone of hemolysis on sheep blood agar

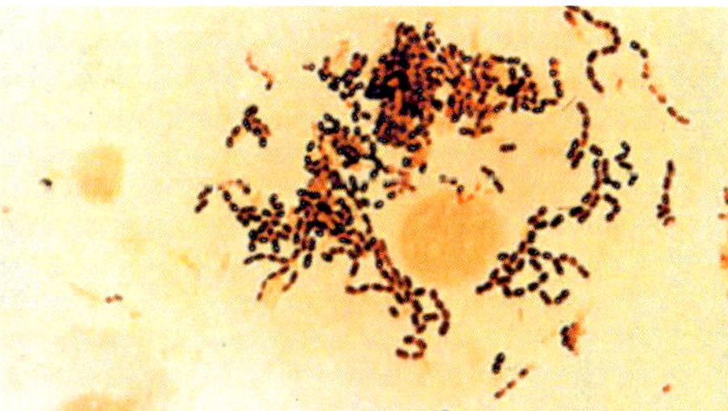

Fig. 17.11: Gram-positive cocci arranged in chains streptococci. Gram stain (×100)

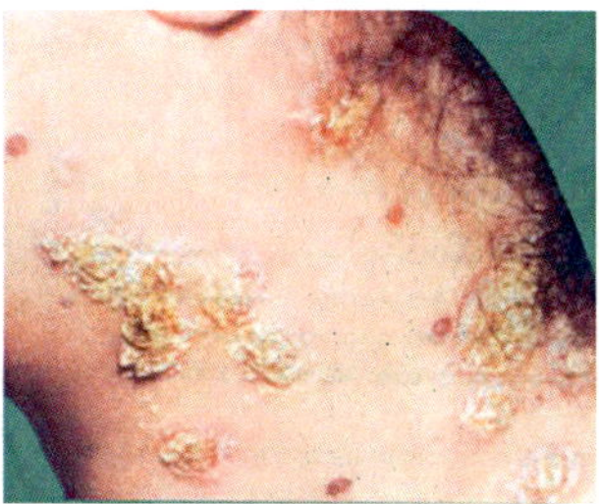

Fig. 17.12: Streptococcal infection

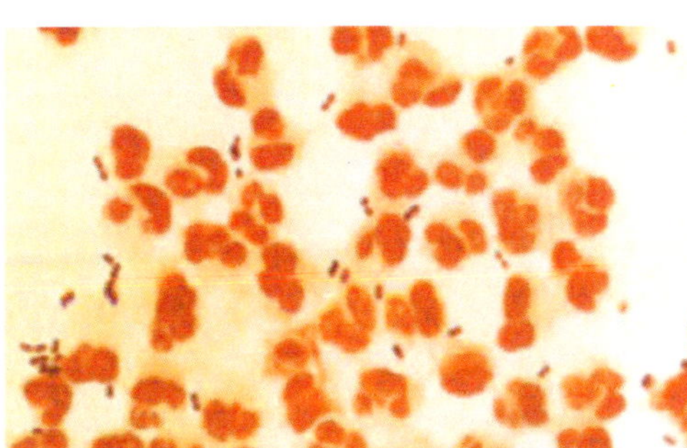

Fig. 17.13: Pus cells with gram-positive cocci in pairs. Pneumococci Gram stain (×100)

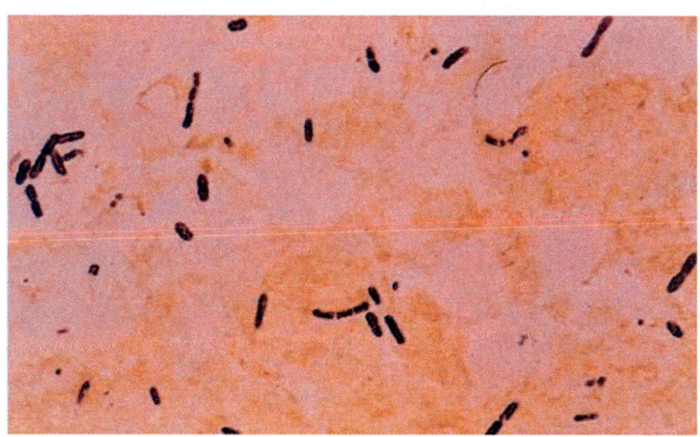

Fig. 17.14: Gram-positive thick bacilli from a gangrene patient. *Clostridium* species (×100)

PLATE 6

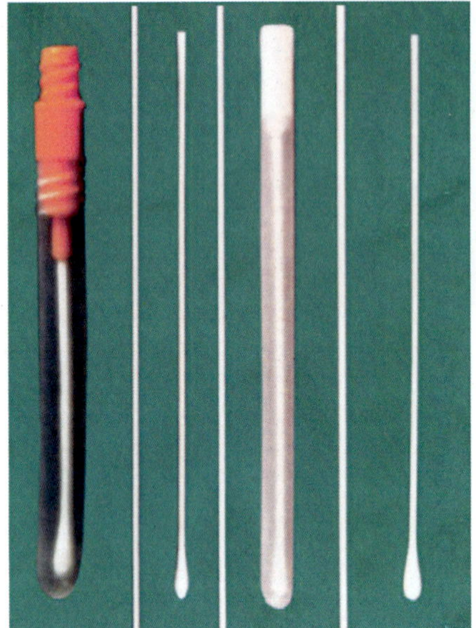

Fig. 21.1: Swabs for the collection of specimens like pus or throat swab, nasal swab, wound swab, etc.

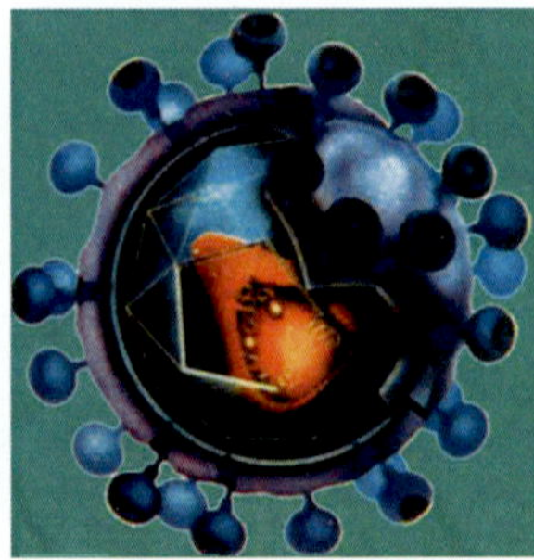

Fig. 22.1: Schematic diagram of hepatitis B virus

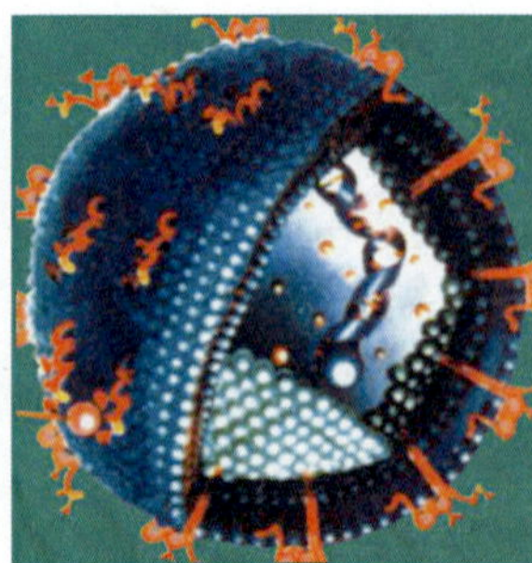

Fig. 22.2: Schematic diagram of human immunodeficiency virus

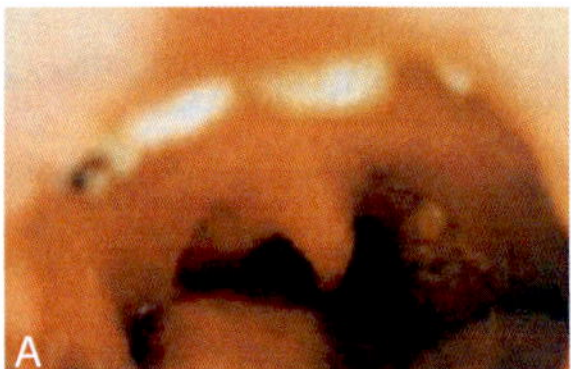

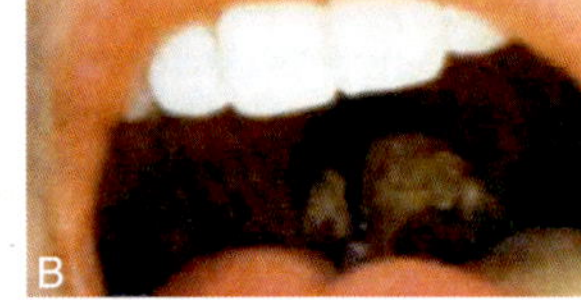

Fig. 22.3: Streptococcal pharyngitis and infectious mononucleosis

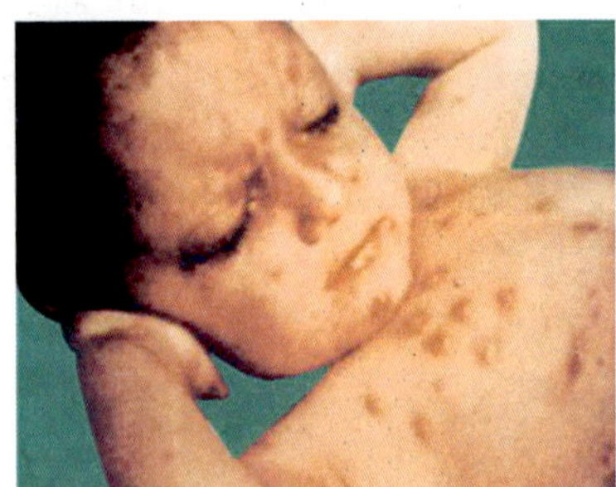

Fig. 22.4: A baby with chickenpox. Note the erythematous papules and pustules mostly on chest and abdomen. Less number on the face

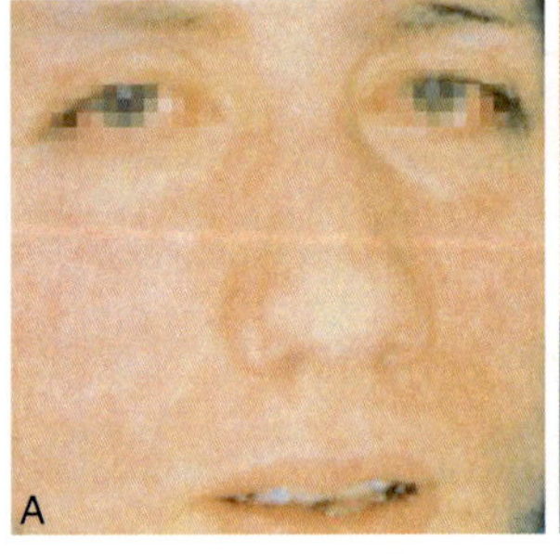

Fig. 22.5: Rash, conjunctivitis, and Koplik's spots due to measles infection

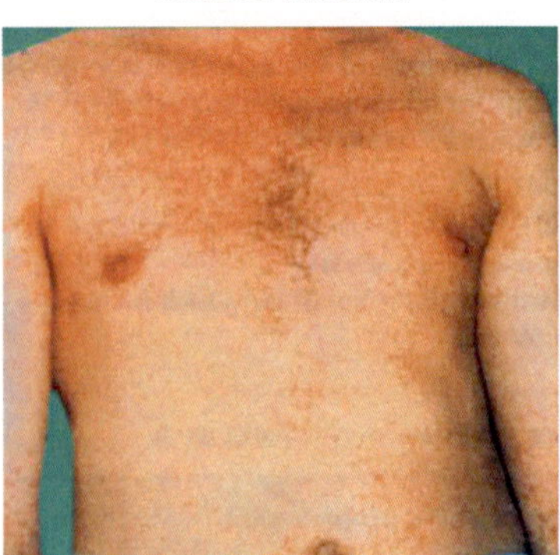

Fig. 22.6: A patient showing skin rash due to rubella infection

PLATE 7

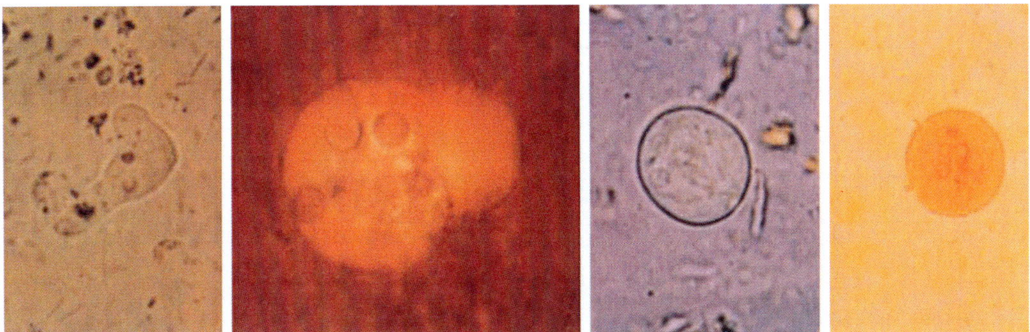

Fig. 23.1: Trophozoite and cyst form of *Entamoeba histolytica*. Note the presence of RBC within the cytoplasm of *E. histolytica* trophozoite form

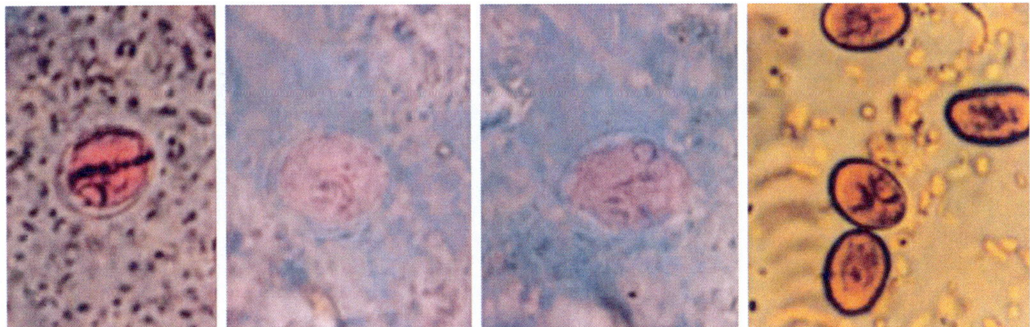

Fig. 23.3: Trophozoites and cysts of *Giardia lamblia*

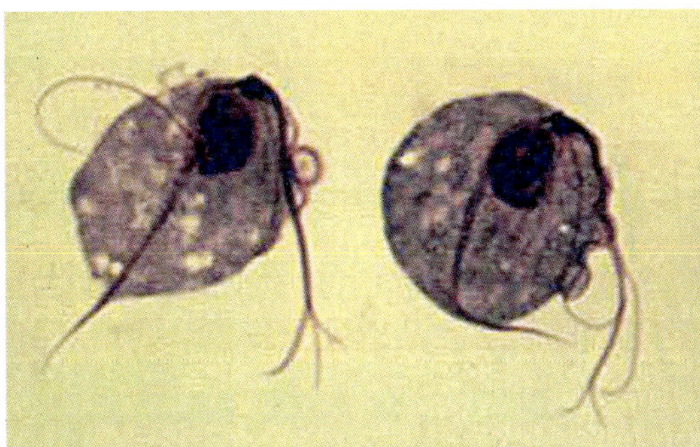

Fig. 23.5: *Trichomonas vaginalis*

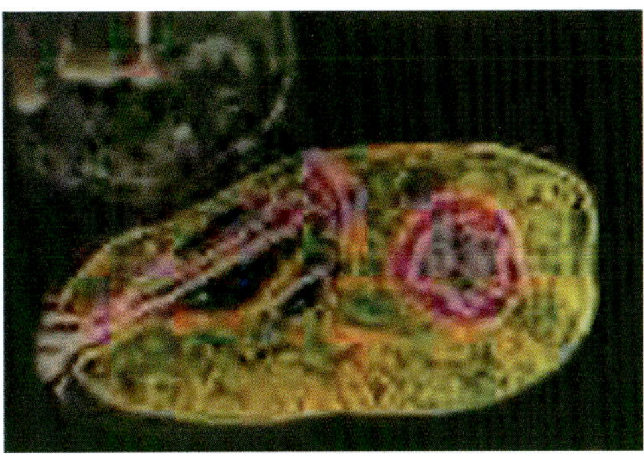

Fig. 23.6: *Leishmania*

PLATE 8

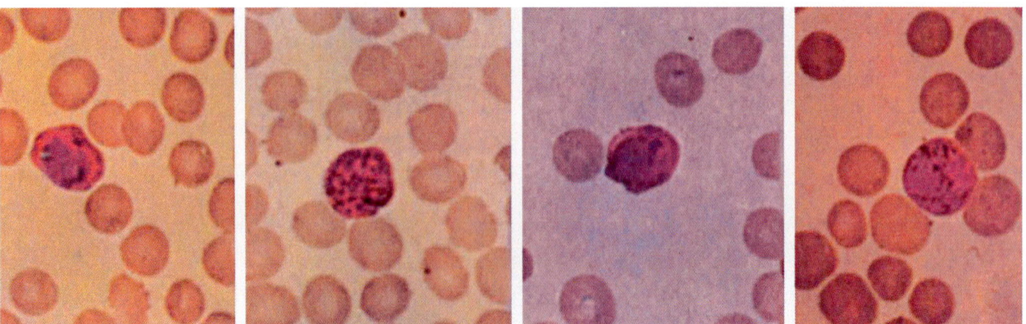

Fig. 23.9: Schizont stage of malarial parasite (*Plasmodium vivax*)

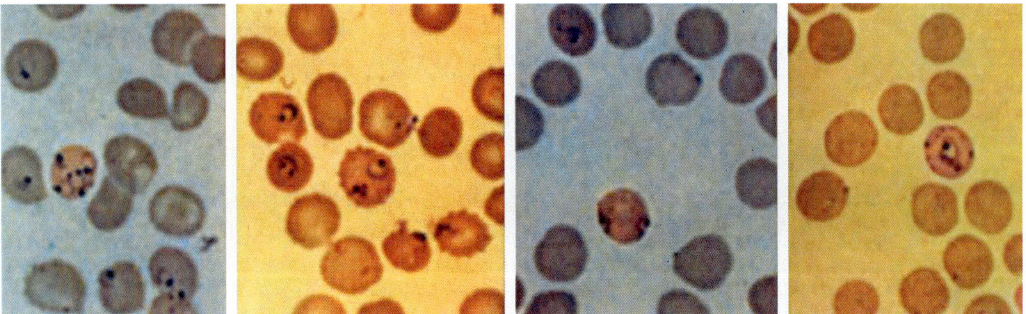

Fig. 23.10: Ring forms and schizont stage of malarial parasite

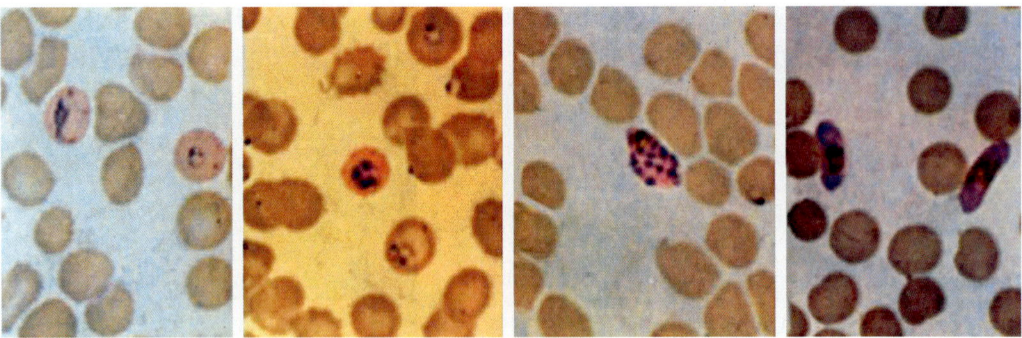

Fig. 23.11: Ring forms and gametocytes of *Plasmodium falciparum*

PLATE 9

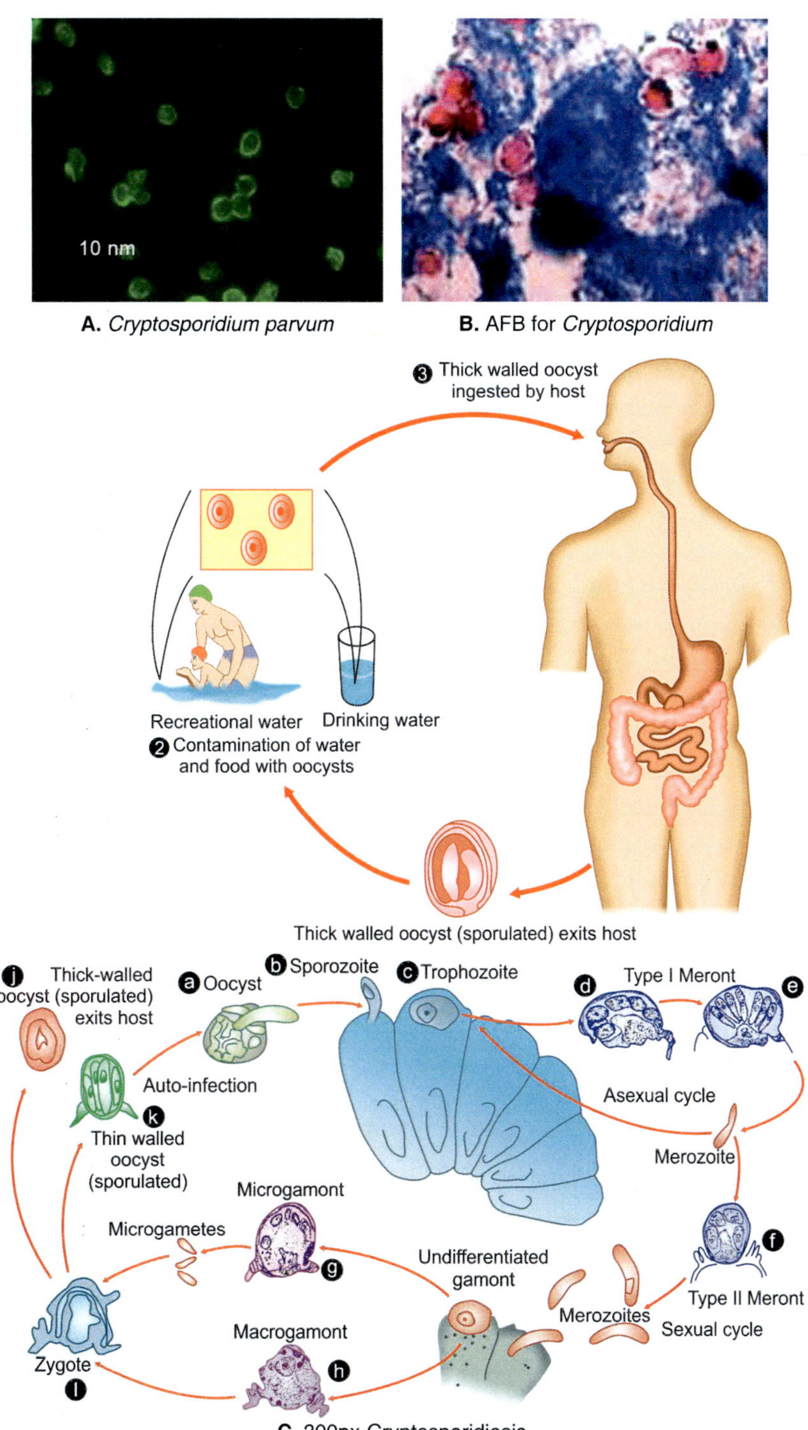

A. *Cryptosporidium parvum*

B. AFB for *Cryptosporidium*

C. 300px-Cryptosporidiosis

Fig. 23.14: Life cycle of *Cryptosporidium*

PLATE 10

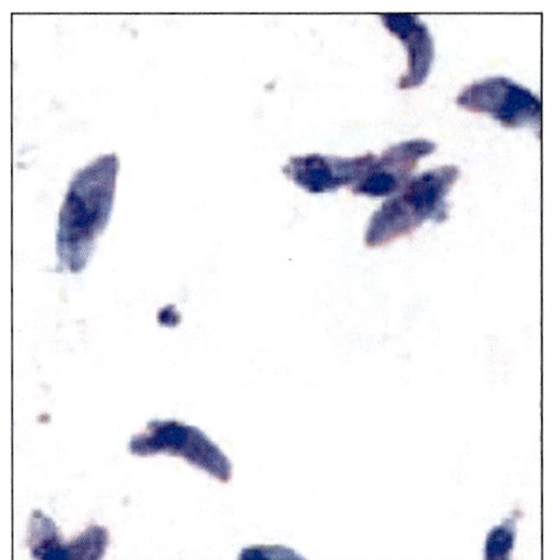

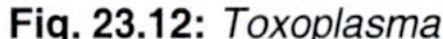

Fig. 23.12: *Toxoplasma*

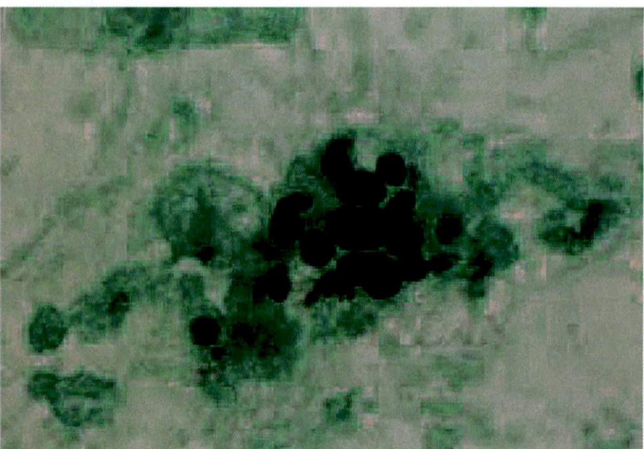

Fig. 23.15: *Pneumocystis carinii*

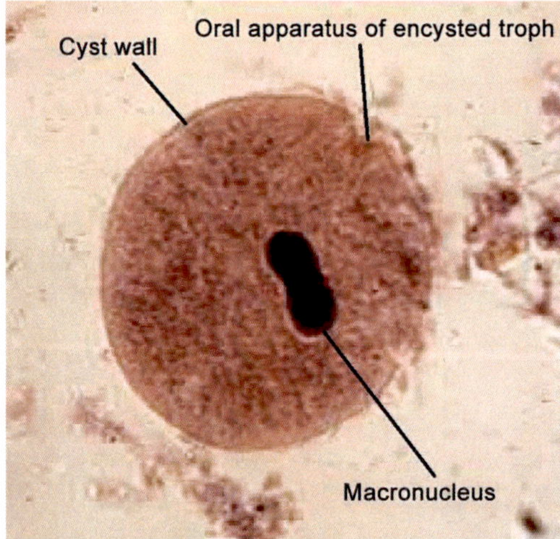

Fig. 23.16: *Balantidium coli*

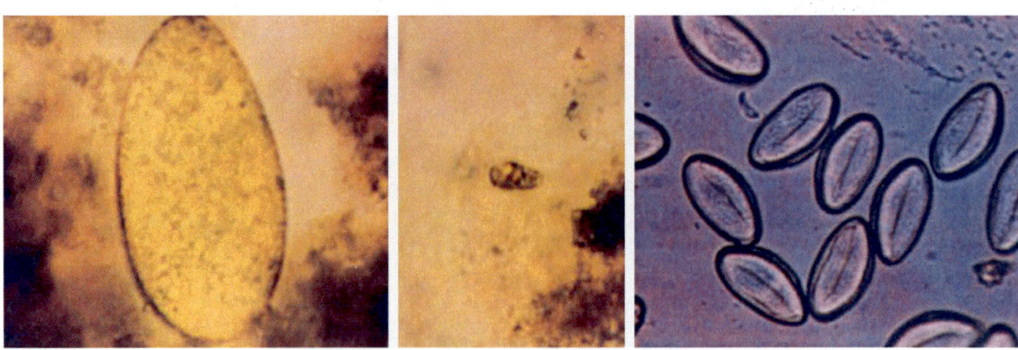

Fig. 23.18: Ova of liver fluke and pinworm (*Enterobius vermicularis*)

PLATE 11

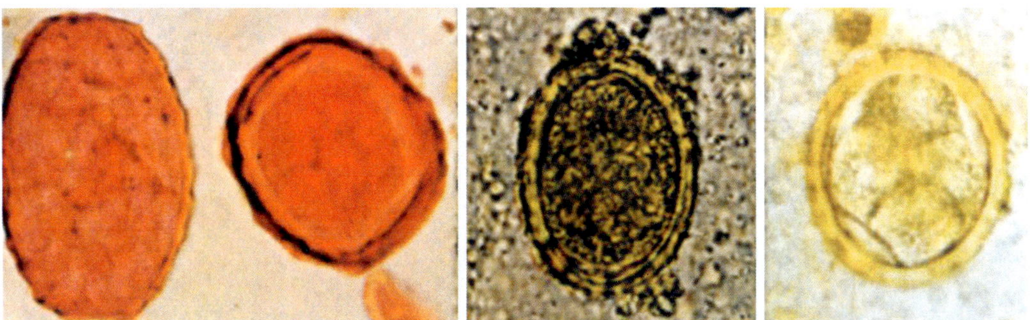

Fig. 23.19: Ova of the roundworm (*Ascaris lumbricoides*)

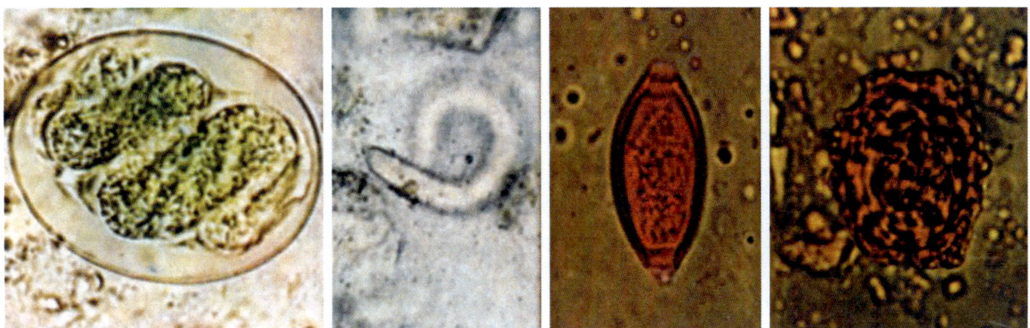

Fig. 23.21: Hookworm embryo and ova of the whipworm (*Trichuris trichiura*)

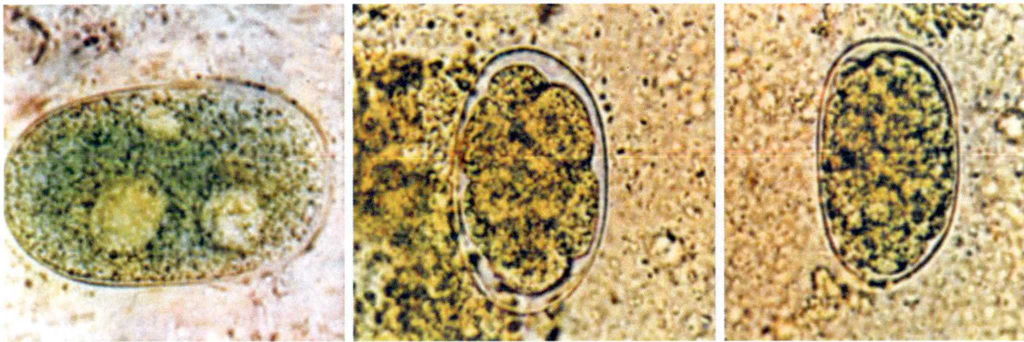

Fig. 23.23: Ova of the hookworm with embryo in different stages

PLATE 12

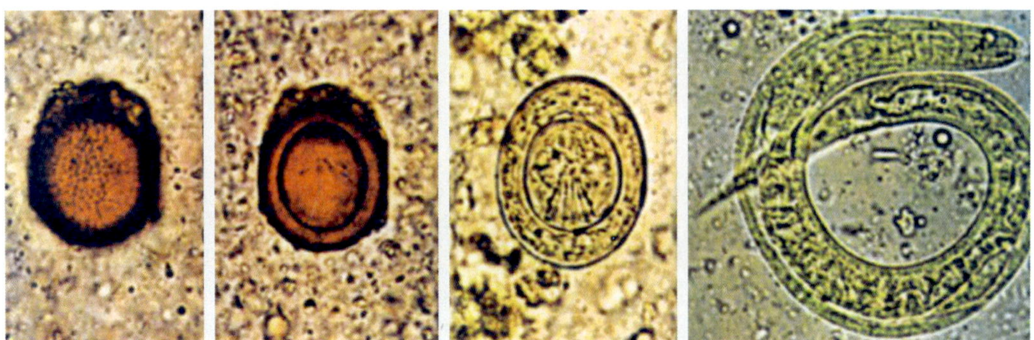

Fig. 23.30: Ova of tapeworm (*Taenia solium*, *T. saginata*, and *Hymenolepis nana*)

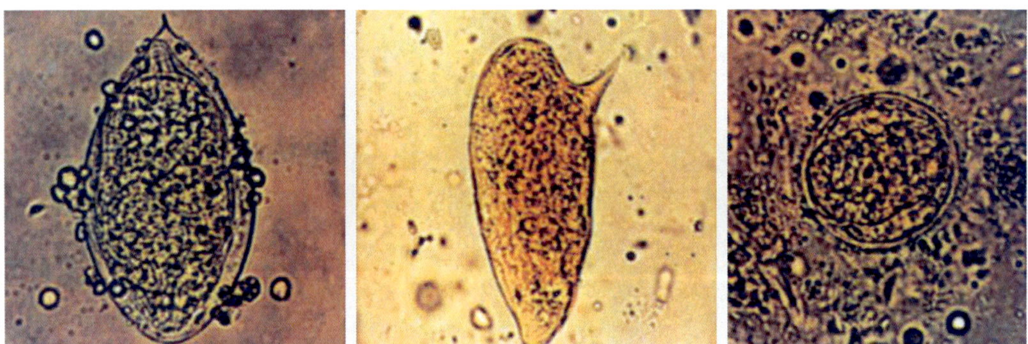

Fig. 23.31: Ova of the blood flukes

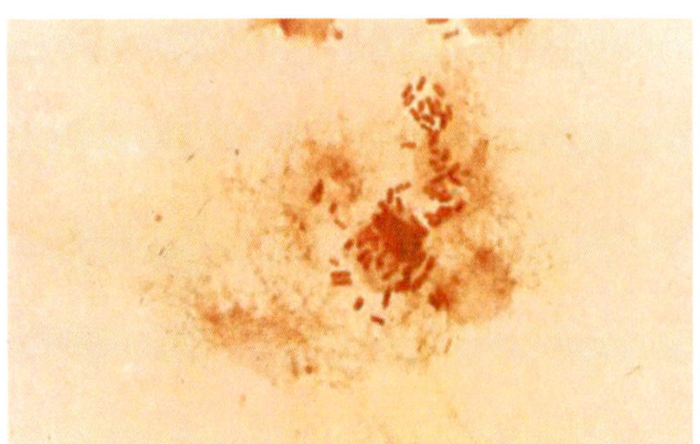

Fig. 25.1: Pus cells with gram-negative bacilli. Gram stain of urine smear (×100)

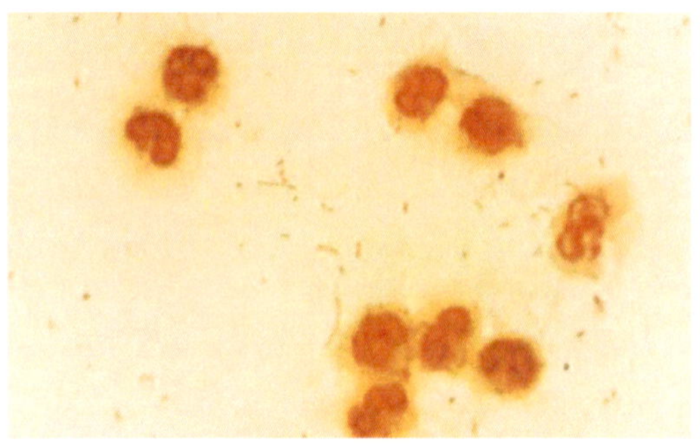

Fig. 25.2: Pus cells with gram-negative bacilli (×100)

PLATE 13

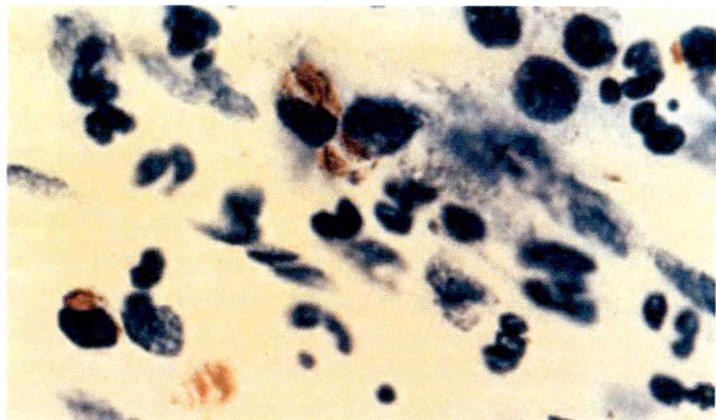

Fig. 25.3: Intracellular acid–fast bacilli. Note bundle of pink-colored slender rods. Z–N stain (×100)

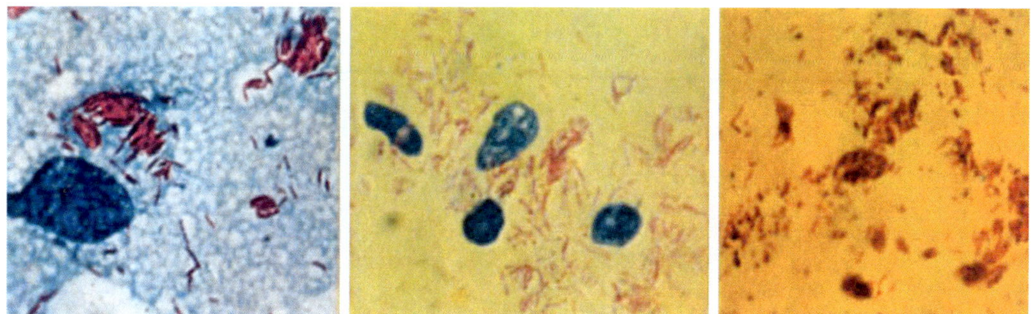

Fig. 25.4: Pink-stained acid–fast bacilli (Z–N stain). Note the different morphological forms

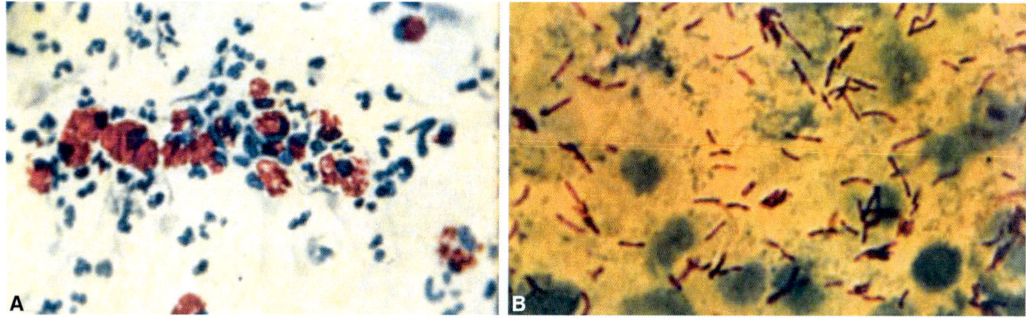

Fig. 25.5: (A) Ziehl–Neelsen stained smear of a nasal scraping from a patient with lepromatous leprosy showing red staining AAFB—*Mycobacterium leprae*—in globi. **(B)** Sputum from a patient with tuberculosis stained by the Ziehl–Neelsen method to show red acid and AAFB—*Mycobacterium tuberculosis*

PLATE 14

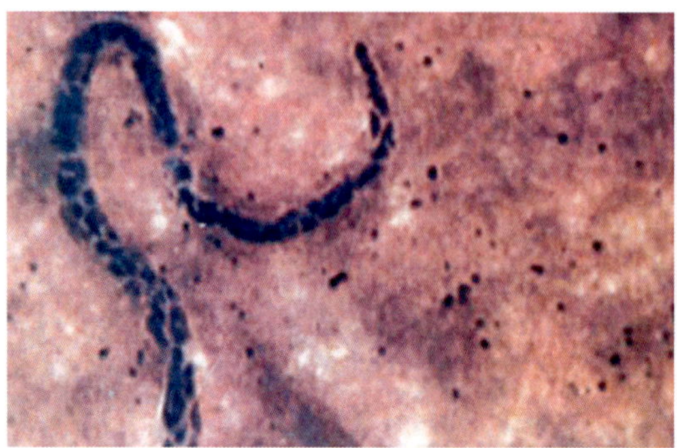

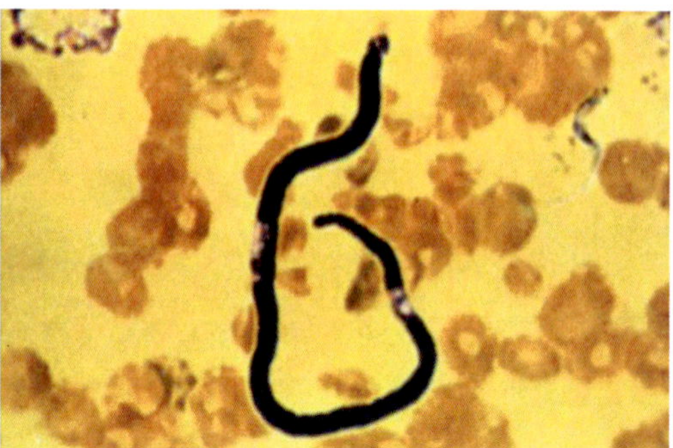

Fig. 25.6: Microfilaria in blood smear

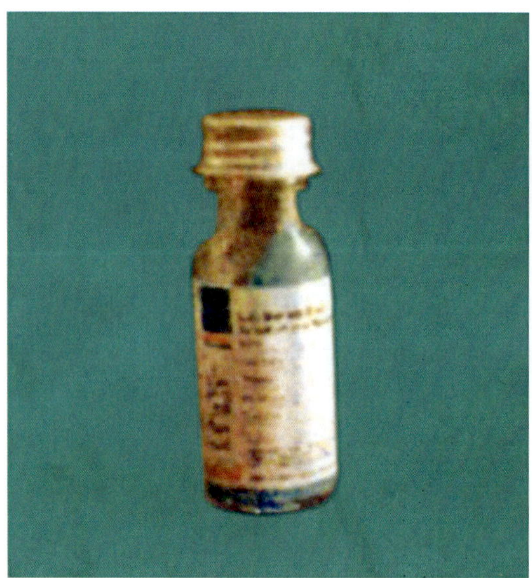

Fig. 25.7: LJ medium bottle used for the cultivation of *M. tuberculosis*

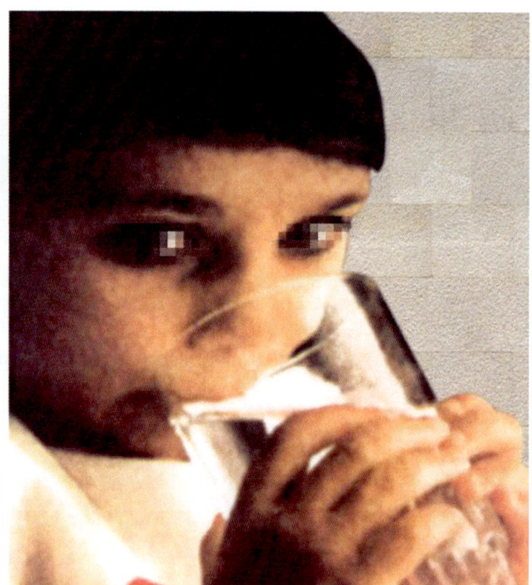

Fig. 26.1: Safe drinking water prevents many infections

Section 1: General Microbiology

Chapter 1

Microbiology as a Science

INTRODUCTION

The cavemen discovered that meat allowed to stand few days was more pleasing to the taste than eaten soon after the kill. The cavemen's earliest descendants learned that intoxicating drinks could be made from grains and fruits. The aging of meat and the manufacture of alcohol were the first unconscious uses of the process now known as *Fermentation*. To primitive men fermentation, putrefaction of dead bodies, souring of milk, different flavors and colors of cheese, yogurt were all a kind of magic. They did not know that they were profiting from the natural activity of tiny living organisms such as molds, yeasts, bacteria, which were nourishing themselves on their food and were producing wholesome chemicals that changed the taste and texture of the food. Apart from these beneficial effects of tiny organisms, ancient people also noticed sudden appearance of infections among the community resulting in high mortality and morbidity. But this was considered as supernatural in origin and sent by the Gods as punishment for the sins of the humans. The treatment and more important the prevention of these diseases were sought by sacrifices and lustrations to appease the anger of the Gods. The concept of contagion (infection) and practice of hygiene was known to some extent to the ancient people. The Old Testament often quoted that leprosy is contagious and can be transmitted by contact. Earlier several philosophers suspected the possible role of invisible creatures in the spread of many diseases. Roger Bacon in 13th century postulated that invisible creatures produced disease. Fracastorius from Vienna expressed the opinion that the seeds of disease passing from one infected person to another caused the same disease in the recipient individual.

LEEUWENHOEK'S MICROSCOPE

Direct observation of these microorganisms was first made by a Dutch lens grinder Antoni van Leeuwenhoek (1632-1732) who invented the microscope. Using the combination of several lenses, he was able to magnify the objects and could see tiny organisms in rainwater, stool samples and described them as 'animalcules'. Later Robert Hook confirmed his observation. Improved microscopes were available due to industrial revolution (Fig. 1.1).

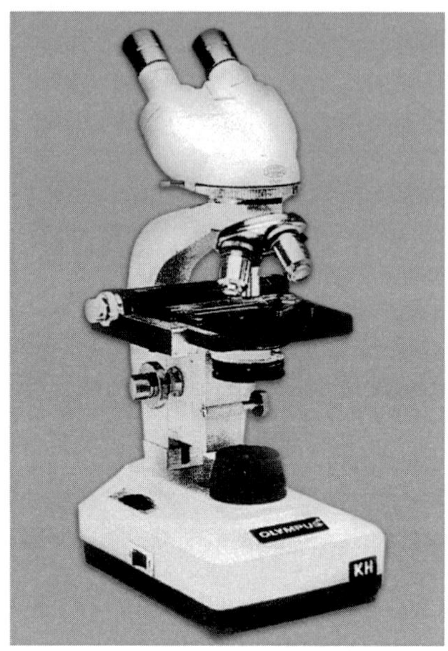

Fig. 1.1: Binocular compound microscope (*For color version, see Plate 1*)

The controversy over the human ability to create life carried over from Greek mythology. Aristotle believed that animals could originate from the soil. For several centuries, people believed that maggots could be produced by exposing the meat to warmth and air. Several workers designed experiments to disprove this concept. It was Louis Pasteur, through his classical experiments, ultimately disproved the concepts and promoted the 'Germ theory of disease'. Louis Pasteur was a French chemist. Pasteur studied the methods and processes that involved the manufacture of beer and wine in order to help the manufactures produce a consistently good product. By examining the samples of beer and wine under microscope, he found that fermentation of fruits and grains resulting in alcohol is brought about by microbes. He also came to a conclusion that in good wine samples one form of microbe was predominated and in poor quality wine another kind was present. By proper selection of the microbe, he was able to produce good quality wine. Pasteur suggested that undesirable microbes might be removed by heating—not enough to hurt the flavor of the first juice but enough to destroy a large number of microbes population. He found that holding the juices at 62.8°C for 30 minutes or at 72°C for 20 seconds the unwanted microbes were killed to a large extent. This process named after him is known as *Pasteurization* which is presently used in fermentation and dairy industries. Pasteur also succeeded in identifying the parasite that was damaging the silk industry. He also tackled the problem of anthrax, a disease of cattle, sheep and sometimes human beings. He was able to develop anthrax vaccine to prevent the disease. One of the most pioneering contributions of Louis Pasteur in medical microbiology was development of vaccine for rabies. Rabies, a deadly disease transmitted by the bite of mad dog. Louis Pasteur collected the saliva from the mad dog and injected into the spinal cord of rabbit. He dried the spinal cord and made it into a suspension and injected first to a 14 years old boy Joseph Meister, who was severely bitten by a mad dog. Pasteur injected 13 subcutaneous injections of increasingly virulent spinal cord preparations to the boy for a period of 10 days. The boy survived thus Pasteur discovered vaccine for rabies before the virus was actually identified and characterized. Pasteur contributions were well recognized all over the world and he was called as Father of Bacteriology (Fig. 1.2). In his honor Pasteur Institute was set up in Paris, which is now one of the well-known institutes for research and contribution.

Later Robert Koch as a student of Henle worked on anthrax and finally isolated the anthrax bacilli in pure form. He, being a meticulous researcher, insisted on the proof that organisms caused disease. For this isolation of the organisms in pure form was necessary.

Robert Koch developed the staining techniques by smearing the bacteria on glass slide and applying aniline dyes for staining. Using these stains Christian Gram differentiated bacteria into gram-positive and gram-negative depending upon the ability of the organisms to resist decolorization with alcohol. Robert Koch developed solid medium using gelatin and on streaking the organisms on this solid media poured in petriplates. He was able to separate various organisms into colonies, which were resulting due to division of single invisible cell. Each colony, which can be seen with naked eye, is composed of several million bacteria of same species. By subculturing the colony into liquid medium, pure culture of the organism could be obtained. Robert Koch later substituted gelatin with agar, the transparent red seaweed extract that solidifies at 43°C and it is autoclavable. It is not metabolized by the microorganisms. Based on his experience with pure cultures, Robert Koch formulated criteria that provided proof that a specific bacterium caused a disease. These are famously known as Koch's postulates (Fig. 1.3).

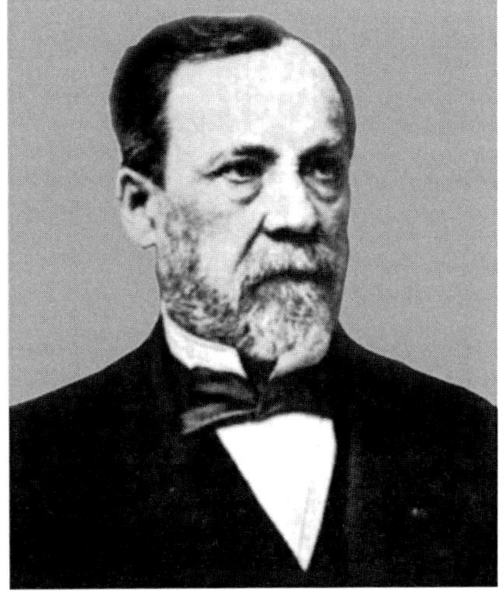

Fig. 1.2: Louis Pasteur (1822-1895)—Father of bacteriology

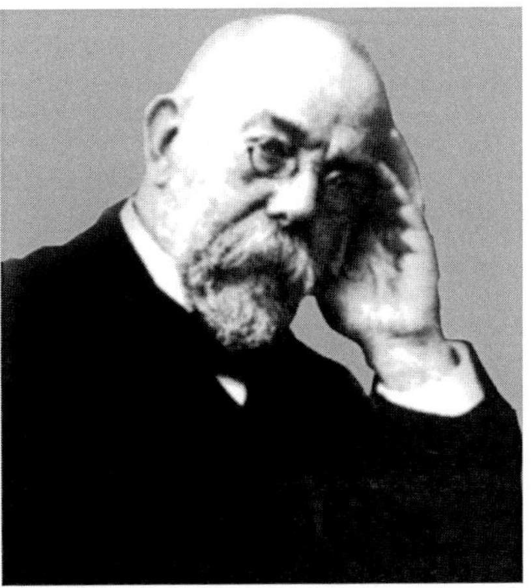

Fig. 1.3: Robert Koch (1843-1910)—Father of modern bacteriology

1. The organism must always be found in a diseased animal but not in healthy ones.
2. The organism must be isolated from the diseased animal and must be grown in pure form away from the diseased animal.
3. The organism grown in pure culture must initiate and reproduce the disease when reintroduced into a susceptible animal.
4. The organism should be isolated from the experimented animal. A fifth postulate that was added later.
5. The organism entering in a susceptible host and producing the disease, should elicit specific antibody response.

Robert Koch further worked on various diseases and discovered organisms like *Mycobacterium tuberculosis,* the causative agent of tuberculosis, *Anthrax* and *Vibrio cholerae.*

Inspired by the fascinating observations of Louis Pasteur and Robert Koch several workers started working to find out the causative agents for various diseases. The 20 years period following Robert Koch work was the golden age of bacteriology. By 1900, organisms of almost all major bacterial diseases organisms such as anthrax, diphtheria, typhoid fever, gonorrhea, tetanus, gas gangrene and syphilis were discovered and the germ theory of disease was firmly established.

However, several times there were failures in isolating the causative agent of many diseases in spite of every possible effort. But the body fluids which were filtered and made bacteria free, when introduced into experimental animals were able to produce diseases. The scientists named them as filterable agents. Ultimately, it was Iwonoski who first crystallized these filterable agents from a diseased tobacco plant and observed under electron microscope, which revealed a new form of living organisms the virus, a name derived from virion means poison. Thus, crystallization of tobacco mosaic virus paved the way for a new branch of microbiology, viz. virology.

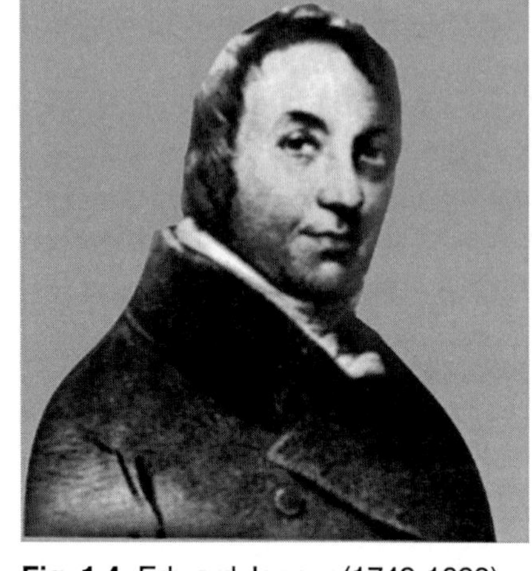

Fig. 1.4: Edward Jenner (1749-1823)—Discovered the efficacy of vaccination against smallpox

While scientists were actively engaged in identifying the causative agents for the diseases, parallelly attempts were made to cure or control these diseases. Paul Ehrlich in 1910 treated syphilis with arsenical and mercurial compounds. In 1935, Domagk showed the therapeutic value of a group of compounds known as sulfanilamides, which are effective against a large variety of microbes. In 1929, Alexander Fleming noticed inhibition of staphylococci on an agar plate that was kept exposed. The inhibition of staphylococcal growth was seen around a mold, which got settled on the agar plate. Further studies on this mold, which was a fungus (*Penicillium* species), yielded the miracle drug penicillin. From then onward intensive search on soil fungi resulted in the discovery of a number of antibiotics, such as streptomycin, tetracycline, chloromycetin and so on and search is still being continued for new antibiotics.

Attempts to prevent infections took a new turn when Edward Jenner (Fig. 1.4) a country physician in England observed that person who suffered from cowpox got protected from serious disease smallpox. So he transferred the material from cowpox lesion from an infected person to the arm of a lad James Phipps. After 6 weeks, the pus from smallpox lesion was inoculated to James Phipps. But he did not develop smallpox. Soon this practice gained popularity as vaccination (*vacca* = cow) and by practicing vaccination smallpox was eradicated. Presently vaccines are available for a number of diseases.

Thus, history of microbiology is very fascinating and study of interaction of these invisible microbes has created many advances in the field of medicine. Although microbes are responsible for diseases, nevertheless, they play an important role in human life. More precisely men and microbes are more friends than foes.

Presently the discipline microbiology expanded and has the following subdivisions, namely bacteriology, virology, mycology, parasitology, immunology and serology.

Chapter 2

Classification and Identification of Bacteria

INTRODUCTION

Bacteria belong to prokaryotic groups of organisms. They do not have nuclear membrane, reproduce by binary fission. They lack 80S type of ribosomes, mitochondria, golgi apparatus and cilia. They are either rod shaped or spherical or spiral or curved organisms. Each bacterium is considered as species and many strains are present in single species. A strain is defined as the progeny of subcultures of a single colony isolate in pure culture. A colony is a cluster of bacterial cells derived from the multiplication of a single bacterium. A colony which contains several thousands of bacteria is visible to the naked eye on a solid medium, whereas a single bacterium cannot be seen by naked eye.

Bacterial species are defined by shape, size, motility, Gram stain reaction and colony morphology, and their biochemical reactions such as fermentation of various sugars (monosaccharides, disaccharides, polysaccharides, alcohols, etc.), end product of metabolism such as acids, amines, aldehydes and other complex metabolites, their physiological requirement such as oxygen, hydrogen ion concentration (pH), temperature requirement for optimal growth, DNA base composition and homology.

Bacterial species contain strains that are interrelated but differ in certain aspects sometimes known as cluster. With each species collection or cluster, a strain is chosen arbitrarily to represent best of that species. This strain is known as biotype and its characteristics are used to describe that particular species. Further subdivision of biotype can be done to know the variation. These variants are known as serotypes, phage types, etc.

All microorganisms have binomial nomenclature, the first name indicates the genus and the second name indicates species. The genus name should begin with capital letter and the species should be written in small letters, e.g. *Staphylococcus aureus* (*Staphylococcus* is the genus and *aureus* is the species name) or *S. aureus*.

The bacterial genetic material or genome or chromosome is made up of purine and pyrimidine bases, namely adenine, guanine, cytosine and thymidine. The base composition is generally constant for each organism and is expressed as G + C percentage. Table 2.1 enlists the microorganisms of medical importance and their identifying properties.

Table 2.1: Selected bacteria of medical importance and their identifying properties

Family, genus species	*Identifying properties*	*Clinical infection*
Section 1. The spirochetes, gram-negative helical bacteria		
Spirochaetaceae	Slender, flexuous, helically coiled, motile with axial filaments	
Treponema pallidum	Host-associated, tightly coiled, probably microaerophilic	Syphilis
Borrelia hermsii	Host-associated, loose, coarse, irregular coils, microaerophilic	Tick-borne relapsing fever
B. bergdorferi	As above	Tick-borne Lyme disease
Leptospiraceae	Flexible, very tightly coiled motile rods, one or both ends hooked, aerobic	
Leptospira interrogans	Parasitic; other properties as above	Leptospirosis
Section 2. Aerobic/microaerophilic, motile, helical/vibrioid, gram-negative bacteria		
Campylobacter fetus	Slender, spirally curved rod, microaerophilic, host-associated	Opportunistic septicemic illness
C. jejuni	As above	Enteritis
Helicobacter pylori	As above, grows at 35°C	Acid peptic disease, gastric ulcers
Section 3. Gram-negative aerobic rods and cocci		
Pseudomonadaceae	Straight or curved rods, motile, oxidase (+), respiratory metabolism	
Pseudomonas aeruginosa	Fluorescent pigments produced; other properties as above	Wound, burn, urinary tract infections
Legionellaceae	Motile, difficult to stain, catalase (+), requires special media	
Legionella pneumophila	As above	Pneumonia (Legionnaire's disease)
Neisseriaceae	Biscuit-shaped diplococci, nonmotile, catalase (+), oxidase (+)	
Neisseria meningitidis	Ferments glucose and maltose	Meningitis
N. gonorrhoeae	Ferments glucose	Gonorrhea
Other genera		
Brucella abortus	Coccobacilli to short rods, nonmotile, facultative intracellular parasite, fastidious growth requirements, catalase (+)	Brucellosis
B. melitensis	As above	Brucellosis
B. suis	As above	Brucellosis
Bordetella pertussis	Minute, nonmotile coccobacilli, mammalian parasites	Pertussis (whooping cough)
Francisella tularensis	Minute, pleomorphic, faintly staining cocci to rods; require enriched media (glucose-cysteine blood agar)	Tularemia
Section 4. Facultative anaerobic gram-negative rods		
Enterobacteriaceae	Small rods, inhabit intestine, catalase (+), oxidase (–), glucose fermented, nitrates reduced to nitrites; genera and species identified biochemically	
Escherichia coli	Motile, mixed acid fermentation, lactose fermented by most strains, H_2 and CO_2 produced H_2S (–), citrate not utilized	Opportunistic infections; some strains cause diarrheas

Contd...

Contd...

Family, genus species	Identifying properties	Clinical infection
Enterobacter aerogenes	Motile, 2,3-butanediol fermentation, lactose fermented with acid and gas, citrate utilized, ornithine decarboxylated	Opportunistic infections
Shigella dysenteriae	Nonmotile, lactose not fermented, no gas from glucose, $H_2S(-)$	Dysentery
Salmonella typhi	Motile, lactose not fermented, no gas from glucose, $H_2S(+)$, indole (–), lysine and ornithine decarboxylated	Typhoid fever
S. species	Acid and gas from glucose	Food poisoning
Klebsiella pneumoniae	Nonmotile, encapsulated, lactose fermented with acid and gas, 2,3-butanediol fermentation, citrate utilized, ornithine not decarboxylated	Pneumonia, urinary tract infections
Proteus mirabilis	Motile, lactose not fermented, urea hydrolyzed	Urinary tract infections
Serratia marcescens	Motile, lactose not fermented, $H_2S(-)$, lysine decarboxylated, citrate utilized, DNase produced, pigment at R°	Opportunistic infections
Yersinia pestis	Cells ovoid to rod-shaped, nonmotile, lactose not fermented	Bubonic plague
Y. enterocolitica	As above	Gastroenteritis
Vibrionaceae	Rigid rods, straight or curved, polar flagella, oxidase (+), catalase (+), metabolism respiratory and fermentative	
Vibrio cholerae	Lactose not fermented, produces toxin; other properties as above	Cholera
V. parahaemolyticus	Lactose not fermented, halophilic, other properties of family	Gastroenteritis from seafood
Pasteurellaceae	Straight rods, nonmotile, organic N sources required, oxidase (+)	
Pasteurella multocida	Small ovoid rod, bipolar staining, other properties as above	Animal bite infections
Haemophilus influenzae	Small pleomorphic coccobacilli to rods, strict parasite, requires nicotinamide riboside and hematin for growth, most strains oxidase (+)	Meningitis, other pediatric diseases
Section 5. Anaerobic gram-negative straight, curved, and helical rods		
Bacteroidaceae	Straight rod with curved ends, pleomorphic with vacuoles, non-sporeforming, major component of intestinal flora	
Bacteroides fragilis	As above	Opportunistic multiple organism anaerobic abscesses
B. melaninogenicus	Produces dark pigment on blood agar	Opportunistic infections
Fusobacterium species	Long slender, spindle-shaped rods, present in natural cavities of man	Opportunistic infections
Section 6. Rickettsiae and chlamydiae, gram-negative		
Rickettsiaceae	Small rods, coccoid and diplococcal, usually intracellular parasites associated with arthropods	
Rickettsia rickettsii	Grows intracellularly in cytoplasm and nucleus	Rocky Mountain spotted fever (Tick typhus)
R. prowazekii	Grows intracellularly in vacuoles	Epidemic typhus
Coxiella burnetii	Grows preferentially in vacuoles, forms endospores, disseminated by airborne aerosols	Q fever

Contd...

Contd...

Family, genus species	Identifying properties	Clinical infection
Chlamydiaceae	Nonmotile, coccoidal, obligately intracellular parasites, developmental cycle in cytoplasm, metabolically limited	
Chlamydia trachomatis	As above	Trachoma, lymphogranuloma venereum
C. psittaci	As above	Psittacosis
Section 7. Mycoplasmas (Cell wall-less bacteria)		
Mycoplasmataceae	Small cell wall-less, highly pleomorphic, gram-negative, require cholesterol for growth, colony has "fried-egg" appearance, penicillin-resistant	
Mycoplasma pneumoniae	Facultatively anaerobic, gliding motility, special structure for attachment to host cell	Primary atypical pneumonia
Ureaplasma urealyticum	Microaerophilic, hydrolyze urea with production of ammonia	Some strain cause nongonococcal urethritis and urinary tract infection
Section 8. Gram-positive cocci		
Micrococcaceae	Spherical cells, divide in more than one plane, catalase (+), nonmotile, no endospores	
Staphylococcus aureus	Often occur in grape-like clusters, facultative anaerobe, coagulase (+)	Suppurative abscesses, toxic manifestations
S. epidermidis	Coagulase (–), otherwise as above	Opportunistic infections
S. saprophyticus	As above	Urinary tract infections in young females
Other genera		
Streptococcus	Spherical or ovoid cells in pairs or chains, nonmotile, homofermentative metabolism, catalase (–), complex nutritional requirements	
S. pyogenes	β-hemolytic on blood agar, bile-esculin (–)	Acute pharyngitis, tonsillitis skin infections, acute rheumatic fever
S. agalactiae	Produces cAMP factor, otherwise as above	Neonatal meningitis
S. pneumoniae	α-hemolytic on blood agar, lancet-shaped diplococci or short chains, bile-soluble	Lobar pneumonia
S. faecalis	Grows in 6.5 percent NaCl, withstands 60°C, bile-esculin (+)	Opportunistic infections
Section 9. Endospore forming gram-positive rods and cocci		
Bacillus	Cells rod-shaped, often peritrichously flagellated, strict aerobes or facultative anaerobes	
B. anthracis	Nonmotile, facultative anaerobe	Anthrax
(Clostridium)	Cells rod-shaped, anaerobes, motility (±), spores distend cell	
C. botulinum	Motile, produce neurotoxins (7 types)	Botulism
C. perfringens	Nonmotile, stormy fermentation in milk, produces exotoxins	Gas gangrene
C. tetani	Motile, terminal spores, single type of neurotoxin	Tetanus
C. difficile	Motile, produces exotoxin (2 types)	Pseudomembranous colitis

Contd...

Contd...

Family, genus species	Identifying properties	Clinical infection
Section 10. Regular, nonsporing, gram-positive rods		
Lactobacillus species	Microaerophilic, fermentative lactate producers, catalase (–), no cytochromes	Dental caries (secondary role)
Listeria	Small, short rods, facultatively anaerobic, catalase (+), oxidase (–)	
L. monocytogenes	β-hemolytic	Meningitis
Section 11. Irregular, nonsporing, gram-positive rods		
Corynebacterium	Straight to slightly curved rods, irregular staining, often produce metachromatic granules, not acid-fast, facultatively anaerobic, produce short chain mycolic acids	
C. diphtheriae	Produces potent exotoxin	Diphtheria
Actinomyces	Nonmotile, nonacid-fast rods, filaments, some branching, facultatively anaerobic, catalase (–), CO_2 required for maximum growth	
A. israelii	As above	Actinomycosis
Section 12. Mycobacteria (acid-fast rods)		
Mycobacteriaceae	Slightly curved or straight rods, gram-positive, acid-fast, nonmotile, aerobic, catalase (+), long chain mycolic acids produced	
Mycobacterium tuberculosis	Very slow grower	Tuberculosis
M. avium–M. intracellulare	Properties as for family; one of mycobacterium species other than tuberculosis (MOTT)	Chronic pulmonary disease, disseminated disease in immunocompromised
M. leprae	Cannot be cultured on artificial media	Leprosy
Section 13. Nocardioforms		
Nocardia	Gram-positive, no endospores, nonmotile aerobic bacillus, filaments, fragmentation into rods and cocci; partially acid-fast, produce medium length mycolic acids	
N. asteroides	As above	Nocardiosis

Adapted from Krieg and Holt (Eds): Bergey's Manual of Systematic Bacteriology, vol 1, 1984, and Sneath, Mair, Sharpe, Holt (Eds); Bergey's Manual of Systematic Bacteriology, vol 2, 1986, Williams and Wilkins.

[a]Only sections have been included that currently contain bacteria of medical importance.

Chapter 3

Structure of Microorganisms

INTRODUCTION

Microorganisms although apparently seem to be very simple, they have complex structure to carry out the metabolic activities. The structure of microorganisms not only helps them to exist in nature even under unfavorable environmental conditions, but also performs a number of activities necessary for their survival.

STRUCTURE OF BACTERIA

Most of the bacteria measure 0.4 μ in size (1 micron = 1/1000 mm). Morphologically, they may look like rod-shaped with rounded or square ends, or spherical or oval-shaped. Some of them are half-moon-shaped or kidney-shaped (Fig. 3.1). They vary considerably in size, length, diameter and this is known as pleomorphism. They are arranged in clusters or long chains, or irregular arrangement. Study of these characters often helps us in identifying the organism. Morphology of bacteria are better studied using light compound microscope or its modification. For studying the structure of bacteria or other microorganisms, the organism are magnified upto one lakh times using a special microscope called electron microscope.

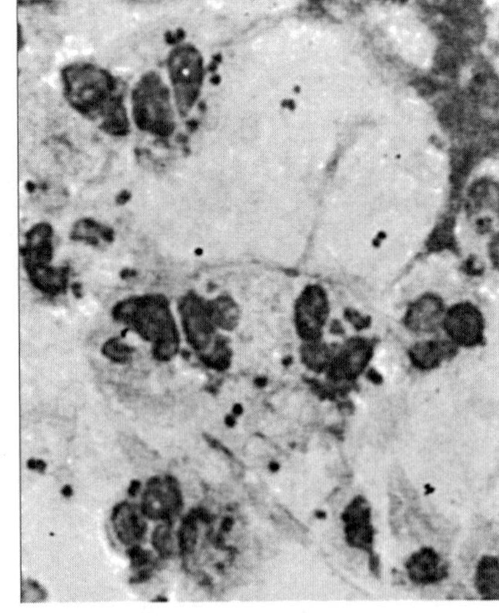

Fig. 3.1: Gram-negative intracellular cocci (meningococci) (×100) *(For color version, see Plate 1)*

Typically a bacterium has cell envelope, which includes an outer cell wall, plasma membrane, specialized proteins and polysaccharide (carbohydrates); the bacterial cell envelope contains transport sites for nutrients and receptor sites. The receptor sites are responsible for attachment of the bacteria to the human cells and initiate infection by a process known as invasion.

Cell Wall

Present in all free-living bacteria except *Mycoplasma* or L-forms of bacteria. This outer layer of the cell protects bacteria from variations in the external environment such as low osmotic pressure and maintains cell shape. The gram-positive bacteria contain techoic acid in the cell wall whereas gram-negative bacteria contain lipopolysaccharides (Fig. 3.2).

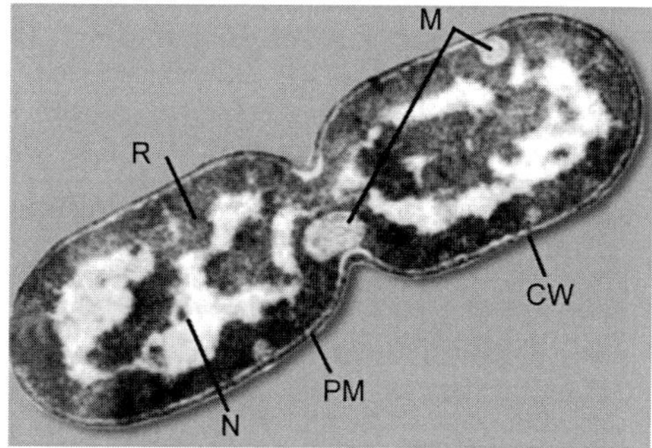

Fig. 3.2: A prokaryotic cells. Achromobacter, a dividing gram-negative bacterium showing cell wall (CW), plasma membrane (PM), nuclear area (N), densely packed ribosomes (R), and mesosomes (M) x 42,0000

Plasma Membrane

Below the rigid cell wall layer and in close association with it, a delicate cytoplasmic membrane or plasma membrane is present which is very important for the bacterial cell. The membrane essentially is made up of protein, carbohydrate and lipid. Various enzymatic activities are associated with plasma membrane, which are required for the metabolic activities of the bacterial cell. The space between plasma inner and outer membrane is known as periplast. This is a gel like substance, more easily seen in gram-negative bacteria and is the source of a number of enzymes and proteins responsible for bacterial metabolic activity (Fig. 3.2).

Mesosomes

These are sac like structures associated with cytoplasmic membrane. These are associated with cell division because it has been seen that DNA and cell membrane attach to mesosomes during the cell division process (Fig. 3.2).

Cytoplasmic Structures

The cytoplasm contains the DNA molecule, which controls the cell function, and it is responsible for transfer of cell properties to the progeny. It is a double stranded helical structure madeup of purine and pyrimidine bases and it occupies 10 percent of the cell volume and represents 2 to 3 percent of the bacterial cell weight. The cytoplasm contains ribosomes, which are necessary for protein synthesis. The number of ribosomes in a given bacterial cells are variable according to the growth conditions and nutrients available. Some of the bacteria show granules known as volutin granules or Babes-Ernst granules. These are reserve food materials for bacteria and they are made up of polymetaphosphates. These are stained by a special staining procedure called metachromatic staining. When stained they appear as purple blue spots under light microscope within the bacterial cell. These are very commonly seen in diphtheria bacilli.

Capsule

Some of the bacteria possess an outer slimy layer known as capsule. Capsulated organisms are more virulent and can cause acute serious infections. Capsule protects the bacteria from white blood cells of the human or animal host, which usually engulf the bacteria and remove from the system. Capsule is made up of polysaccharide but in some bacteria it is made up of protein. Capsule appears as an halo of light surrounding the bacteria if the bacteria are mixed with India ink and observed under microscope. The capsule can also be seen under phase contrast microscopy. The capsular polysaccharide reacts with a protein present in the human serum and forms a precipitate. The protein is known as C-reactive protein. Special stains are used to demonstrate capsule around the bacterial cell.

Flagella

Some of the bacteria move from place to place with the help of special filamentous structures known as flagella (Flagellum is singular). These thread like or thin filaments are made up of proteins. Depending upon the number of flagella and their position on a bacterial cell, they can be called as monotrichous (single flagellum at one pole of the bacterial cell), amphitrichous (one flagellum on each of the ends of the bacterial cell), lophotrichous (a bunch of flagella at one end of the bacterial cell), peritrichous (flagella all around the bacteria cell). With the help of flagella, bacteria can move from place to place in search of nutrients or they can move away from any toxic substance that may cause damage or death of the cell. Apart from flagella, bacteria also have small thin filamentous structure known as fimbriae. These fimbriae help the bacteria to attach to the cells and help in invasion or penetration of bacteria into the human cells. Some bacteria like spirochetes do not have flagella but they are motile due to rotation of the cell around the structure known as axial filaments; these organisms exhibit corkscrew type of movement.

Bacterial Spores

Under unsuitable environmental condition some bacteria produce specialized structures called spores. These spores may be located centrally or terminally or subterminally in the bacterial cell. They are highly resistant to heat, drying, chemicals and starvation. The spores are highly refractile and seen as round or oval structure within the bacterial cell. The chemical composition of bacterial spore is very much different from the bacterial cell, from which it is formed. Under favorable conditions these spores germinate and produce the parent bacterial cell known as vegetative form.

Bacteria ordinarily lyse in water or serum if the rigid cell wall present on the outer surface is removed by chemicals or enzymes like lysozyme. However, if they are stabilized by chemical like sucrose, a cell wall free osmotically sensitive spherical body called spheroplast is liberated. If the cell wall is retained but it is weak (not rigid) the cell is called protoplast. Gram-positive bacteria can be generally converted into protoplast and gram-negative bacteria as spheroplasts.

STRUCTURE OF VIRUSES (FIG. 3.3)

The name *virus* is derived from *'virion'* means poison. Viruses are ultramicroscopic organisms (not seen by ordinary light microscope), contain either DNA or RNA that multiply within the living mammalian cells and use the cell machinery for their replication.

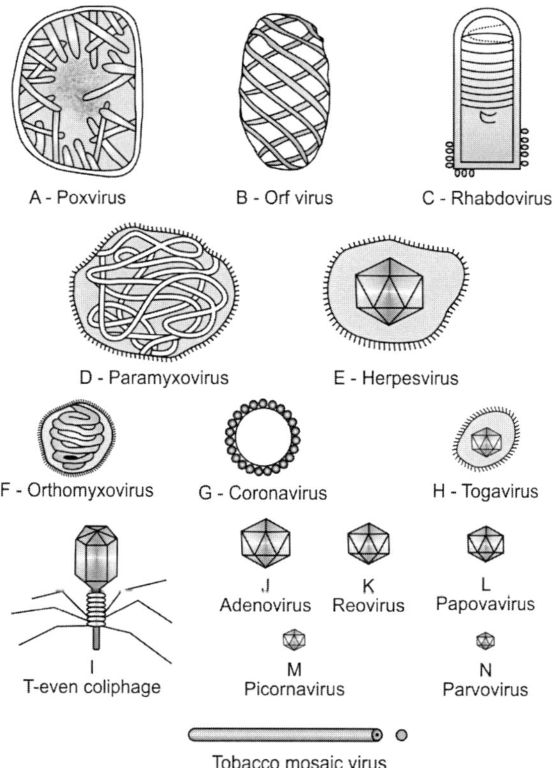

Fig. 3.3: Morphology of viruses

The size of the virus particle is measured in nanometers ($1/10^9$th part of a meter) directly using electron microscope, or by passing them through filter having different size of pores or by their rate of settling when centrifuged at a high speed, usually at 1,00,000 rpm (revolutions per mintue). They can multiply only in living cells. Outside the cells though viable, they are metabolically inert. They do not have any energy yielding enzyme system. The viral DNA or RNA enters the living cell, and directs the cell DNA to prepare viral DNA or RNA copies and necessary proteins required for envelope and these are assembled. These assembled virus particles are released from the cell by the lysis of the cell or by passive release from it.

The virus particles vary in size from 20 to 300 nm. They are generally spherical or rod shaped consisting of a central core of nucleic acid (DNA or RNA) surrounded or closely associated with a protein coat known as capsid. The capsid is made up of small identical subunits (usually proteins) known as capsomeres. These capsomeres are arranged in a specific symmetry, namely cubical, helical or complex. In viruses with cubical symmetry, the capsomeres are arranged in such a way to form 20 equilateral triangles and this type of arrangement is called icosahedron symmetry. This is seen very commonly in many viruses. Some viruses show helical symmetry wherein the capsomeres are arranged along the spiral shaped DNA or RNA. The complex symmetry is difficult to define. Probably it is a combination of both cubical and helical symmetry. The viruses with complex symmetry have

Table 3.1: Classification of viruses

DNA viruses	*RNA viruses*
1. Poxviruses	1. Orthomyxoviruses
2. Herpesviruses	2. Paramyxoviruses
3. Adenoviruses	3. Picornaviruses
4. Parvoviruses	4. Rhabdoviruses
5. Papovaviruses	5. Coronaviruses
	6. Arenaviruses
	7. Togaviruses
	8. Reoviruses

All DNA viruses are double stranded except parvoviruses.
All RNA viruses are single stranded except picorna viruses and reoviruses.
All DNA viruses have cubical symmetry except poxviruses.
The RNA viruses may have either cubical symmetry or helical symmetry.

brick shaped particles with finger like projections giving an appearance of a woollen ball. Some viruses have an extra-coat made of lipids and such viruses are called enveloped viruses. These enveloped viruses are sensitive to ether because the lipid coat is ether soluble.

Viruses are classified as DNA and RNA viruses (Table 3.1).

Most of the viruses are heat sensitive. They can survive at low temperature like – 70°C or – 196°C. They are soluble in ether or chloroform and become noninfectious. They can be easily inactivated by a number of disinfectants like chlorine, sodium hypochlorite, tincture iodine, formaldehyde, hydrogen peroxide, etc. They are resistant to antibiotics. They can withstand pH ranging from 5 to 9. Many viruses cause agglutination of a wide variety of human and animal red blood cells. This phenomenon is called hemagglutination.

STRUCTURE OF FUNGI

Fungi occur in two forms in nature: (i) yeast like budding cells (Fig. 3.4) or (ii) mycelium, i.e. hyphal filaments arranged irregularly and appear like cotton wool. The hyphae are short or long with or without septa. Mycelial forms of fungi are multicellular and filamentous. The filaments are branching cylindrical tube like structure known as hyphae (singular hypha). Some hyphae are divided into cells by septa or cross walls. Cytoplasm continuity is maintained both in septate and nonseptate hyphae. Some fungi grow as yeast like cells at 37°C whereas at 28°C they grow as mycelium. This feature is known as dimorphism. Based on the size and shape of spores, they produce, fungi can be characterized. The spores of fungi are known as conidia. Some fungi produce pigmentation like red, violet, yellow, greenish yellow or black. Some fungi especially the yeast like cells possess capsule made up of polysaccharide. The fungal cell wall is thick and protect the fungal cells from external environment. The cell wall composition

Fig. 3.4: Yeast-like budding cells along with pseudomycelia *Candida albicans* (×100) *(For color version, see Plate 1)*

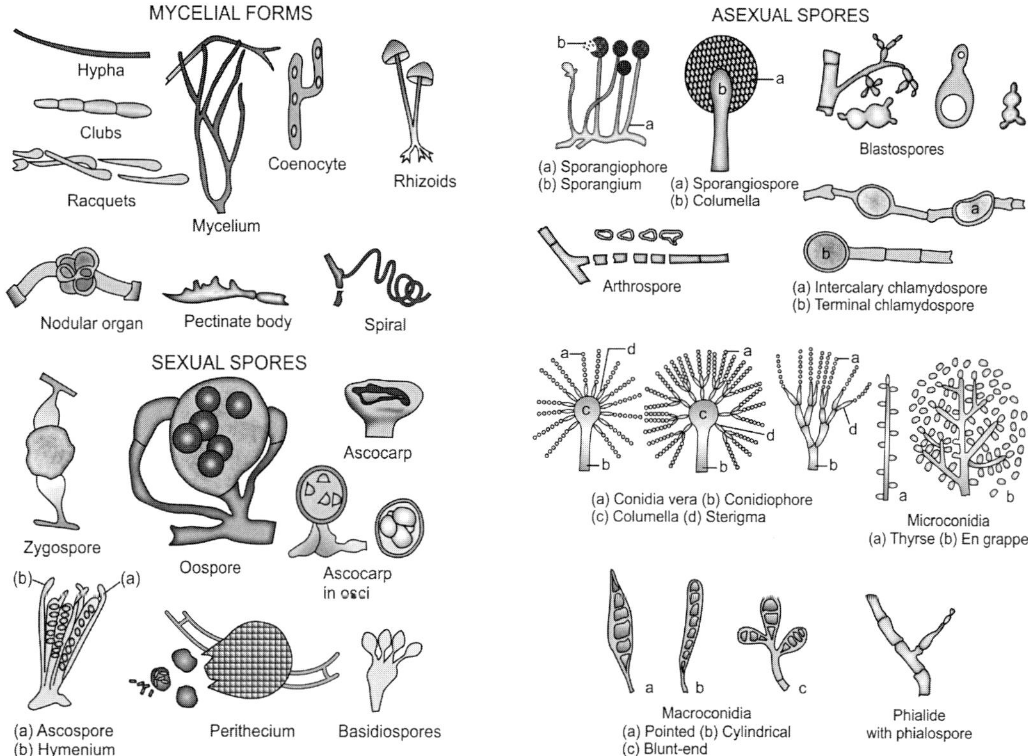

Fig. 3.5A: Mycelial forms and sexual spores of fungi

Fig. 3.5B: Various types of asexual spores produced by fungi

varies and may contain chitin, cellulose, glucan or mannan. Fungal cell wall also contain protein and glycoprotein. The fungi have bilayered cell membrane similar in structure of eukaryotic cells. The cell membrane protects cytoplasm and regulates the transportation of nutrients. The cell membrane contains phospholipids and sterols. The cytoplasm contains nuclei, mitochondria and vacuoles. Fungi reproduce both sexually as well as by asexual process (Figs 3.5A and B).

Definition and Terms

1. Mycetes: Fungus
2. Mycosis: A disease caused by fungus.
3. Thallus: The vegetative or growing form of fungus.
4. Mycelium: Cotton wool like mass of interwoven hyphae.
5. Coenocytes: Multinucleated arising from mycelium.
6. Club: The swollen end of hyphae.
7. Spores: Reproducing body resulting from fusion of two similar gametes.
8. Zygospore: Sexual spore resulting from fusion of two similar gamestes.
9. Oospore: Sexual spore resulting from fertilization of male and female cells.
10. Ascocarp: Fruit bodies containing asci.

11. Ascospores: Sexual spore enclosed in ascus.
12. Sporangiospores: Asexual spores that are endogenous.
13. Thallospores: Spores arising from the vegetative cell.
14. Blastospores: Spores arising from budding.
15. Arthrospores: The old mycelia become thicker and show segmentation. They may be intercalary, i.e. along the course of hyphae or terminal (at the end of the hyphae).
16. Chlamydospores: Spores formed by the bulging of hyphae.
17. Conidia: A sexual spores. Two types: Microconidia. These may be sessile, spherical or subspherical. Macroconidia or fusiform, spindle shaped or club shaped. They are either lateral or terminal. These are seen in fungi causing superficial skin infection, e.g. dermatophytes.

STRUCTURE OF PARASITES

These are broadly classified as protozoa and metazoa.

1. Protozoa: They are unicellular organisms whose further morphology is characterized by the presence or absence of locomotory organs such as pseudopodia, cilia, flagella and undulating membrane. The cell is having outer cytoplasmic membrane. The nucleus is covered by nuclear membrane and contains chromatin. The karyosome is either central or eccentric. Some protozoa contain axostyle. The number of flagella are variable. They may contain vacuoles and food particles within the cytoplasm. The cytoplasm is granular.
2. Metazoa: These are multicellular organisms and classified as cestodes, trematodes and nematodes (Table 3.2).

Table 3.2: Classification of metazoa

Cestodes	*Trematodes*	*Nematodes*
• Tape like segmented. Each segment acts as a single unit	Leaf like unsegmented	Cylindrical
• Monoecious	Monoecious except schistosoma	Dioecious (Sexes are separate)
• Mouth parts contain suckers with or without hooks	Suckers without hooks	Well-developed buccal capsule
• No alimentary canal	Incomplete alimentary canal	Complete alimentary canal

Chapter 4

Bacterial Nutrition and Growth

INTRODUCTION TO NUTRITION

All living organisms whether it is a unicellular microorganism like bacteria, or a higher living beings like plant or an animal show two important functions, i.e. (i) growth and (ii) multiplication. In order to achieve these two aims they have to build up to the structural units, from simple substances. In this process, they essentially require: (i) water, (ii) carbohydrates, (iii) proteins, (iv) lipids, (v) minerals, and (vi) vitamins. These essential food materials, either they must be able to synthesize using simpler substances with the help of enzymes and other cellular machinery they possess or they should obtain from the environment. In this aspect all the living beings behave more or less in a similar way and that is called "unity of biochemistry" and all the chemical changes that occur in effect of catabolism and anabolism. Catabolism comprises of breaking down of larger molecules, and these smaller substances are later on polymerized into cell wall proteins, cytoplasm nucleic acids, etc. This requires adenosine triphosphate (ATP) consumption.

Bacteria can take up simpler substances like nitrogen, or CO_2 and build up complex food materials using sunlight as energy—autotrophs or lithotrophs.

By Using Organic Compounds

These are called heterotrophs. All medically important bacteria are heterotrophs, and they live as parasites and multiply at the expense of host food materials.

Once these simpler substances in the form of building blocks enter the cell, they are processed through different enzymatic pathways such as glycolytic pathway or Krebs' cycle, pentose pathway to liberate the energy or through pathways of biosynthesis to build up complex substances required for the formation of cell wall components, ribosomes, flagella and other structural constituents of the bacterial cell. During these processes they may liberate some of the complex molecules into the environment surrounding them and they may act as toxins and produce disease in the host.

During the process of the breakdown of these nutrient substances they may be completely converted to CO_2 and water using oxygen as the terminal acceptor and such bacteria are aerobes and the process is oxidative phosphorylation.

Those bacteria, which cannot use oxygen as terminal acceptor of electrons, are anaerobes but use nitrates and sulfates. Bacteria which require very low concentration of oxygen and a little more concentration of CO_2 are called microaerophillic.

Fermentation

Where organic compounds act as electron donors and electron acceptors. Bacteria may grow on simple substances, may require supplementation of amino acids, minerals, vitamins, animal proteins and some directly require preformed ATP.

Apart from these nutritional requirements other factors responsible for the growth and multiplication are oxygen, carbon dioxide, etc.

Moisture and desiccation kills organisms like gonococci, *Treponema*.

pH and osmotic pressure are also to be maintained for optimum growth of bacteria.

GROWTH OF BACTERIA

Let us suppose that a known number of bacteria are placed in a suitable environment providing all required nutrients and measure their rate of multiplication in relation to time. If we plot a curve, we get a bacterial growth curve (Fig. 4.1) which comprises of the followings:

Lag Phase

No multiplication, increase in size and adaptation to new environment, synthesis of new enzymes or origin of mutants.

The duration of lag phase depends upon: (i) number of cells originally inoculated (ii) type of bacterial species, (iii) state of the bacteria cell at the time of placing them in the medium.

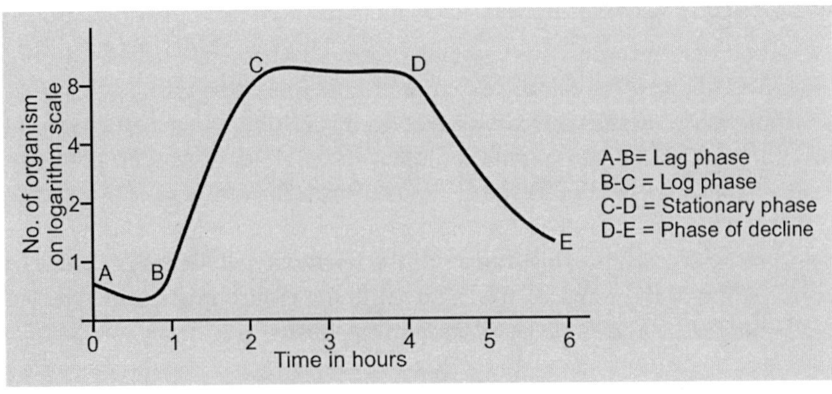

Fig. 4.1: Bacterial growth curve

Log Phase

Increase in number of cells in geometric progression. Hence, we get almost a straight line indicating a direct relationship between multiplication and time.

The log phase of a given species of bacteria depends upon:

i. Optimum temperature
ii. Nature of the medium
iii. Aeration of the medium
iv. pH of the medium
v. Nature of the organism.

IMPORTANCE OF LOG PHASE

If the organism is rapidly multiplying disease process may be very severe and body may not defend itself and hence it suffers. In this phase, transformation of DNA from one bacterial cell to other bacterial cell can occur.

Stationary Phase

Once the nutrients are exhausted or once toxic substances accumulate, the bacteria will neither multiply nor decrease in number, i.e. their total number will be constant state of "suspended animation". At this stage the metabolic activity is slow. In this stage cells can show a wide range of variation or morphology, the reserve food materials accumulate. Gram-positive organism may become gram-negative.

They may release secondary metabolites such as toxins, enzymes, lysins that act on the host cells and contribute to the severity of the disease. Sporulation can start at this stage.

Phase of Decline

Once the stationary phase is prolonged, the cells will begin to die, and even if you transfer these cells which are in very late stages of stationary period, they will not be able to multiply further and further the cells get lysed due to liberation of autolytic enzymes.

Now by this above growth curve study, we infer that by continuous supply of nutrients in a suitable medium it is possible to grow the bacteria continuously and we can get actively growing, pure yield of good number of cells. By applying this principle various instruments like chemostat or turbidostat are developed which are very much useful in producing vaccines, drugs, and many useful products on large-scale.

Chapter 5

Bacterial Variations: Genetics vs Drug Resistance

BACTERIAL VARIATIONS

Imagine that you have treated 100 cases of typhoid fever with the choice drug, i.e. chloramphenicol. Among these 100 cases say 60 did not respond whereas 40 got cured. If you isolate the typhoid bacilli from all these 100 cases, it will be found that 60% of them are resistant, i.e. they can grow even in the presence of chloramphenicol. Let us take another example, staphylococci when grown in a suitable medium containing blood usually show visible colonies which are small, opaque and show golden yellow pigments and hemolysis of the blood. But sometimes we do get staphylococcal colonies which are large, do not show any pigments or hemolysis. Another classical example is imagine that you have injected sputum of a patients suffering from acute lobar pneumonia, into mice. If this sputum contains pneumococci, usually mice die within 6 hours. But sometimes even though pneumococci are present in the sputum, the mice may not die or the organisms can show a change in their morphology, i.e. organisms can lose their capacity to kill the host.

Such deviations from the normal behavior of the bacteria are called bacterial variations. Now the questions are:

1. Whether these variations are temporary or permanent?
2. Whether they are heritable or nonheritable. That means whether these changes can be transmitted to their progeny or not?
3. How frequently these variations are encountered?
4. What are the factors which influence these variations?
5. What is their significance in medicine?

Let us try to answer one by one.

The answer to the first question is that we can encounter both temporary and permanent variations. We can study these variations as:

Morphological Variations

Variations in size, shape of the bacilli can be seen in during late lag phase or stationary phase of the bacterial growth. Capsule production by an organism depends upon the nutrients or nature of the medium, e.g. capsule production best seen in medium containing milk. Sporulation depends again on the environmental conditions.

Cultural Variations

Size of the colony, pigment production, shape of the colony all are determined by the composition of the medium, temperature at which they have grown, moisture, etc. An organism that may not produce pigment at room temperature may produce pigment at 37°C. Those which do not produce pigments on nutrient agar may produce pigments on milk or blood. This shows that organism is genetically capable of producing pigment but because of the influence of the external environment, it is temporarily not expressed.

All bacterial characters determined by the influence of external environment are called phenotypic characters. Whereas all the bacterial characters that are genetically determined or mediated through genes of the chromosome are called genotypic characters.

Variation in Biochemical or Physiological Characters

Young cultures are easily killed with disinfectants whereas old ones are more resistant. Temporary suppression of enzymatic activity of the bacteria can occur due to environmental influence or presence of inhibitors.

All these above variations are temporary variations.

Permanent or Hereditary Variations

Hereditary variation can occur due to:
1. Mutations
2. Transformations
3. Conjugation
4. Transduction
5. Lysogenic conversion.

Mutations

Mutations were first discovered by Luria and Delbruck and Lederberg in 1930. A sudden permanent change in the genetic composition is called mutation. This may occur due to loss or gain of genes. In bacteria mutation occurs at the rate of 10^{-4} to 10^{-10}, i.e. in 10,000 or 1:10,000,000 and can be exhibited in the form of:
1. Development of resistance to a drug to which it was previously sensitive.
2. Failure to grow in a normal medium in which it was growing previously.
3. In the form of failure to ferment a given sugar.
4. In the form of change in the protein, lipid, carbohydrate, concentration of the bacteria.
5. In the form of changes in the morphological features such as loss of flagella.

Mutations are usually irreversible; sometimes very rarely the bacteria can gain a character that it has lost previously. This is called back mutation. This can occur 1:10^{15} cells/generation.

Mutations can be induced in bacteria by agents like ultraviolet rays, γ-rays, chemicals like acriflavine, nitrous oxide when they are used in sublethal doses.

Bacterial mutants can be isolated or studied using replica plating method of Lederberg.

Transformation

Bacteria can gain new genes due to entry of chromosome of one bacterium into the chromosome of other bacteria of the same species. This usually occurs during late stage of stationary phase of growth when the old cells get autolyzed and liberate their DNA. This sometimes enters the other cells and transforms their genetic character. This is better seen in organisms like pneumococci, *H. influenzae*, etc.

Conjugation

Conjugation is another method by which one bacterium donates complete or part of its chromosome to another bacterium. Those bacteria which donates the chromosome is called the donor and the one that receives it, is called recipient. Only those bacteria, which have special structure, called pili can donate the chromosome.

Plasmids are small, circular, extrachromosomal pieces of DNA that are capable of self-replicating and transfer one cell to another. There are many types of plasmids like F factor, plasmids for drug resistance, plasmids for toxin production, plasmids for fermentation, plasmids for fimbriae production, like that. Some of these plasmids can be transferred to other cells autonomously—such ones are called autotransmissible plasmids. The other requires a separate factor called transferable factor and only with its help they can be transferred to other cells. Such ones are called nonautotransmissible plasmids.

Sometimes, these plasmids become integrated with bacterial chromosome and in such instances they can transfer the chromosome to other bacterium in a very high frequency such strains are called Hfr strains.

When the bacteria containing plasmids are mixed with bacteria without plasmids, first a bridge will be formed between them and through this either the plasmid or the plasmid with bacterial chromosome will be transferred to the recipients. With this process, the bacteria can gain new genes and have new characters such as drug resistance, toxin production, etc.

Transduction

Just like we get infection from viruses, bacteria also sometimes get infected with viruses. These viruses are called bacteriophages. When bacteria are infected with virus, two things can happen. The virus may multiply inside the bacteria and cause lysis of the cell, (such phage are virulent phages) or its DNA may be incorporated into bacterial DNA and it is passed on to progeny. Such phages are called prophages. Sometimes these prophage get activated due to some chemical changes, and they come out of the bacterial DNA. During this process, they take out some of the bacterial genes. When this virus carrying bacteria, genes infects other bacteria they can transduce the genes and thus the second bacterium gets new characters.

Lysogenic Conversion

Some bacterial phages induce new properties to bacteria when they get incorporated into the bacterial DNA and these new properties persist as long as the virus exists in the incorporated stage, if by any chance the virus gets out of the bacterial DNA, the bacteria lose the properties, which it was exhibiting previously. For example, diphtheria bacilli, which contain the phage only produce toxin, whereas other diphtheria bacilli are not. This is one method by which bacteria gain new characters and then deviate from the normal behavior.

ANTIMICROBIAL AGENTS

1. Drugs acting on cell wall: Penicillin, cephalosporin.
2. Drugs acting on cell membrane: Polymyxin B.
3. Drugs acting on ribosomes: Tetracycline, gentamicin, kanamycin.
4. Drugs acting on nucleic acid: Nalidixic acid, actinomycin, streptomycin, fluoroquinolone 5-fluorouracil, mitomycin.
5. Drugs acting on biosynthetic pathways: Sulfonamides, trimethoprim, vancomycin, erythromycin.

Bacteria gain resistance through one of the genetic alteration. They exhibit resistance:

i. By inactivating the drugs with enzymes.
ii. By altering their cell permeability.
iii. By altering the receptors for the drugs.
iv. By altering their biosynthetic pathways.

Prevention of Drug Resistance

Prevention depends on proper use of the drugs, proper selection of the antibiotic, administration of complete course, control of the spread of drug resistant strains, etc. Some of the antibiotics like tetracycline are known as growth factors for cattle, poultry. So usually they are incorporated into poultry or cattle feed in low doses. This results in development of drug resistance in the intestinal flora of these animals, which may spread out to cause human infection. So such uses must be discouraged.

BACTERIAL DRUG RESISTANCE

Before we consider the actual mechanisms of drug resistance, first let us know the various antimicrobial agents available for treatment. We have:

1. Drugs acting on cell wall: Penicillin, penicillin derivatives, cephalosporins.
2. Drugs acting on cell membrane: Polymyxin A, B, C.
3. Drugs acting on ribosome: Tetracycline, aminoglycosides, erythromycin, vancomycin, chloramphenicol, lincomycin.
   Experimental stage: Streptogramin, kasugamycin, sparsomycin, oxazolidones, etc.
4. Drugs acting on the biosynthetic pathways: Sulfonamides, trimethoprim.
5. Drugs acting on DNA and RNA: Actinomycin D, mitomycin C.

Mechanisms of Drug Resistance

1. Enzymatic detoxification.
2. Alteration of the finding site of the drug.

3. Genetic alteration of protein that binds the drug.
4. Alteration of the structure of ribosome.
5. Alteration in the permeability of cell membranes.
6. Changes in the transport system of a drug.
7. Increased production of a substance that neutralizes the action of the antibiotic changes in the biosynthetic pathways.

All these above mechanisms are mediated by one of the methods that has already mentioned, i.e. either by mutation, transformation or conjugation or by transduction.

Among these methods, conjugation or plasmid mediated drug resistance is the most common form that we come across in our practice. The plasmids carry the genes of drug resistance for one or sometimes more than one drug. One plasmid sometimes carry genes for as many as 5 to 10 antibiotics and such bacteria are called multiple drug resistant bacteria.

Bacteria showing drug resistance were first isolated in Japan. In the year 1959, there was an outbreak of bacillary dysentery and the cases were first treated with sulfonamides. Initially the response was good, but soon, it was found that the bacteria causing dysentery were resistant to sulfonamides. Within short-time, they acquired resistance to other antibiotics like tetracycline, streptomycin, chloramphenicol, etc. Later on by experiments, it was shown that the resistance exhibited by these bacteria causing dysentery could be transmitted to other bacteria also. Soon it was found that multiple drug resistance was found in almost many bacteria causing disease. Because this is transferable from one bacteria to another. It was called infectious drug resistance.

Reasons for Multiple Drug Resistance

1. Selective pressure of antibiotics: Because of the heavy usage of antibiotics bacteria became acquainted to the drug and develop a sort of tolerance and start nullifying its action.
2. During the antibiotic therapy, the pH, the electrical potential on the surface of the bacteria may alter and may become favorable for transfer of the drug resistance from one cell to another.
3. Antibiotics act as growth factors for cattle and poultry. So these are mixed in their feeds in low concentrations. Under this low concentration, the bacteria present in the guts of these animals develop resistance to the antibiotics.

Presently multiple drug resistant strain are commonly encountered in:

1. Urinary tract infections.
2. Postoperative wound infections.
3. Hospital acquired pneumonias.

In India the first chloramphenicol resistant typhoid fever was reported during 1970s in Calcutta. Later on it started spreading and now more than 80 percent of typhoid fevers are chloramphenicol resistant. The typhoid bacilli are also resistant to ampicillin and furazolidone.

Majority of staphylococci are nowadays penicillin resistant. Fortunately streptococci so far did not develop resistant to penicillin although there is tolerance.

Multiple drug resistant bacterial infections are more common in hospitals because of the conglomeration of the different patients.

Multiple drug resistant bacteria also exhibit resistance to metallic salts and various disinfectants.

Preventive Measures

1. Minimize the use of antibiotics. Antibiotics should not be prescribed for minor illnesses.
2. Proper selection of the antibiotic based on the laboratory sensitivity tests on the isolated bacteria from the patients suffering from infection.
3. Complete administration of the full course of antibiotics.
4. Restricted use of type of antibiotics to particular type of infection. For example, chloramphenicol should be used only for typhoid fevers (which are sensitive to chloramphenicol) and not for other infections, unless the laboratory tests indicate that the particular bacterium is sensitive to chloramphenicol but not to others.
5. Combined therapy based on laboratory tests may reduce the chance of origin of multiple resistant bacteria.
6. The use of antibiotics as animal foods must be discouraged.
7. The antibiotics used for treating the animal diseases must be separated from that used for treating human infections.
8. Each hospital should have an antibiotic policy in which it should be clearly specified which antibiotics should be used for empirical treatment (before the laboratory results are available), and which should be used for prophylaxis (prevention of infections). Surgical prophylaxis with antibiotics should be restricted to only for 24 to 48 hours.

Chapter 6

Culture Media

INTRODUCTION

So far we knew about the metabolic activity and nutritional requirements of most of the disease producing bacteria. Since they are all heterotrophs, one needs:

1. A nutritive substance derived from organic source.
2. Water and electrolytes to maintain the isotonicity.
3. Optimum temperature and oxygen, H^+ concentration to grow these organisms in the laboratory and to study them. Such preparations of complex nutritive substances to grow the organisms in laboratory by providing them all the conditions which closely resemble that of the body environment are called culture media. They are better defined as a natural, synthetic or semisynthetic complex substances which support the growth of an organism in the laboratory, i.e. outside the body.

CLASSIFICATION

Culture media are classified as under:

According to Consistency

a. Liquid
b. Semisolid
c. Solid.

Depending upon their Use and Function

Simple Media

They contain minimum required nutrients necessary to support microorganisms, which are not fastidious. They consist of mainly some proteins, carbohydrates, few mineral salts and water. They are provided in the form of (Fig. 6.1):

- *Peptone*: Water soluble, yellowish granular powder, hygroscopic prepared by acid hydrolysis of cheap protein or meat and contains proteases, amino acids, minerals and other essential nutrients. It is commercially available and various biological firms supply it. Depending upon their nutritive value various grades are there like bacteriological peptone, casein hydrolysate neopeptone, etc.

- *Meat extract*: This is prepared by mixing the meat and boiling it with the presence of a little alkali and we get thin extract and if we concentrate it by evaporation, we get a thick, black, semisolid substance, which contains proteins, carbohydrates, fats, minerals, vitamins, etc. This is also commercially available.

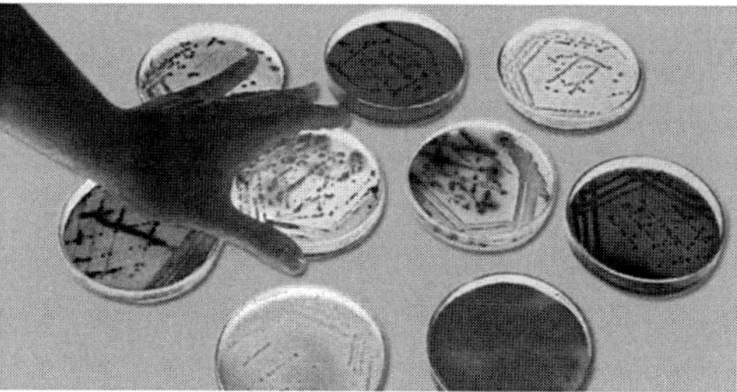

Fig. 6.1: Various types of nutrient media which support the growth of bacteria (*For color version, see Plate 1*)

If you add agar which is inert, polysaccharide melts at 98°C, solidifies at 42°C, available in the form of powder or shreds to the peptone or meat extract. It provides a soild medium on which organisms can be cultivated.

The agar is of two types: New Zealand agar used in concentration of 1.5 percent and Japanese agar used at two percent concentration.

Selective Media

By adding chemicals or antibiotics, which specifically allow the growth of some bacteria but at the same time, suppress others, which are not wanted, e.g. *Salmonella*, *Shigella* agar, Wilson-Blair medium, desoxycholate citrate agar.

Enriched Media

By addition of animal proteins such as blood, egg albumin, egg yolk, serum, ascitic fluid to a simple nutrient medium; the medium is made rich with proteins and other nutrients required for the growth of the organism. Such type of media support the growth of a number of bacteria responsible for disease, e.g. blood agar, chocolate agar (blood agar heated to 80°C), Brain heart infusion agar. Casein hydrolysate medium.

Synthetic Media

By adding all essential amino acids, minerals, and vitamins one can prepare media that promote the growth of microorganisms, e.g. tissue culture media like Eagle's medium, Dubeccos medium, RPMI 1640 medium.

Differential Media

Certain bacteria utilize sugars like lactose and produce acid. The acid production is detected by a suitable indicator or which changes its color in acid conditions, e.g. MacConkey agar.

This contains lactose and neutral red as indicator organisms which ferment lactose and produce acid show pink colored colonies on the medium. Whereas those which do not ferment lactose show pale or colorless colonies.

Enrichment Media

These are liquid selective media mostly used to isolate pathogenic bacteria from diarrheal stools or from food materials, which are suspected for contamination as in cases like food poisoning. These types of media suppress the growth of normal flora, so that the pathogenic bacteria remain viable even though their number is low, e.g. Selenite-F broth, tetrathionate broth, Leedlam's medium.

Transport Media

These media contain essential salts and low concentration ratio of nutrients so that bacteria are not multiplied before they are examined in the laboratory. Transport media are mainly used to collect the specimens with sterile swabs and bacteria present in such swabs are maintained by putting the swab in the transport medium before they are dispatched, e.g. Amies charcoal medium, Stuart's medium, Hajna's medium, Cary-Blair medium.

Assay Media

These media are useful for studying the activity of biological products. By trial and error we have developed a wide variety of media, which support the growth of disease, producing bacteria, and one can use them for growing the specific bacteria depending upon requirements.

More or less one medium is developed for one bacterium and so far about 500 well recognized formulae for various media are available.

Once the media is prepared according to the prescribed formula, pH is adjusted, autoclaved and it is distributed into test tubes or Petri dishes or screw capped bottles or conical flasks. Most of the media can be stored at refrigerator temperature for about a week. Prolonged storage of media (or old media) causes deterioration of the essential nutrients. Hence, such media are not useful.

Once the media are prepared accordingly and they must be inoculated with the material obtained from the patient suspected of suffering from disease. This method is called inoculation (Fig. 6.2). If it is a liquid medium and if the specimen contain bacteria, the whole liquid become turbid, granularity, turbidity pellicle formation should be studied. On solid media, colonies appear. Study the morphology of the colony, size, shape, surface, edge, and pigment, hemolysis of RBC. Study whether they are uniform or not, pickup do Gram's stain, study motility, characterize the organism by biochemical reactions, conduct animal experiments, agglutination with specific antibodies to identify the organism.

Bacteria requiring anaerobic conditions for growth can be cultured in a special equipment called McIntosh Fildes jar.

- *Isolation of pure cultures*: Plating, examination and pick up the colonies. Use of selective, enrichment, indicator media. Use of selective growth conditions, selective treatment of the specimen. Animal inoculation.
- *Disposal of the cultures*: Disinfectant, autoclaving.

Preservation: Agaslopes, egg medium, liquid medium with paraffin seal, freeze-drying.

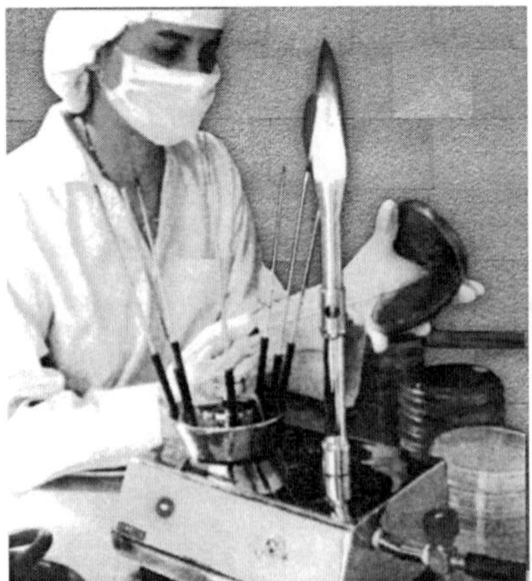

Fig. 6.2: Inoculation of specimen on culture media (*For color version, see Plate 3*)

SELECTED EXAMPLES OF MEDIA FOR PRIMARY ISOLATION OF MICROORGANISMS

General Purpose Media—Enriched

Blood Agar (5% sheep blood added to blood agar base such as nutrient agar, brucella agar, etc.)

Enriched medium used for the primary recovery of most commonly encountered microorganisms.

Chocolate Agar (Enriched)

Hemolyzed blood agar with supplements that serves as an enriched medium for recovery of such fastidious organisms as *Neisseria gonorrhoeae* and *Haemophilus influenzae*. Heating the blood agar gradually to a temperature of 80°C causes lysis of red blood cells, and the contents of red cells are released. The medium turns into chocolate color. Hence it is called chocolate agar.

Blood Agar (Anaerobic)

Nonselective blood agar used to recover anaerobic bacteria from clinical specimens. Contains sheep blood supplemented with yeast extract, hemin, vitamin K_1 and L-cystine. Kanamycin and vancomycin may be added for selective purposes. May or may not be held anaerobically before inoculation.

Enteric Media (CL 1 to 6) (Fig. 6.3)

MacConkey Agar, Eosin Methylene Blue Agar, Tergitol 7, or Desoxycholate Agar

Differential medium for the recovery of gram-negative bacilli. Most gram-positive bacteria are inhibited.

Salmonella-Shigella (S-S) Agar, or Hektoen Enteric (HE) Agar or Xylose-Lysine-Deoxycholate (XLD) Agar, Deoxycholate-Citrate Agar

Media more selective than MacConkey or eosin methylene blue agar, designed specifically to recover species of *Salmonella* or *Shigella* from feces or other body fluids or secretions. SS agar is not recommended for the isolation of *S. sonnei* but is helpful for the isolation of *Y. enterocolitica*.

Bismuth Sulfite (BS) or Brilliant Green (BG) Agar

One-purpose media for the isolation of all *Salmonella* sp. including *S. typhi* (BS) or for *Salmonella* sp. other than *S. typhi* (BG).

Gram-negative (GN), Selenite F Broth, or Tetrathionate Broth

Enrichment broths for concentration of pathogenic *Salmonella* or *Shigella* from contaminated clinical specimens, particularly feces.

CIN Agar

One-purpose medium for the isolation of *Yersinia enterocolitica*.

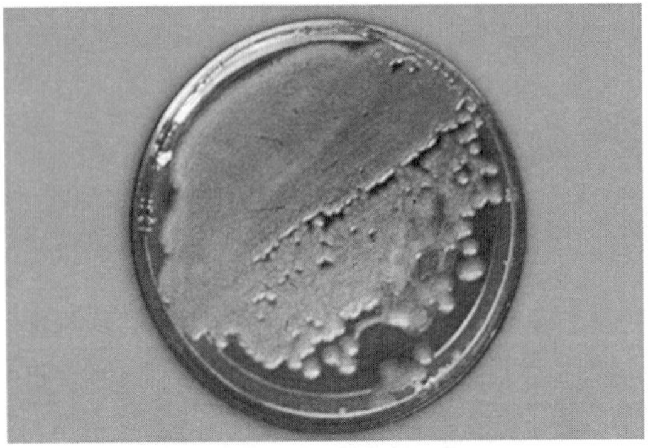

CL 1: Agar plate showing mucoid colonies of *Klebsiella pneumoniae*

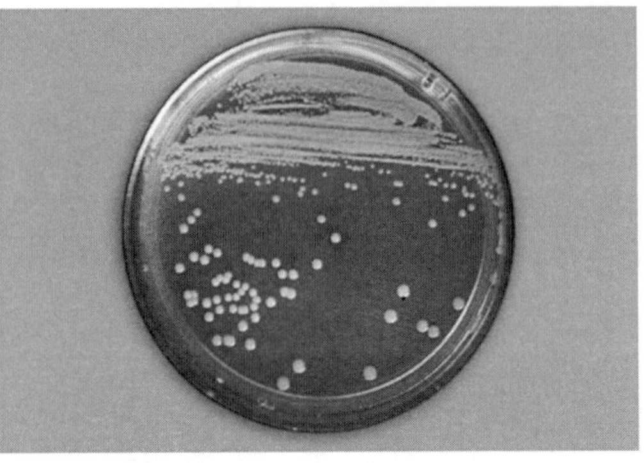

CL 2: Agar plate showing discrete colonies

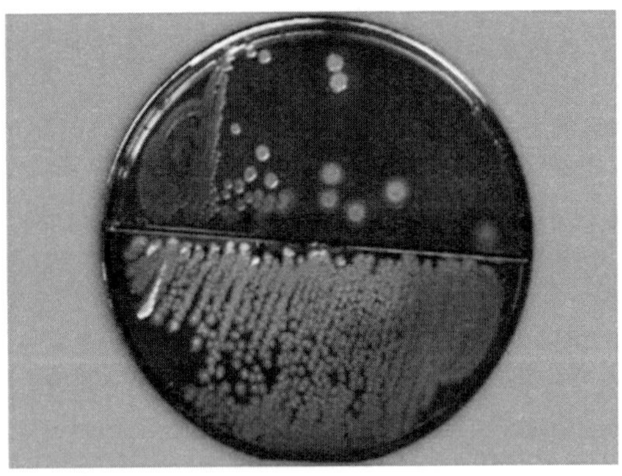

CL 3: Colonies of blood agar and MacConkey/ CLED agar

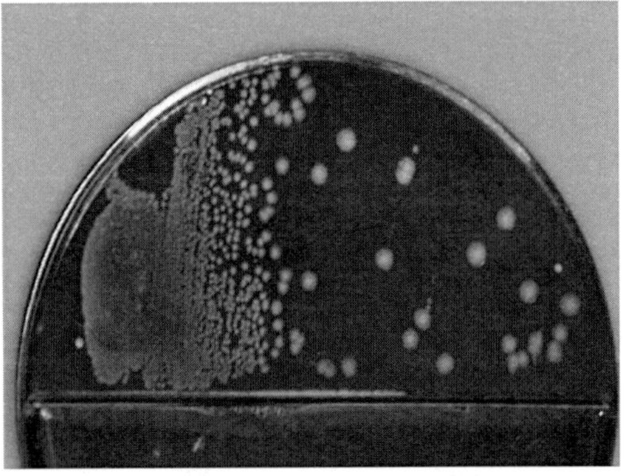

CL 4: Blood agar showing colonies of staphylococci

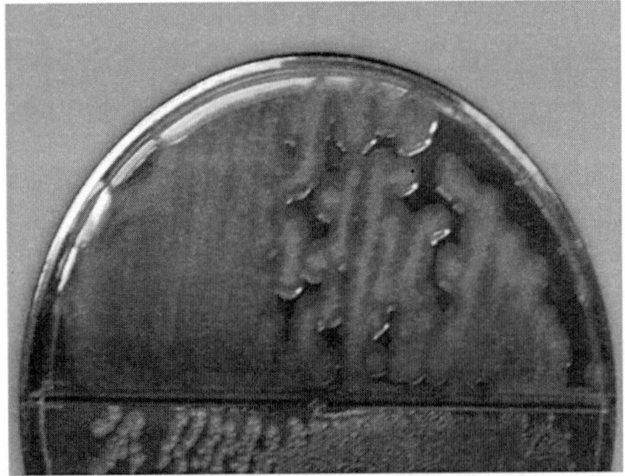

CL 5: MacConkey agar showing pink colored mucoid colonies of *Klebsiella pneumoniae*

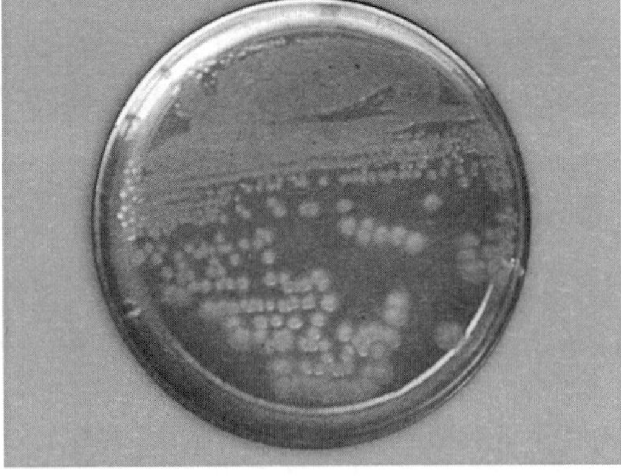

CL 6: CLED agar plate showing yellowish colored colonies due to lactose fermentation

Fig. 6.3: Enteric media (CL 1 to 6) (*For color version, see Plate 2*)

Inhibitory Media—Special Use

Blood Agar (Phenylethyl Alcohol)

Selective medium for the isolation of gram-positive organisms, especially for specimens heavily contaminated with gram-negative organisms, such as *Proteus* sp. which are inhibited by this medium.

Lowenstein-Jensen (LJ) Agar, Middlebrook 7H10 or 7H11 Agar

Primary recovery of mycobacteria. Growth on LJ medium needed to demonstrate niacin accumulation. Middlebrook agar is transparent and used for microscopic examination of colonies.

Mannitol Salt Agar

Selective medium for the isolation of staphylococci.

Peptone Water (Alkaline pH 8.4), Thiosulfate-Citrate-Bile salts-Sucrose Agar (TCBS)

Primary recovery of *Vibrio cholerae* from fecal or other contaminated material.

Regan-Lowe Medium

Selective medium containing cephalexin in a charcoal agar base used for culture of *Bordetella pertussis*.

Skirrow's Campy BAP, Other Selective Media for Isolation of Campylobacter

Special media with a variety of antibiotics that are designed to inhibit normal fecal flora but not affect growth of *Campylobacter jejuni* when incubated at 42°C. All liquid stools should be routinely screened for *C. jejuni*.

Modified Thayer-Martin Agar (MTM)

A modified chocolate agar containing enrichments and the antibiotics vancomycin, colistin, and nystatin to inhibit growth of bacteria other than pathogenic *Neisseria* species. In the modified formula, trimethoprim lactate has been added and the agar concentration increased to two percent to inhibit the spreading of *Proteus* species. The carbohydrate concentration has also been increased to 0.25 percent to enhance growth. Other modifications are available.

Broth Media

Thioglycollate broth (enriched with Hemin and vitamin K) or chopped. Meat broth designed for recovery of anaerobes from clinical materials.

Trypticase Soy Broth or Tryptose Phosphate Broth

General nutrient broths used for recovery of fastidious bacteria, for subculturing colonies of bacteria or for preparing the standard inoculum for the Bauer-Kirby susceptibility test, for various antibiotics.

Table 6.1: Specimen processing in bacteriology

Type of specimen	Media and conditions	Normal flora	Common pathogens	Comments
Throat	Blood agar 35°C aerobic	Alpha and gamma streptococci; Commensal *Neisseria* *Staphylococcus epidermidis* Diphtheroids *Streptococcus pneumoniae* Anaerobes *N. meningitidis*	Group A, beta-hemolytic Streptococci (*Corynebacterium diphtheriae*) *(Bordetella pertussis)*	Chocolate agar should be used if *Haemophilus influenzae* is suspected. Should not be routine. The epiglottis should not be swabbed in suspected cases of epiglottitis.
Respiratory	Blood agar Chocolate agar 35°C, CO_2 MacConkey (aerobic) Anaerobic media	Larynx, trachea, sinus, sputum: *S. epidermidis* Non-beta streptococci Diphtheroids Commensal *Neisseria* Haemophilus Transtracheal and Bronchial: None	Group A, beta streptococci *H. influenzae* *S. aureus* Enterobacteriaceae *Pseudomonas* sp. *S. pneumoniae*	Gram stain: Sputum All aspirates
Urine Clean catch specimen colony count Catheterized or aspirated	Blood agar MacConkey 35°C, aerobic	None	*Escherichia coli* and other enterics Enterococci *Pseudomonas* sp. Staphylococci	
Feces	MacConkey xylose-lysine-deoxycholate Selenite-F 35°C, aerobic Selective medium for *Campylobacter* 42°C, 5% O_2	Anaerobes Enterobacteriaceae Enterococci	*Salmonella* sp. *Shigella* sp. *Yersinia enterocolitica* *Campylobacter jejuni* *E. coli* (enterotoxigenic, enteroinvasive)	
Genital for GC only	Modified Thayer-Martin (MTM) 35°C, CO_2	Lactobacilli Diphtheroids Alpha streptococci Enterobacteriaceae Enterococci	*Neisseria gonorrhoeae* Inhibited on MTM	Gram stain

Contd...

Contd...

Vaginal, cervical, routine genital	Blood agar Enriched chocolate MTM 35°C, CO_2 MacConkey-aerobic	Lactobacilli Diphtheroids Enterococci *Enterobacteriaceae* Non-beta streptococci Anaerobes *G. vaginalis*	*N. gonorrhoeae* *Candida albicans* Group A and B streptococci *Listeria monocytogenes*	Culture for *G. vaginalis* is of questionable value
Genital—surgical or aspirates	Blood agar Chocolate agar MTM 35°C, CO_2 MacConkey-aerobic	None	Same as above plus anaerobes	Gram stain
Sterile body fluids CSF, joint fluid, pleural fluid, peritoneal fluid, etc.	Blood agar Chocolate agar 35°C, CO_2 MacConkey agar Thioglycolate 35°C, aerobic Anaerobe blood agar (except for CSF)	None	Identify all isolates *S. pneumoniae* *N. meningitidis* *H. influenzae* Gram-negative rods	Gram stain
Blood	Submitted in two bottles: one 35°C aerobic and one 35°C anaerobic	None	Any isolate potentially significant	
Wound (superficial) includes eye and ear	MacConkey agar 35°C, aerobic Blood agar Chocolate (eye) 35°C, CO_2	*S. epidermidis* Diphtheroids Commensal *Neisseria* Anaerobes Other skin flora	*S. aureus* Beta-hemolytic streptococci *P. aeruginosa* *H. influenzae* biotype III (*H. aegyptius*) Enterobacteriaceae	Gram stain
Wound (surgical or aspirate) Tissue specimens	Same as above plus anaerobic blood agar KV blood agar* Thioglycollate	None	Same as above plus anaerobes Any isolate is potentially significant	Gram stain

*Kanamycin-vancomycin Blood agar

Transport Media

Transport Medium: Stuart's, Amies, or Carey and Blair

A transport medium should be available in all laboratories to maintain viability of microorganisms in specimens which must be forwarded to reference laboratories (see Chapter 8).

SUPPLEMENTAL PRIMARY CULTURE MEDIA FOR RECOVERY OF SPECIAL FASTIDIOUS ORGANISMS

Medium and Purpose

Bordet-Gengou Potato Infusion Agar

Selective medium for recovery of *Bordetella pertussis*. Inoculation of medium with a nasopharyngeal swab is recommended instead of the use of a cough plate.

Brucella Agar

Enriched peptic digest casein medium designed for recovery of *Brucella* species from clinical specimens and other infected material.

Fletcher's Semisolid Medium

Basal medium used with serum enrichments for the recovery of *Leptospira* species.

Loeffler Medium and Tellurite Medium

Used for inoculation of nasopharyngeal cultures for recovery of *Corynebacterium diphtheriae*. Also used to prepare methylene blue stains of suspicious colonies. Various specimen processing procedures are discussed in Table 6.1.

Chapter 7

Disinfection and Sterilization

DISINFECTION

Disinfection is defined as destruction or removal of an article of all organisms, capable of giving rise to infection. A disinfectant is one, which kills the organisms outright. An antiseptic is a substance, which prevents the growth of microorganisms as long as it remains in contact with them and it is relatively bland and nontoxic for superficial application to living tissues. Disinfectants are potent microbicidal but relatively strong substances and toxic to living tissues. They rapidly kill all the vegetative forms of all pathogenic organisms. They are suitable for application to inanimate objects. Disinfection is carried out where absolute sterility is not essential or not practicable. The terms disinfection is generally used in the meaning of chemical disinfection, but the articles which are suitably treated by heat and other physical agents can also be referred to as disinfected. Thus, disinfection can be achieved by:

1. Chemical methods
2. Physical methods
3. Natural methods.

Chemical Methods of Disinfection

To begin with substances with strong deodorant property were employed to nullify the smell of putrefying matter in a belief that infectious diseases arose from the putrefying material. Early in the 19th century hypochlorites came into prominence. Lord Lister successfully used carbolic acid in the control of wound infection and paved the way for the antiseptic surgery. Budd advocated the use of phenol compounds for preventing the spread of typhoid fever. Robert Koch made the comparative study of the germicidal effect of different disinfectants. Later on several workers like Nyman, Chick studied the factors influencing the action of disinfectant and they concluded that the action of disinfectants on bacteria obeyed the law of unimolecular chemical reaction.

Classification of Disinfectants

Many chemical are recognized as disinfectants and they can be grouped as:

1. Oxidizing agents: H_2O_2, $KMnO_4$ (potassium permanganate).
2. Halogens: Chlorine, hypochlorites, chloramine T, iodine, iodoform.
3. Acids and alkalies: Boric acid, benzoic acid, salicylic acid, mandelic acid, chromic acid, potassium hydroxide, sodium hydroxide.
4. Alcohols: 70% alcohol (ethyl), isopropylalcohol.
5. Aldehyde: Formaldehyde, glutaraldehyde
6. Metallic salts: Silver, copper, mercury.
7. Dyes:
   a. Azodyes: Scarlet red, pyridium, prontosil
   b. Acridine dyes: Acriflavine, proflavine
   c. Fluorescent dyes
   d. Phenolphthalein
   e. Triphenyl methane dyes: Gentian violet, brilliant green
   f. Methyl thionine or methylene blue.
8. Phenol derivatives: Phenol, cresol, Dettol, Lysol, creosote, guiacol, resorcinol
9. Detergents:
   Anionic detergent: Soaps
   Cationic detergents: Quaternary ammonium compounds like: Cetrimide, Benzalkonium chloride.
10. Miscellaneous: Alkaloids of quinine, volatile oils, nitrofurazone, scabicides like sulfur, benzyl benzoate. Fungicides like caprylic acid, undecyclic acid derivatives, salicylic and benzoic acid chrysarobin.

Mode of Action of Disinfectants

Many disinfectants in general are protoplasmic poisons. Simple chemical reactions such as neutralization of free acidic or basic groups on bacterial proteins bring about the metabolic disturbance and subsequently causing the death of the organism.

Anionic antiseptics or acid dyes function through interaction of their acidic ions with the basic groups of bacteria to form feebly ionized compounds. Some disinfectants such as mercurial salts inhibit the bacterial growth by combining with sulfhydryl groups of metabolites. Others groups act on the surface by adsorption. They accumulate on the surface of the organism. So that the cell is surrounded by the dense layer of the disinfectant.

Disinfectants such as formaldehyde acts by forming complexes with free amino groups of bacterial proteins. The halogens and hypochlorites, act both by halogenating the amino groups, through a direct oxidizing action. Chemicals like H_2O_2, ozone act as oxidizing agents. Some disinfectants like ether, act as a lipid solvents and cause disruption of the organism.

Dyes such as neutral red, proflavine, toludine blue bind to the guanine base of nucleic acids and thereafter exposure to fluorescent light the dye absorbs the energy and these may cause breaking of the stands of DNA. This is referred as photodynamic action.

Other methods by which disinfectants act on microorganism are alteration in the electrophoresis mobility, modification of the permeability of the cell wall with leakage of the constituents of the cell or abnormal penetration of the substance to the cell, cellular lysis, irreversible coagulation of the cell protein.

Factors Influencing the Action of Disinfectant

The activity of a disinfectant is modified by the following factors (Fig. 7.1).

1. ***Temperature***: The microbicidal action of infectants is usally increased by heat in the limits of the thermostability of the chemical. So, it is advised to use disinfectants under warm conditions rather than in cold. But when an organism is suspended in a favorable medium. The effect of temperature on inhibition of growth may be opposite to that of disinfection. Higher concentration of the disinfectant is required to inhibit the growth at 37°C than at lower temperatures.
2. ***Duration of contact***: In general, germicidal activity is exerted with time and sufficient exposure is necessary for efficient disinfection. Disinfection is usually considered as a process in which bacteria are killed of time within reasonable length.
3. ***Concentration of the disinfectant***: Many disinfectants function only at high concentration. But some salts of heavy metals kill the bacteria in a very low concentration (Oligodynamic reaction). There is also tendency of poisonous relation of reagents to stimulate biological processes in a very low concentration.
4. ***Nature of the medium***: Some antimicrobial effects are correctly dependent on the pH of the disinfectant. High acidity or alkalinity increases the action of the disinfectant. The hardness of water may markedly interfere with the disinfecting action of surface active agents. It is noted that H ions are more toxic than OH ions in similar concentration. At pH bacteria are negatively changed. pH also determines the ionic capacity of disinfectants.
5. ***Presence of organic matter***: Greatly influence the action of many disinfectants. Organic matter should be removed before applying any disinfectant.

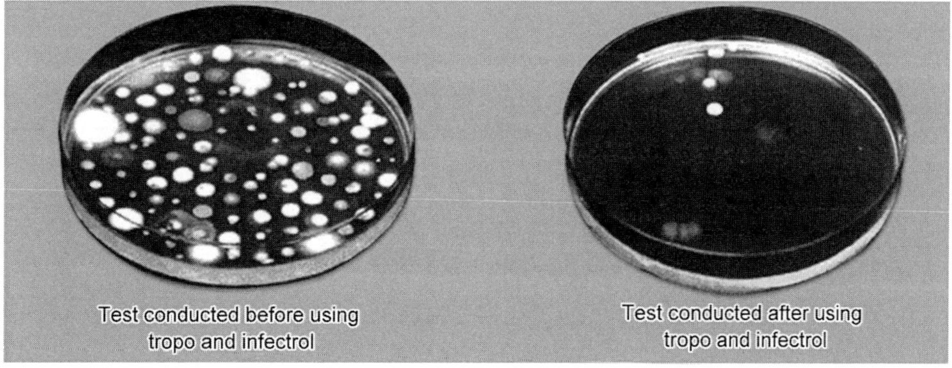

Fig. 7.1: Nutrient agar plates showing the effect of disinfection. Note the number of colonies have reduced after disinfection (right side) (*For color version, see Plate 1*)

6. ***Number and nature of the organism*:** Larger the number of organism greater will be the time taken for disinfection of bacteria. Spores are exceptionally resistant to many disinfectants.
7. ***Standardization of disinfectants*:** It is desirable to have some method to measure their relative germicidal effect of various disinfectants.
   i. *Koch's thread method*: Suitable organisms such as anthrax spores are dried on silk threads subjected to the action of disinfectant and subsequently washed and transferred to a solid medium to ascertain whether all the spores had been killed. But in this method presence of disinfectants may inhibit the growth.
   Kronig and Paul replaced the silk threads by garnets, and made the test quantitative by planting out the washing from the garnets and counting the number that developed.
   ii. *Rideal-Walker drop method*: In this method, similar quantities of organisms are submitted to the action of varying concentration of phenol and the germicide to be tested. Subculture is made into broth every 2½ minutes upto 15 minutes, and the tubes incubated 37°C for 3 days. The dilution of the disinfectant in test which sterilizes the suspension in a given time is divided by that of phenol, which sterilizes. The same suspension in the same time and this is called phenol coefficient.

The ***Chick-Martin test:*** Rideal-Walker test compares the action of the antiseptic with that of phenol on *S. typhi* in distilled water. Hence, it does not give any indication of the disinfecting power under practical condition where much organic matter is usually present. Accordingly Chick-Martin test has been advocated in which the disinfectant is tested in the presence of organic matter which is heat sterilized liquid feces containing 10 percent solids is mixed with twice its volume of disinfectant.

Garrod has devised the modification of Chick-Martin test with five percent yeast extract instead of feces.

Uses of Disinfectants

In bacteriology

1. For the disposal of cultures (usually 3% lysol or 1% sodium hypochlorite is used).
2. To prepare some selective media such as Dettol agar for the isolation of *Pseudomonas;* Phenol to suppress—antigen in culturing the *Salmonella typhi* for the preparation of 'O', H antigen.
3. For preservation of sera, e.g. addition of chloroform.
4. For the preservation of vaccines:
   - 0.5 percent phenol
   - β-propiolactone
   - 50% glycerol.

In surgical procedure

1. To wash hands before conducting any operative procedure.
2. To clean the area of operation.

3. To collect blood under aseptic precaution (70% alcohol or tincture iodine is used).
4. For safe disposable of infected materials such as excreta or surgical dressings.
5. Cleaning of the wounds, e.g. H_2O_2, alcohol.
6. For disinfection of used instruments.

In hospital

1. Disinfect the operating rooms.
2. To control the spread of cross-infection.
3. To disinfect the linen and surgical dressings.

In public health services

1. For providing safe drinking water (chlorination).
2. Disinfection of the sewage before disposing it into the fields.

Disinfection by Physical Methods

The commonly used physical methods by which the articles rendered or disinfected are as follows:

1. *Dry hcat*: Direct flaming of the articles such as scalpels, forceps, bacteriological loops, mouths of the tubes, render then sterile. The more common apparatus used fur sterilizing the articles like glass ware is hot air oven. In this the articles are subjected to heating at 160°C for 1 hour.
2. *Moist heat*: Boiling, steaming and autoclaving are another methods in which moist heat is used as the sterilizing agent.
3. *Irradiation*: Ultraviolet rays or γ-rays. They interfere with DNA replication. Just as many factors influence the chemical disinfections, disinfection by physical methods is also affected by many factors such as time, temperature, nature of the medium, presence of number of bacteria and the nature of bacteria. Adequate displacement of air before applying moist heat for sterilization.

All the equipment used for the physical methods of sterilization should be monitored for the temperature, air circulation, air displacement, and for cooling the article.

Disinfection is most readily obtained by simple procedure of washing, cleaning and ventilations which if done thoroughly destroy majority of the pathogenic organisms. More effective disinfection is obtained by application, though less degree of the same kinds of procedures as are used for sterilization.

Types of Disinfection

1. Concurrent disinfection: This is the immediate destruction of microorganisms present in the infected material throughout the course of illness. The disease agents are destroyed as soon as they are released from an infected person and in this way further spread is stopped, e.g. disinfection of urine, feces, vomitus, dressings, etc.
2. Terminal disinfection: Disinfection of infected material after the death or recovery of the patient, e.g. disinfection of rooms, article used by the patient.
3. Prophylactic disinfection: Chemical treatment of water, boiling of water, pasteurization, washing of hands.

Recommended Disinfection Procedures

1. *Feces and urine*: Collected in impervious bags. Treat with a disinfectant for 2 hours. The disinfectants used are bleaching powder, formalin, cresol, and phenol.
2. *Sputum*: Five percent cresol or autoclaved.
3. *Room:*
   a. First wash with soap water.
   b. Mopping with five percent phenol or 2.5 percent cresol.
   c. Spraying of formalin 500 mL/1000 cu ft.
   d. Expose to formaldehyde vapor for 24 hours.
4. *Linen*: Boiling, steam disinfection, exposure formalin gas.
5. *Dead bodies*: Ten percent formalin or five percent phenol.
6. *Instruments*: Three percent lysol.

STERILIZATION

So far, we were discussing about the various methods to grow the organisms under artificial conditions and study their properties. Let us consider the other side of it, i.e. how to destroy the microorganism? The rendering of any article free from bacteria, fungi and their spores and viruses is called sterilization. This is an absolute term. You can say only whether an article is completely sterile or not; there are no relatively sterile or partially sterile terms.
The purpose of sterilization in medicine is as follows:

1. In bacteriology or microbiology, all the glassware, media used for cultivation and study of microorganisms must be rendered sterile before they are inoculated with specimens.
2. In all surgical procedures, all the instruments needles, catgut, surgical dressings must be sterile before they are used.
3. The drugs administered for treating the diseases must be sterile, IV infusions, etc.
4. In canning industry where tinned food is prepared or in dairy industry, the milk, cheese, butter must be made free from organisms before it is served for consumption.
5. The operating rooms, the places where vaccines are prepared must be made free from bacteria (at least pathogenic). Added to this there are many more purposes where it is necessary to make the conditions free from bacteria. To achieve this task, we have 4 major methods:
   - Physical methods
   - Chemical methods
   - Filtration
   - Irradiation.

Physical Methods

By far the cheapest and the most reliable method of sterilization is by heat. Before we know the various procedures of heat sterilization, let us see the factors responsible for sterilization by heat.

1. ***Temperature:*** Higher the temperature, shorter is the time required for sterilization.
   Example:

• *Dry heat*	*temp*	*time*	
		120°C	8 hr
		140°C	2½ hr
		160°C	1 hr
• Moist heat	100°C	20 hr	
		110°C	2½ hr
		115°C	50 min
		121°C	15 min

The lowest temperature required to sterilize completely a given suspension of bacteria in a given time is called thermal death point. The shortest time required to sterilize given suspension under a known temperature is called thermal death time.

In practice all articles, which are sterilized by dry heat, must be heated upto 160°C for 1 hour and all articles, which are sterilized by moist heat must be heated upto 121°C for 15 minutes.

2. ***The number of microorganisms*:** More the number, more temperature and longer time is required for sterilization. That is the reason all the articles must be cleaned thoroughly with detergents to minimize the number present on it before they subjected to sterilization.
3. *The species, strains and spore forming ability.* The sterilizing temperature varies with each organism. If it is a spore forming one, longer sterilizing temperature and time are required.
4. *Presence of organic material* like air, fats, pus, protein, blood, protect the bacteria from killing. Hence must be removed before the article is sterilized.

Dry Heat

Dry heat kills the microorganisms by destructive oxidation. Commonly used methods are:

1. *Red heat*: Sterilize the article by putting it into flame till it becomes red-hot, e.g. needles, wires, forceps, scalpels, spatulas, etc.
2. *Flaming*: Place all the contaminated articles in an enamel bowel and put spirit till they are immersed. After 5 minutes, burn off all the spirit. Not a good procedure.
3. *Hot air oven*: This is a very widely used instrument for sterilizing many article like glassware, pipettes, flasks, Petri dishes, bottles, swabs, syringes.

This is a metal made rectangular box with racks in side. The electric coils are placed below the perforated plate and they are heated by electricity. There is a thermostat control mechanism by which one can adjust the temperature upto 160°C (Fig. 7.2).

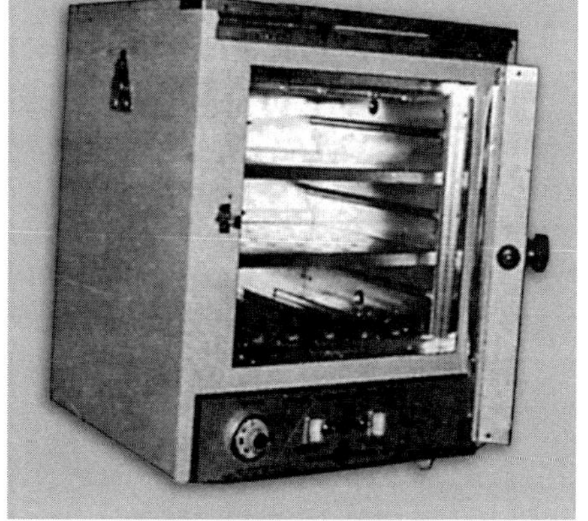

Fig. 7.2: Hot air oven

All the articles requiring sterilization are first cleaned with soap and water, thoroughly and dried, then they are all wrapped in a paper separately. All the mouths of test tubes or flasks, must be plugged with cotton. Then these are placed in the hot air oven and close the doors of it and start heating. It takes at least 2 hours to reach the temperature of 160°C; keep the temperature for 1 hour by thermostatic regulation. After 1 hour (that means totally 3 hours), switch off the coil and allow the oven to cool and reach the room temperature otherwise, there is every chance of breaking of the glassware because of the sudden contraction of the expanded material due to entry of cool air. Hot air oven can also be used for sterilizing fats, oils, and powders, but they must be placed in small quantities.

Infrared Radiation

The infrared rays are directed onto the article and usually a temperature of 180°C can be obtained. In vacuum we can attain 200°C and many of the surgical instruments can be sterilized. Oxidation can be prevented by admitting nitrogen into the chamber.

Moist Heat

Heating an article in the presence of moisture causes the death of microorganisms due to denaturation and coagulation of cellular proteins.

Most of the pathogenic organisms die at 60°C in 10 minutes with moist heat. Rarely they can tolerate temperature upto 80 to 90°C for ½ hour. But the spores of the bacteria are viable at 121°C upto 10 minutes. *Clostridium botulinum* spores are can be viable at 100°C for 8 hours and at 115°C upto 1 hour.

Moist heat can be conveniently employed for killing the bacteria in 3 forms:

1. Heating below 100°C
2. Heating at 100°C
3. Heating above 100°C under pressure.

Heating below 100°C

1. Pasteurization of milk
   a. Holder method 63°C for 10 minutes.
   b. Flash method 72°C for 20 seconds.

   Ensures killing all pathogenic bacteria but not spores.
2. Vaccines: For sterilization of vaccine. Heat the vaccines to 60°C for 1 hour. This ensures killing of the organisms and at the same time protect its potency.
3. Heating at 80°C: Utensils, clothing, can be conveniently made free from pathogenic in hot water for 10 minutes.

Heating at 100°C

1. *Boiling*: Glass syringes, scalpels, can be made safe for use by boiling them for 5 to 10 minutes. It does not destroy spores and also repeated boiling causes loss of sharpness of blades or needles.
2. *Intermittent exposure at 100°C*: This is usually carried out for heat sensitive substance like sugar solutions which should not be exposed to high temperature. The sugar solutions are heated upto 100°C for 20 to 40 minutes. Then it, is taken out and incubated at 37°C. The process is repeated for 3 days. The reason behind it is at 100°C the vegetative bacteria are killed but not the spores. But the spores are placed in suitable environment.

Hence, they germinate producing bacteria, which are killed on exposure to heat on the next day. This intermittent heating is called tyndalization.

3. *Inspissation*: This is a type of sterilization in which the substances are slowly coagulated and sterilized in the presence of moisture. The media containing serum egg yolk are placed in a special instrument called inspissator, which is nothing but a rectangular box with water jacket inside. The water jacket is heated to 80°C and the steam comes out through small holes. This maintains the moisture of the medium and at the same time slowly coagulates the medium. The heating is continued for 30 to 45 minutes and the process is repeated for 3 days.

Heating above 100°C using steam under pressure: Normally water boils when the vapor pressure is equal to the atmospheric pressure. If the water is boiled under pressure, the temperature at which it boils raises. For example,

- 5 lb/sq in 108°C
- 10 lb/sq in 115°C
- 15 lb/sq in 121°C
- 30 lb/sq in 130°C

The advantage of steam heating under pressure are:

1. It is quicker in heating hence less time is required.
2. It penetrates more quickly than air.
3. When the steam condenses over an article, it liberates its latent heat and hence the article gets heated up very quickly. As the steam condenses to water, it draws more and more steam till the article is heated.
4. The condensation of water ensures moist conditions.

   The instrument by which sterilization under pressure is carried out is called autoclave. Many types are there:

   1. Simple nonjacketed
   2. Steam jacketed
   3. High pressure autoclave
   4. Automatic vacuum operated autoclaves.

Radiation

Radiation means energy travelling through space. Many forms exist in nature and many other forms are produced naturally. Radiations which have shorter wavelength than visible light exhibit the most pronounced lethal effect. (Wavelength is expressed in Angstrom (Å) = 1/10,000 μm or 1/254,000,000 of an inch).

1. ***Ultraviolet rays:*** Ultraviolet rays of wavelength 2,650 Å are having highest bactericidal activity. But most of these rays of shorter wavelength of the type are filtered out by atmosphere. Hence sunlight though effective as a bactericidal agent has limited value. Many lamps emiting the rays of 2600 to 2700 Å are available. Hence are widely used to reduce the microbial population in operating rooms, pharmaceutical industry. One disadvantage is that these rays are not penetrable, so only useful for surface sterilization.

2. ***X-rays:*** These are extremely penetrating and lethal to microorganisms. They are:
   i. Expensive.
   ii. Difficult to utilize efficiently.
   iii. Harmful to human beings.
3. ***Gamma rays:*** These are emitted from radioactive substances like isotopes of cobalt. These are of shorter wavelength and penetrate more. Because of their penetrability they can be used to sterilize prepacked material such as disposable plastic syringes, catheters, IV sets, etc.
4. ***Electron beam radiation:*** It consists of exposure to a beam of electrons. At high intensity it is microbicidal. A special instrument called electron accelerator is nowadays used to sterilize surgical supplies, drugs, etc. This is used for prepacked articles at room temperature.

Filtration

Filtration is a method by which the heat sensitive biological fluids such as serum, plasma, liquid broth cultures, toxins, etc. can be made bacteria free and at the same time preserving the biological properties of these fluids.

Available Filters

1. Earthenware candles: Berkefeld, Chamberland L_1, L_2, $L_3 \ldots L_{13}$
2. Asbestos filters: Seitz filter K, N, EK.
   Cellulose membrane filters:
   - Gradecol membranes
   - Millipore filters
3. Sintered glass filters: Finely ground glass fused sufficiently to make the particle adhere.
   All these filters should not allow the passage of *S. marcescens*.
   All above filters can be sterilized either by hot air oven or an autoclave. Commonly used filter in bacteriology is Seitz filter.

Chapter 8

Collection and Transportation of Specimens

INTRODUCTION

"If a physician is dependent upon microbiology laboratory data for helping to save his patients the one who collects the specimen may determine the course of the patient recovery."

One of the main tasks of the laboratory incharge of a clinical microbiology laboratory is to provide detailed guidelines for the collection and transportation of the specimens obtained from the patient. Improper collection and delay in transportation may result in overgrowth of normal microbiota prevailing at the site of collection, outgrowing of opportunistic flora and death of labile, fastidious but more virulent organisms which are in fact might be the cause of the infection.

Paradoxically, medical students become acquainted with the molecular biology and genetics of microbiota but are less likely to even suspect the role of microorganisms in the pathogenesis. They enter the clinical arena of learning and order to laboratory tests without an appreciation of the importance of proper collection and transport or even of the reasons for the procedure. Harold C Neu has termed "Fear medicine" which encompasses the unassessed degree of compromise of the individual patient and results in the excessive submission of specimens from every available body site. The information obtained may be ignored since 'patient is doing well'. Hence, a continuing educational efforts are mandatory, explaining and insisting the need for the proper collection of appropriate specimen. This chapter mainly deals with specimen selection, collection and rationale.

GENERAL CONSIDERATIONS

1. Collect before antibiotic therapy whenever possible.
2. Collect the specimen where the suspected organism is likely to be found.
3. Absolute aseptic precautions should be observed while collecting the sample.
4. Consider the stage of the disease.
5. Instruct the patient clearly.
6. Use proper containers and/or suitable transport media.
7. Specimen should be delivered to the laboratory as soon as possible.
8. Sufficient and relevant information should be provided to the laboratory.

Open the lines of communication with all persons potentially involved in the specimen handling process.

The requisition form should contain patients name, age, sex, patient location (ward, room number or address), name of the treating physician, nature of the specimen, specific anatomic culture site, clinical diagnosis, procedure used in obtaining the specimen, name of the individual transcribing the orders, antimicrobial therapy if any patient is receiving. This preliminary information is necessary for proper selection of the nutrient media for culturing the pathogens, and to communicate, if any problems concerning the culture request arise. The specimens should be properly labeled containing the name of the patient, location, treating physician's name, culture site, date and hour of collection. Specimens requiring emergency handling or which may contain pathogens of potential danger should be appropriately marked.

Collection Times

The optimal time for collecting the specimen depends to certain extent the type of infectious disease process and the ability of the laboratory staff to process the sample. The microbiology laboratory may not be having adequate staff during 'off' hours, and specimens collected late in the evening may not produce adequate growth by the next morning. However, provisions must be made by the laboratory chief to handle 'urgent' samples after the usual working hours. Consultation with supervisory personnel is highly recommended.

Twenty-four-hour specimen collections must be discouraged. The first early morning sputum or urine specimens are optimal for recovering acid-fast bacteria. Early morning specimens are more concentrated and more likely to contain large number of the etiological agent.

Timing of the blood cultures should be determined by the clinical condition of the patient (Table 8.1). Physicians should always indicate the collection schedule. A blood culture is defined as draw of at least 10 mL of blood divided between two 50–100 mL culture bottles—one incubated aerobically and one anaerobically (Figs 8.1 and 8.2).

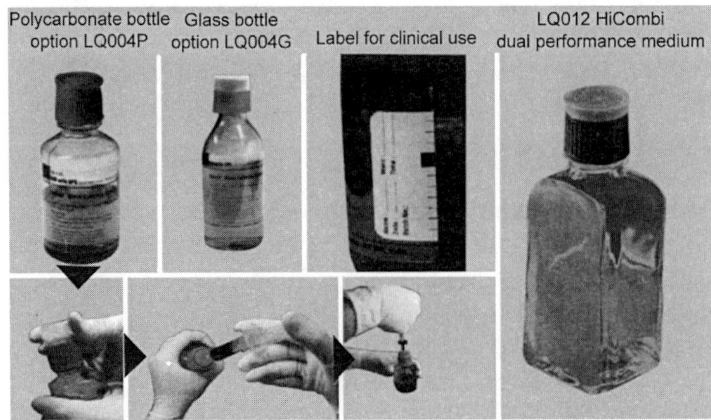

Fig. 8.1: Blood culture bottle and collection of blood for culture under aseptic conditions. LQ—Liquid medium store between 2–8°C, SPS—Sodium polyanethol sulfonate (liquid) (*For color version, see Plate 3*)

Table 8.1: Blood culture collection

Clinical conditions	*Collection protocol*	*Remarks*
Adults and adolescents		
a. Severe septicemia, meningitis, osteo-myelitis arthritis, pneumonia	• Two cultures prior to therapy	• 10–20 mL blood sample from each arm.
b. Subacute bacterial endocarditis	• Three cultures within 24 hr	• Space each collection at least 1 hour apart. Two should be collected at beginning of fever spikes.
c. Acute bacterial endocarditis	• Three cultures within 1–2 hr before therapy	
d. Low grade intravascular infection	• Three cultures within 24 hr	• Same as 'b'
e. Bacteremia of unknown origin	• 4–6 cultures within 48 hr • Patient on therapy	• Specimen blood
f. Febrile episodes	• Not more than three cultures	• Bacteremia may precede fever and chills by about 1 hr
Younger children	• 1–2 mL	• Two cultures are usually sufficient for diagnosing bacteremia in newborn

In infections like endocarditis, typhoid fever, brucellosis, and other uncontrolled infections, the bacteremia is continuous thus making the time of collection less critical. In conditions where bacteremia is likely to be intermittent, one should strictly adhere to the above cited protocols. The recovery rate after three negative cultures in 24 hours is extremely low, except when a sudden fever spike is observed.

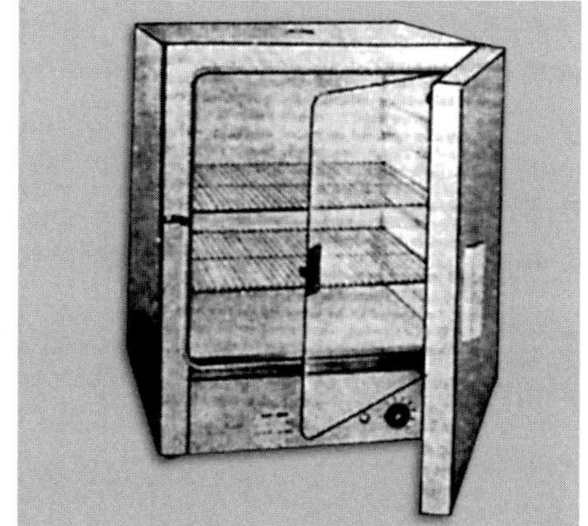

Fig. 8.2: Incubator

All specimens must be collected in appropriate containers. It is the responsibility of the laboratory director that sterile containers which are leakproof are made available. However, nowadays ready to use disposable containers are available in the market which can be used for general purposes. For specimens requiring appropriate transport medium the laboratory should be contacted.

Anaerobic cultures are best collected by aspirating the fluids with sterile disposable needle and syringe and transported to the laboratory with the needle cap *in situ*. The submission of swabs for anaerobic culture should be discouraged, but if swabs must be used they should be immediately placed into the suitable transport medium provided by the laboratory.

Sputum

Sputum specimens must contain lower respiratory secretions. Patients must be instructed to cough deeply. Postural drainage is useful in getting the appropriate secretions. The mouth should be rinsed with water or gargle, dentures should be removed before the collection of the sputum. Induced specimens or transtracheal aspirations are recommended for adult patients who cannot produce sputum. It is futile to process sputum samples if there is no productive cough. Bronchial washings should be transported immediately and should be processed as soon as it is received. Currently, there is no documented support to the use of enrichment medium for bronchial washings for isolation of *M. tuberculosis*. Usually 2 mL of properly expectorated sputum is sufficient (Fig. 8.3).

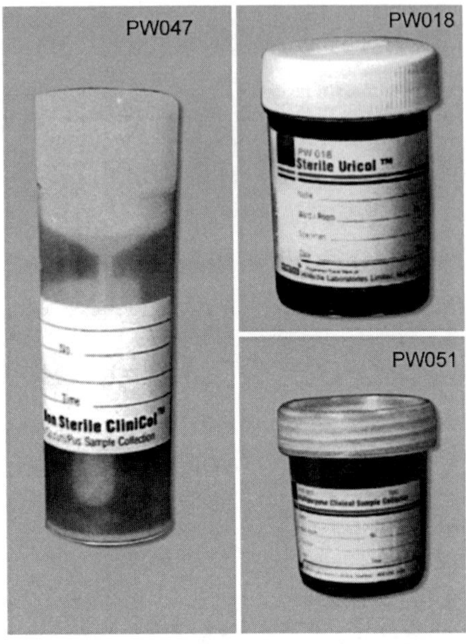

Fig. 8.3: Specimen collectors for urine, feces, and sputum (*For color version, see Plate 3*)

Urine

The clean-catch or midstream collection of urine samples must not be left to chance. Ideally the specimen should be collected by a nurse or an aide. The patient should be given specific instructions such as, retraction of prepuce and cleaning the urethra in males, and retraction of labia in females. It is advisable to print these instructions on card and be given to the patient in the language with which he/she is familiar. For illiterate patients verbal instructions are must. Anaerobic cultures should not be performed on clean-catch specimens. Urinary tract infections due to anaerobes are very rare. If an anaerobic infection is suspected, suprapubic aspiration of the bladder should be performed (Fig. 8.3).

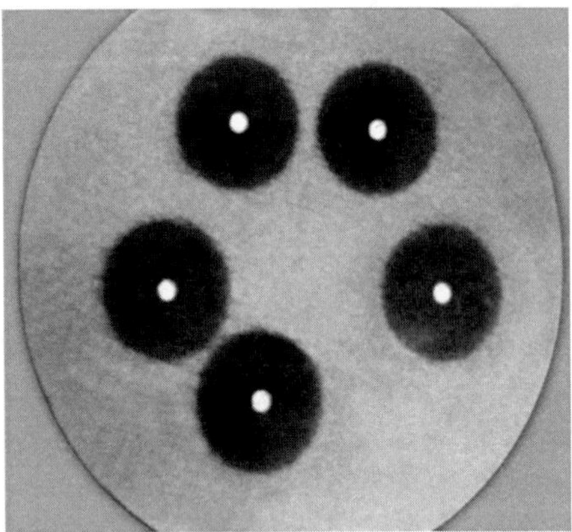

Fig. 8.4: Antibiotic sensitivity testing. Note the clear zone around the antibiotic disk indicating that the organism is sensitive to that antibiotic (*For color version, see Plate 3*)

Foley's catheter tips should not be accepted for culture because it invariably gets contaminated with urethral flora during the removal.

Urine samples collected from in dwelling bladder should not be cultured. For catheter specimens, cultures are to be taken from the catheter with the help of a needle and syringe (i.e., by puncturing the catheter) (Table 8.2).

Table 8.2: Urine culture decisions

Cultures pure or mixed	*Clean-catch specimen from*		
	Asymptomatic patient	*symptomatic patient*	*Suprapubic aspirates*
1. Gram-negative bacilli	A	B	E
2. Enterococci	A	B	E
3. *Staph. aureus*	A	B	E
4. *Staph. saprophyticus*	A	B	E
5. Commensals	D	C	C
(*Staphylococcus epidermidis, Neisseria, Diptheroids,* L-hemolytic or nonhemolytic streptococci, lactobacilli)			

A: Identify. Perform antibiotic susceptibility testing if CFU/mL exceed 10^5/mL. If mixed or less than 10^5/mL. Report as mixed flora and the number of commensal types.

B: Identify and report antibiotic sensitivity pattern when the CFU/mL Exceed 10^4/mL in symptomatic patient.

C: Report as mixed flora and the number of commensal types.

D: Do not identify. Report number and type only.

E: Identify and perform antibiotic sensitivity testing even though the count is very low (Fig. 8.4).

Wound Cultures

Surface lesions must be sampled carefully. The lesion must be opened and the advancing edge of the lesion must be firmly sampled. Pus must be expressed onto the swab. Sometimes culturing the pus may yield sterile reports because the encased organisms may be dead. Surface lesions are unsuitable for anaerobic studies. Dry swab should never be used. Anaerobes are abundant on skin surface and are common surface wound contaminants. Scrub the area around the wound carefully before sampling. Wound cultures requiring anaerobic work up should be transported in appropriate transport medium. Wound site should be clearly mentioned with specific reference to the anatomical land markings, because cultures are to be interpreted in relation to the bacterial flora at that particular anatomical site. The physicians should use clinical judgment when ordering anaerobic cultures because they are quite expensive and requires special setup and expertise. Gas production, foul smell, copious pus formation are clinical indications of anaerobic wound infection.

Spinal Fluids

At least 5 mL fluid is necessary for bacteriological examination. Spinal fluids should be transported immediately because delay affects the viability of fastidious organisms or nutritionally varying phenotypes.

Throat and Nasopharyngeal Cultures

Throat cultures should be looked for β-hemolytic streptococci only. Organisms other than β-hemolytic streptococci do not cause primary acute pharyngitis. Staphylococci may cause tonsilar abscess. *H. influenzae* may cause constrictive epiglottitis and *C. diphtheria* causes membraneous pharyngitis.

Recovery of *H. influenzae* from throat cultures should be discouraged. Antibiotic sensitivity testing should not be performed on throat cultures. β-hemolytic streptococci are universally sensitive to penicillin. Other organisms are not considered pathogenic in the absence of specific complications.

Coliform bacilli in throat cultures are not usually reported. Coliform bacilli can colonize the throat and form a reservoir for respiratory infections. These coliform bacilli are often acquired during hospitalization. Susceptibility tests should not be performed except on request for nosocomial purposes.

Vaginal and Endometrial Cultures

In general, vaginal cultures yield minimum information and hence they should be discouraged. In suspected cases of gonorrhea, cultures should be obtained directly from uterine cervix. Anaerobic cultures should not be performed except on aspirated abscess, other infections due to *Trichomonas, Candida, Gardenella vaginalis* can be diagnosed by direct smear examination. Endocervical cultures can be processed anaerobically by using proper transport medium. In postpartum infections group-B streptococci and lysteria monocytogenes should be kept in mind, while processing the sample.

Tissue

Biopsy specimens should represent the infected portion. Tissue specimens should be processed only after proper mincing using suitable sterile equipment. Anaerobic cultures are set-up on tissue specimens only when there is suspicion (like foul smell, change in color, etc.).

Gastric Specimens

In general, gastric specimens do not give us meaningful results except in infants with intestinal obstruction or sepsis. Bacterial counts in such specimens are of limited value. The presence of large number of bacteria in gastric aspiration indicates alkaline pH due to regurgitation from the duodenum. Gastric aspirates are neutralized before processing for mycobacteria identification in smear or culture of the specimen.

Other Body Fluids

Other body fluid should be aspirated aseptically and inoculated in the enriched media. Direct Gram-smear examination is very useful. Body fluids with high protein content may become clotted before they are transported to the laboratory. Hence, proper sterile container with a suitable anticoagulant should be used. It is ideal to use enriched fluid media to isolate pathogens from the body fluids. Usually large volumes of 20 to 50 mL are ideal for processing.

Specimens that can be Refrigerated before Inoculation

Urines, feces, respiratory exudates, wound specimens.

Table 8.3: Environmentally fragile organisms

Organisms	Most likely specimens	Remarks
• *H. influenzae*	CSF, eye, ear, throat	Sensitive to cold
• *Shigella* species	Feces	Sensitive to cold
• *N. gonorrhoeae*	Genital	Sensitive to cold, 10% CO_2
• *N. meningitidis*	CSF	—do—

Specimens that should not be Refrigerated

1. Spinal or other body fluids.
2. Genital/cervical specimens for *Gonococcus* isolation (Table 8.3).
3. Blood culture bottles.

Specimens Suitable for Anaerobic Cultures

1. Aspirated abscess material
2. Blood
3. Bone marrow
4. Lung aspirate or transtracheal aspirate
5. Suprapubic urine aspirate
6. Endometrial and endocervical specimens
7. Aseptically collected tissue
8. 'Sulfur granules' from any specimens
9. Aspirated body fluids which are transported immediately
10. Bile
11. Placenta—Cesarean section (CS)
12. Culdocentesis
13. Ovary
14. Bartholin's gland.

Urethral, prostatic fluid and seminal fluid are not cultured for anaerobes.

Specimen Priority

As far as possible, all the specimens should be processed without delay. However, for convenience the specimens can be given the following priority:

1. ***Urgent:*** Specimens received from patients with potentially life-threatening infections so that the preliminary information may be given to the physician within 1 hour. Such specimens are: (i) blood, (ii) spinal fluid, (iii) transtracheal aspirate, (iv) endophthalmitis, (v) pericardial fluid, (vi) peritoneal fluid, (vii) specimens from lower respiratory tract of patients admitted in ICU, (viii) joint fluid, (ix) surgical specimens from ICU, etc.
2. ***Routine:*** Specimens received from patients with no immediate life-threatening sequelae but that represent a potentially important infectious event requiring diagnostic

confirmation or preventive observation: Throat cultures, pleural fluids, burns, eye infections, urine (Catheter or clean-catch), female genital, surgical (from operating theater), lower respiratory specimens if diagnosed of pneumonia, peritoneal fluid.

3. ***Elective:*** Specimens requiring fastidious handling and the information obtained is more of a confirmatory value rather than an emergency diagnostic procedure. All other specimens.

Specimens Requiring Gram Stain

Cerebrospinal fluid, eye specimens, urine, pus, sputum and tracheal aspirate, tissue, urethral smears. The following disease states are often rapidly diagnosed by Gram's smear: (a) meningitis, (b) brain abscess, (c) pneumonia, (d) endocarditis, (e) peritonitis, (f) gas gangrene, (g) diphtheria, (h) necrotizing fasciitis, (i) intra-abdominal infection, (j) gonorrhea, (k) Vincent's angina.

When to Suspect Mycobacterial Infection

a. With all respiratory infections.
b. When smears reveal poorly stained diphtheroid like organisms but culture negative within 48 to 72 hours.
c. Cervical lymphadenitis.
d. Negative routine bacteriology cultures.
e. When cultures for anaerobic or microaerophillic bacteria are negative even after prolonged incubation in a suitable nutrient medium.
f. Failure to respond to usual course of antimicrobial agents.
g. Negative serological tests against suspected pathogen.

When to Suspect a Fungal Infection

a. Body fluids showing lymphocytosis with negative smears for Gram's stain and acid-fast stain.
b. A negative gram stain report on aspirated pus.
c. Sputum cultures showing insignificant bacterial cultures in an immune compromised host.
d. Patients showing negative blood cultures and deterioration for unexplained reasons.
e. Cultures showing moulds or yeasts.
f. When a specimen is a skin biopsy of granulomatous lesion.

Chapter 9

Host–parasite Relationship

INTRODUCTION

So far we were dealing with the behavior morphology, isolation, identification, and their variations and methods of sterilization, etc. But what happens when a human body is invaded by bacteria or microorganisms. How the host tissue responds to such type of invasion? Let us take an example. Imagine there is a village with 1000 population. The source of water supply to this village is, say, well. During rainy season imagine there is an outbreak of cholera in this village. Let us assume first it started in the members of the one house and soon within 3 to 5 days it started spreading to other houses, i.e. they also started having the disease. After 10 days, say, the infection is completely subsided. At the end if you analyze. Let us suppose that totally 200 people got infected with cholera and of them 50 died. Now we have many questions to analyze.

1. How the infection started first?
2. How it spreaded to other houses?
3. Why only 50 people died?
4. How the rest of the 150 people recovered from infection?
5. And lastly to our surprise, why the rest of the 800 people did not suffer from infection at all?

Answers to these questions has created a special branch in microbiology, i.e. immunology.

Now if you go to cell level, usually bacteria cannot infect a normal cell. That means normal cell has got some defense mechanisms against the invasion. What are those defense mechanisms? We can classify them broadly into two groups:

- Nonspecific defense mechanisms
- Specific defense mechanism.

NONSPECIFIC DEFENSE MECHANISMS

The skin forms a protective layer for the internal organs. Normal intact skin cannot be penetrated by bacteria. But organisms can enter sweat or sebaceous glands. But sweat and sebaceous secretion by virtue of their acid pH and presence of unsaturated fatty acids usually kill the bacteria and tend to eliminate pathogenic organisms. Enzymes like lysozyme are also present in skin, which usually dissolve the cell wall of the bacteria. Skin resistance varies with age.

Mucous Membranes

Membranes of the respiratory tract usually contain cilia and mucus secretions, which constantly drive away the bacteria entering the system.

Secretions

Secretions of the respiratory tract, GIT, tears, and saliva contain hydrolytic or proteolytic enzymes which usually digest the bacteria that are accidentally taken or inhaled. The gastric juice contains hydrochloric acid, which is a powerful bactericidal agent. So usually bacteria cannot cause infection of the GIT unless the acid level is lowered; it is neutralized by the presence of food and other agents.

Presence of Normal Flora

The upper respiratory tract and genitourinary tract are usually colonized by commensal or harmless bacteria. These bacteria usually do not allow the entry and establishment of pathogenic organisms. Such a phenomena is called interference phenomena.

Phagocytosis

Human body contains a variety of phagocytic cells such as neutrophils, eosinophils, macrophages, and these are present in all organs of the body. Any microorganism which if enters by accident, these organisms are engulfed by one of these cells and inside the cells the bacteria are digested with the help of digestive enzymes secreted by the phagosomes.

Reticuloendothelial System

The phagocytic cells of the blood, lymph nodes, liver, lung, spleen, constitute reticulo-endothelial system and these organs or the cells present in these organs like Kupffer cells, macrophages, act as filters of microorganisms and they trap out any bacteria or particulate matter if they enter into the body by accident.

Biochemical Tissue Constituents

These constituents contain soluble substance present in blood like opsonins (proteins which enhance phagocytes), bacteriolysins, properidin, certain polypeptides cause lysis of the bacteria or help the cells to cause rapid lysis of invading organisms.

Inflammatory Response and Any Injury to the Tissues

Invasion by bacteria, and due to the multiplication of bacteria in the tissues, or physical as well as chemical agents evokes what is called inflammatory response. This is characterized by vasodilatation of the local arterioles and capillaries, leading to exudation of plasma and tissue fluid and migration of phagocytic cells at the site of injury (chemotaxis). The phagocytes engulf the bacteria and digest them soon there will be alteration of the pH at the local site of injury, and this leads to the release of phagocytes more enzymes which act on bacteria. Once all the bacteria are killed, the dead bacteria and leucocytes are liquefied and that is called pus, this pus points toward the least site of resistance and it will be drained off. The cavity now left out will be filled up with new cells coming from the surrounding tissue. This is called granulation tissue and finally healing takes place.

The severity of the inflammatory response depends upon the individual response, the nutritional status, the age and the nature of the organism, or the agent responsible for tissue injury.

Fever

Some people consider fever as a nonspecific protective mechanism. If the temperature is above 37°C, the environment is usually not suitable for the multiplication of bacteria. Fever results due to interaction of various substance present on the surface of bacteria as well as on the tissue of the host leading to production of substance called "pyrogens". These pyrogens stimulate the thermoregulatory center, resulting in increase of body temperature.

SPECIFIC DEFENSE MECHANISMS

The above-mentioned factors are nonspecific and they try to stop the invasion of the bacteria irrespective of the nature of the organism. That means these factors contribute to protect the tissue from all types of infections. These mechanisms are also called Ist and IInd line of defense mechanisms.

If the bacteria succeed in breaking through these defense mechanisms even then the host tissue may not get infected, because of the specific defense mechanism and it is called immunity. Immunity may be defined as resistance to specific microorganism or we can say the properties of the host that center resistance to specific infectious agent. Immunity may be natural or acquired.

Natural Immunity

This is inherent or genetically mediated property that is not influenced by previous infection or contact with the bacteria causing such infection. This is again of the following types:

Species Immunity

Avian tuberculosis affects birds but not humans. Anthrax bacilli infects humans but not chickens. Mouse is very much susceptible to pneumococci but not rabbit. Gonococci infect only humans or chimpanzees but not other animals.

In short, we can say some diseases does not occur under natural conditions in resistant animals.

Racial Immunity

Within same species there may be marked racial and genetic difference in susceptibility. For example, American Indians are more easily infected with tubercle bacilli. Persons who have G6PD enzyme deficiency are resistant to malaria infection. Some mice are more easily infected with viruses.

Individual Immunity

Resistance to infection varies from person to person within the same race and within the same area. This may be due to the difference in their metabolic, hormonal activity and nutritional status.

Age is also another important factor, which contributes to susceptibility. Extremes of age infections are common.

Acquired Immunity

Acquired immunity is defined as the immunity to a specific infectious agent that results due to previous experience with the same infectious agents. We have:

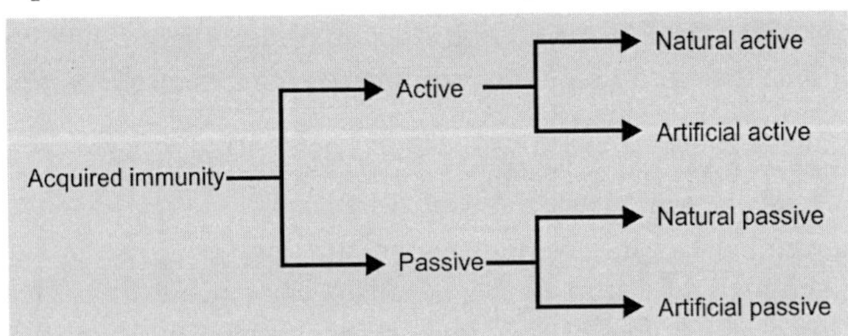

Natural Active

This type of immunity results after the person actually suffering from particular infection. For example, a person who suffered from smallpox in his childhood will be resistant to smallpox reinfection. A child who has suffered from diphtheria will be resistant to reinfection due to diphtheria.

Some infections give us lifelong immunity. That means once you suffer and recover from it you will not get the same infection for the second time, whereas some infections give us only short-lived immunity. Whether a particular infection gives you a lifelong immunity or temporary immunity depends upon many factors.

Artificial Immunity

This is obtained by deliberately exposing a person to a infection agent that is rendered harmless but at the same time it possesses the capacity to induce immunity. Such a preparation of an infection agent is called vaccine. We have mainly three types of vaccines:

i. *Live vaccine*: The bacteria are alive but by submitting them to some chemical processes or prolonged subculturing by repeated passage into new medium or repeated by inoculating the culture obtained from one animal of same species into the other animal of same species they are made harmless, e.g. BCG vaccine.

ii. *Killed vaccine*: It is a suspension of bacteria that is made harmless by killing the bacteria either by heat or by using chemicals, e.g. typhoid vaccine, cholera vaccine, plague vaccine, etc.

iii. *Vaccines prepared from bacteria metabolites*: For example, the toxin liberated by bacteria are rendered safe by adding chemical and they are administered, e.g. DPT, tetanus toxoid.

Persons who are rendered immune by administering these artificial bacteria products will be resistant to infection even though they contact it.

Natural Passive

Whenever a person suffers from any infection, certain soluble protein substances are produced in the body, which antagonize the infectious agent and protect him/her from that infection. Such substances are called antibodies. These antibodies can be transmitted to a fetus by its mother either through placenta or through milk, and you can actually recognize such antibodies in infants blood soon after his birth, even though he or she has not suffered from such infection. These antibodies protect the infant, till the infant develops his own immune system. These antibodies usually persist upto 6 months afterbirth.

Artificial Passive

It has been found that the γ-globulin of a person who has recovered from an infection can be separated from the rest of the blood and can be administered to another person if you want to protect him from a particular infection. For example, if a child is suffering from diphtheria, the progress of the disease can be arrested by administering γ-globulin rich in antibodies against diphtheria toxin. Such type of γ-globulin is available for various specific infections like (i) rabies, (ii) measles, (iii) mumps, (iv) jaundice due to hepatitis virus, (v) tetanus, etc.

Herd Immunity

Whenever there is an epidemic of any infection, only certain percentage of people will suffer and show clinical signs and symptoms, whereas majority suffer a subclinical infection, and they become immune to that infection subsequently. This is called herd immunity.

Infection Immunity

Immunity obtained by suffering and recovering from an infection.

Chapter 10

Infection

INTRODUCTION

Infection by bacteria is successful invasion on the host tissue and such bacteria causing infection are called pathogens. There are natural pathogens or true pathogens which have got the inherent capacity to invade a normal tissue also whereas an opportunistic pathogen can cause infection only when the host defense mechanisms are altered or lowered.

FACTORS INFLUENCING VIRULENCE

The successful invasion on the tissue by bacteria depends upon the virulence of the bacteria (defined as the degree of invasive capacity). The factors, which influence the virulence of the bacteria, are:

Toxicity

Some organisms produce poisonous substance called toxins. These are two types:

i. *Exotoxins:* These are liberated into the medium as secondary metabolites. They are proteins, heat labile and highly toxic. By adding formalin they can be converted into harmless or nontoxic substance called toxoids. These toxoids when they are administered they give rise to resistance to infection.
ii. *Endotoxins:* These are liberated due to autolysis of the bacteria. They are lipopolysaccharides and are heat resistant. They can cause variety of effects like fever, intravascular coagulation, shock, endothelial damage cell degeneration, inhibition of enzyme activity or enzyme synthesis.

Enzymes

Many bacteria secrete enzymes like hyaluronidase, lecithinase, lipases, collagenase, coagulase, which act on the host tissue and cause dissolution of the basement membrane of the cells or phospholipids of the cells or the connective tissue of the host and such damage to the tissue render the bacteria to invade the host more easily.

Hemolysins

Some bacteria produce a variety of protein substances that cause lysis of the RBC. This again facilitates the spread of infection.

Capsule

The bacteria that are capsulated or resistant to phagocytosis, capsular material can cause damage to the living tissue.

FACTORS INFLUENCING INFECTION

Tissue Affinity

Different bacteria show different affinity towards tissue. For example, typhoid bacilli—Peyer's patches of intestine; diphtheria—pharyngeal or laryngeal epithelium; streptococci; gonococci, mucous membranes.

Change of their Normal Habitat

Bacteria, which are usually commensals in particular area, become pathogenic when they enter other tissues.

Hypersensitivity

Some bacteria sensitize the host tissue and infection due to such bacteria will lead to severe, generalized infection. For example, streptococci can sensitize the heart and cause rheumatic heart disease.

Infective Dosage

The number of organisms required to cause infection is called an infective dose. This depends on the nature of the organism.

Portal of Entry

Not only the dosage but the portal or route of entry of a microorganism is also important. The microorganisms can gain entry into the body either by: Ingestion, inoculation, and inhalation, through an abrasion in the skin or by inoculation (introduction of malarial parasite by the bite of mosquito).

Communicability

Spread of a particular infection from person to person depends upon, the rapidity by which the bacteria are transmitted. This usually occurs by:

i. Direct contact with an infected patient.
ii. Flies, mosquitoes, which can spread infection. They are called vectors of infection.

Contact with infected article like clothing, beds, food, and water, droplet infection, which spread due to coughing or sneezing, animal bites, etc.

- Contact
- Airborne
- Food and water
- Insect-borne.

Thus in conclusion, the development of infection depends upon a number of factors: cofactors, bacterial virulence, factors influencing the infection, etc.

Host factors	*Bacteria factors*
Resistance	Infection

Epidemic

Epidemic among the people is unusual incidence of disease in a community.

Pathogenicity

Ability of a parasite to gain entrance into a host and produce disease.

Infestation

Infests are disturbed or hostile. Presence of large number of microorganisms on the body of the host. It does not imply any damage to the host. Infestation by certain arthropods like lice, ticks and fleas and itch mite (causing scabies) on the superficial surfaces causes irritation, itching and due to constant scratching abrasion are formed in the skin which leads to secondary by opportunistic pathogens.

Chapter 11

Antigens

INTRODUCTION

An antigen is a substance of high molecular weight with a surface composed of specific determinant groups of small size and when injected parenterally is capable of eliciting antibody response in a living tissue. The antibody that is produced combines specifically with the antigen and neutralizes its effect on the tissue, or the complexes of antigen and antibody are engulfed by phagocytes and are removed from the body.

PROPERTIES

An antigen is capable of evoking antibodies only if it is foreign to the living tissue (immunologically competent). Failure to develop antibodies to its own antigens by the living tissue is called self-recognition or tolerance, which is usually present upto the 3rd month of gestation in a fetus. Tolerance once developed, persists throughout the life of an individual. If immunologically competent tissue begins to produce antibodies to its own antigen, the result is immunological crippling, a feature which is seen in certain autoimmune diseases.

Most of the antigens, distributed in the nature, are in the forms of proteins or polysaccharides. Polymers of α-amino acids can elicit antibody response whereas that δ-amino acids are completely devoid of antigenicity.

Certain chemicals which when combined with a carrier protein, become immunogenic and elicit antibody response from a living tissue. Such chemicals are called haptens. Haptens are capable of combining specifically with their antibody but fail to produce them, unless they are coupled to a carrier, protein (e.g. metals, arsenic acid, drugs, solvents, and dyes).

There are two types of haptens: (i) simple, (ii) complex.

Most of the naturally occurring antigens are of high molecular weight ranging from 40,000 to more than 1,00,000. Materials of low molecular weight may be weakly antigenic.

Most of the soluble protein antigens are rapidly metabolized and excreted when they are injected intravenously. Fifty percent of the injected protein is excreted within 1 hour and 70% in 24 hours under normal conditions. The excreted antigenic material is quite heterogeneous with respect to physical properties and much of it is associated with RNA. The rapid breakdown of the antigen is brought about by proteolytic enzymes and also by intracellular digestion by macrophages, and granulocytes. Most of the antigen apparently plays no part in the production of antibody. The antigen is quickly digested into fragments of smaller but variable size. Each of the fragments contains some specific determinant groups against which antibody is produced. It appears that phagocytosis and the phagocytic enzymes play an essential role in the processing of antigenic information to the immunologically competent cells. Substances, which cannot be metabolized by the body, are devoid of antigenicity.

Antigens are composed of certain localized specific groups against which only antibodies are produced but not against entire surface area of the antigen. These are called determinant groups and usually their number per antigen molecule ranges from 5 to 200. Valence or the number of determinant groups per antigen molecule is proportional to its molecular weight. The determinant groups of an antigen molecule generally consists of penta- or hexapeptides of small length and the determinant group consists of tetrapeptide or a trisaccharide. Within the determinant group, a particular amino acid or sugar residue is often responsible for the binding affinity of the antibody. That residue which shows high affinity toward the antibody is called immunodominant group. Not only the terminal amino acids but sometimes interior residues of an antigen molecule may act as immunodeterminant group. They may act directly as such or indirectly by maintaining particular shape of the antigen or conformation among the adjacent residues in the determinant groups. Certain antigens are distributed in many species of animals and cross react. Such antigens are called 'Forssman' antigens and the antibodies produced are known as 'heterophile antibodies'.

MONOVALANT HAPTENS

Hapten is a determinant group that is artificially introduced by covalent linkage into the surface structure of a carrier protein. Haptens are incapable of inducing antibody formation but they readily combine with the antibody produced against hapten-protein conjugate but does not form a precipitate. This is called hapten-inhibition. Haptens, in addition, confer new specificity to the carrier protein. Haptens are important in clinical medicine. Numerous haptens like metals, solvents, dyes, plant products to which man is naturally or artificially exposed may conjugate with epidermal or plasma proteins and thus forming functional antigens. These functional antigens stimulate production of specific antibodies and the interaction between the two may lead to hypersensitivity reactions or autoimmune diseases.

Chapter 12

Immunoglobulins

DEFINITION

Immunoglobulins are proteins of animal origin endowed with known antibody activity and certain other proteins related by chemical nature and hence antigenic specificity.

DISTRIBUTION

They are found in plasma, lymph, urine, spinal fluid, saliva, tears, bile, nasal intestinal secretions, lymph nodes, spleen and bone marrow.

CLASSES

Five classes of immunoglobulins are known; they differ in their, physicochemical properties like electrophoresis mobility, sedimentation coefficient, diffusion coefficient, molecular weight and the amino acid content. The five types are IgM, IgA, IgG, IgE and IgD. Each immunoglobulin molecule has two light chains and two heavy chains and can react specifically with the determinant group of antigen.

TYPES

The light polypeptide chains are common to all classes of antibodies. These are of two types: K and L. A given immunoglobulin contains either two K chains or two L chains but not one of each type.

SUBCLASSES, SUBGROUPS, AND SUBTYPES

Each polypeptide chain of the immunoglobulin molecule has got one variable region and one constant region. Differences involving the small genetic changes in the constant region of heavy chains of a given class are the basis for separating immunoglobulins into subclasses.

Changes in the variable region of a light chain of given type are used as a basis for defining groups. These are designated by Roman numerical. Subtypes represent the variable subgroup with its associated constant region.

CONCENTRATION, METABOLISM, AND DISTRIBUTION

Total concentration of immunoglobulins in normal human plasma is 1.26 g%. IgG is the predominant class of antibody in human plasma. It is five times as high as IgA, 15 times as high as IgM. The total concentration of IgD and IgE put together is usually less than one percent of the total.

Regulation of the catabolic rate is a function of Fc (crystallizable fragments of the immunoglobulin) fragment of the heavy chains. IgG is synthesized and its activity is longer than the other. One molecule of IgM is synthesized for every 4 molecules of IgA and 20 molecules of IgG. IgD has got shortest life period.

Except for IgG the rest are synthesized and catabolized at a constant rate irrespective of their blood concentration. Whereas the catabolic rate or IgG is directly proportional to its concentration in the blood.

IgG is distributed uniformly between extravascular and intravascular components of the body fluid. IgM is firmly bound to tissues for several weeks.

IgA is of two types: Secreting and circulating. Small lymphocytes destined to form plasma cells synthesizing IgA are predominantly located in the interstices of salivary glands and in the submucosal layers. After the synthesis of IgA by the plasma cells, the monomeric units are released into the blood or sometimes the monomeric units pass through the epithelial cells lining the mucous membrane forming dimers by acquiring a secretory piece in the process. Thus, by this mechanism IgA is specially concentrated in saliva, tears, nasal mucus, tracheal and bronchial washings, gastrointestinal, genital, urinary, and mammary secretions. The attachment of the secretory piece, a glycoprotein with a molecular weight of 50,000 confers on IgA an increased resistance to digestion by proteolytic enzymes. Following antigenic stimulation of mucous membranes, secretory IgA production can occur in the absence of demonstrable circulating IgA.

PHYSICOCHEMICAL PROPERTIES

The immunoglobulins show a broad range of mobility. IgG has got the widest range; IgM, IgA, IgE show narrower range and generally migrate with the β globulins and fast moving γ-globulins.

SEDIMENTATION CONSTANT

Generally IgG, IgD, IgE have coefficient of sedimentation of 7S. IgM has a value of 19S; IgA values ranges between 7S and 14S depending upon the state of polymerization.

MOLECULAR WEIGHT

The molecular weight ranges from 1,50,000 to 9,00,000; IgG has got a molecular weight of 1,50,000, IgM is 9,00,000, IgA has got a molecular weight of 1,50,000 to 4,00,000, the molecular weight of IgD and IgE is approximately 2,00,000.

SIZE AND SHAPE

This is observed by low angle X-ray diffraction and by electron microscopy in antigen-antibody complexes. IgG is a slender symmetrical tight Y-shaped molecule with antigen binding sites located on the two arms, which are flexibly hinged to each other near the base. After combining with two molecules of antigen, the two arms of the antibody open to a variable degree including full extention to a T-shape. Thus, antibody molecules form bridges between antigen molecules thus building a large number in soluble lattice.

Even though the base of the antibody is digested away (Fc) by pepsin, the molecule retains the property of forming bridges between the antigen molecules and forms an insoluble complex. But after removal of the Fc fragment completely, the antibody molecules lose their important properties like ability to bind complement to release anaphylatoxin, to cross placenta and to attach firmly to tissue cells.

IgM is a polymer composed of 5 units each of which contains two heavy chains and two light chains. The Fc portion of alternate heavy chains are linked with sulfhydryl bonds to produce a central shallow cylindrical portion with five radiating arms. These IgM molecules appear spherical.

Circulating IgA despite having two combining sites on each molecule, which can bind two molecules of antigen, fails to extend to a T-shape. The heavy chains of IgA are held together and impede the formation of a complex lattice. Similarly, IgD and IgE cannot form insoluble lattices with antigen.

CHEMICAL COMPOSITION

Chemically these are glycoproteins, which contain 2 to 14 percent carbohydrate and 86 to 98 percent amino acids. IgG has low carbohydrate content. The rest other have got a carbohydrate content of 10 to 14 percent. Significance of carbohydrate is uncertain.

STRUCTURAL AND FUNCTIONAL COMPONENTS

i. Fragments: The term antibody fragment indicates the portion of the molecule that are obtained as a result of cleavage of peptide bonds.

Fragment	*Produced by digestion with*
• $F(ab)_2$ antigen binding	Pepsin
• F(ab) antigen binding	Papain
• Fc crystallizable	Papain
• Fd heavy chain portion of the F(ab)	Papain

ii. Diagrammatic representation (Fig. 12.1): Each molecule of IgG is made up of two light chains and two heavy chains having molecular weight of approximately 25,000 and 50,000 per chain.

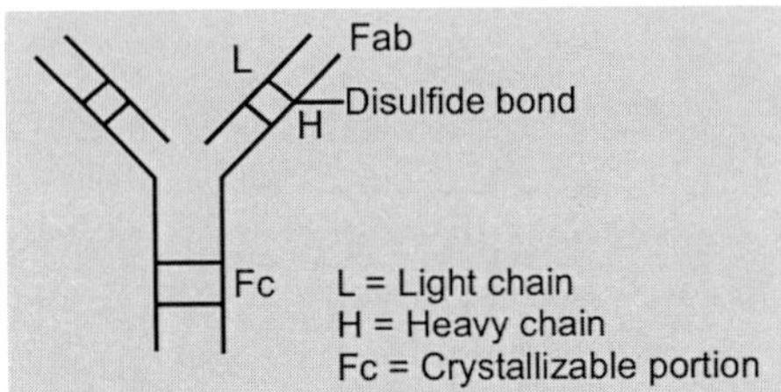

Fig. 12.1: Schematic diagram of IgG molecule

The both chains differ in their amino acid sequence and in their determinant groups.

The polypeptides are held together primarily by disulfide bonds which link the light chain to heavy chain and the heavy chain to each other.

Under ideal conditions papain hydrolyzes IgG into three fragments.

Fc fragment contains the COOH terminals of heavy chain, which are held together by disulfide bonds.

The two F(ab) portions contain the light chain and the NH_2 terminal of the heavy chain.

The F(ab) fragment combines with the specific antigen molecule while the Fc fragment is devoid of antibody activity. On reduction and alkylation, the F(ab) fragment yields a light chain and the NH_2 terminal portion of the heavy chain (Fd fragment).

If pepsin at pH 5 is used to digest IgG, a fragment $F(ab)_2$ is obtained with a sedimentation constant of 5S which gives precipitation with antigen so it is called 5S antibody. On reduction $F(ab)_2$ gives two F(ab) fragments which will recombine when oxidized. Some of the F(ab) fragments obtained from IgG contain K chain and some contain λ chain. Intact K molecules of IgG as well as that of F(ab) fragment are more positively changed than λ molecules.

iii. Structure of other immunoglobulins: IgM is a polymer of 5 units. It consists of monomers of 7S. It has got 10 combining sites. But the monomers are devoid of agglutinating and precipitating property. IgD, IgE and circulating IgA have got similar structure as that of IgG. Secretary IgA is a dimmer + glycoprotein secretory piece. IgA myeloma proteins usually occur in plasma as polymers 2, 3, 4 or more monomers. On treatment with reagents IgA breaks down to its monomers.

COMBINING SITES

Valence: The number of combining sites on the surface of the antibody molecule is referred to as the valence. Except for IgM and IgA (rarely) all other antibody molecules are divalent. IgM has got 10 combining sites and IgA at times polymerizes to have 4, 6, 8 combining sites.

Size: The approximate size of the combining sites is about 25 to 35 Å and molecular weight of 400 to 1000.

Chapter 13

Antigen–antibody Reactions

INTRODUCTION

Whenever an antigen (whole bacteria, or part of it such as cell wall, lipopolysaccharide, proteins of the cell membrane or metabolites such as toxins or any foreign protein (e.g. egg albumin is a protein and it is not present in our body) enters through parenteral route, it can initiate antibody production, combine with corresponding specific antibody and produce mainly five types of reactions:

1. Precipitation
2. Agglutination
3. Neutralization
4. Opsonization
5. Complement fixation.

These reactions are called antigen–antibody reactions. The general features of these reactions are:

1. They are specific.
2. They are reversible at times.
3. There is no alteration in the chemical nature of antigen or the antibody.
4. They combine in multiple proportions.

The antigen-antibody reaction can be measured either by:

1. Estimating the nitrogen content of the complex formed.
2. By determining the highest dilution of the antibody which can give us an observable reaction. This is expressed in titers. Titer is defined as the reciprocal of the highest dilution which shows visible antigen-antibody reaction.

PRECIPITATION

Precipitation is an antigen-antibody reaction in which the antigen is in soluble form and when corresponding antibody is added it gets precipitated and the complex of antigen and antibody settles down at the bottom of the test tube leaving a clean supernatant fluid, with its corresponding antibody only when they are combined in optimum proportions, which varies from antigen to antigen, and precipitation will not occur when there are excess antibodies or excess antigen. The occurrence of maximum precipitation at optimum ratios is called zone phenomenon. The optimum concentration required for maximum precipitation of any antigen with its corresponding antibody is called zone of equivalence. Whereas if the antibodies are in excess, it is called prozone, and if antigen is excess, it is called post-zone (Fig. 13.1).

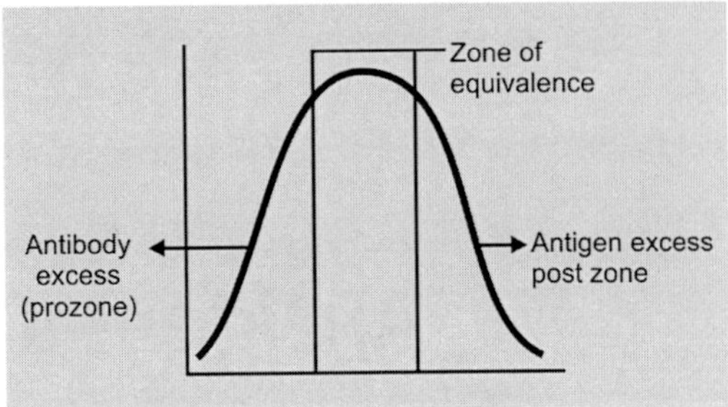

Fig. 13.1: Precipitation curve

Because antibodies are bivalent (i.e. they can combine with two antigen molecules) and antigens are multivalent, (i.e. they can combine with many antibody molecules) large lattices are formed when they combine in optimum proportion and that is the basis of precipitation.

1. Application: Precipitation reaction is very sensitive and it can detect the antigen upto a concentration of 1 µg.
2. Uses:
   a. Identification of blood and seminal stains in medicolegal cases.
   b. For the detection of adulterants in the food.
   c. For the detection of antigen or antibody in diagnosing the infectious diseases.
3. Methods
   a. Ring test: Take the solution containing antigen into a test tube and carefully add corresponding antibody. A formation of white ring indicates precipitation of antigen (Fig. 13.2).
      Used in diagnosis of:
      i. Anthrax
      ii. Streptococcal infection, detection of C-reactive protein elevated in rheumatic fever. The same can be done on a slide or in tube, e.g. VDRL test for syphilis or detection of diphtheria toxin.
   b. Agar gel diffusion: Mix serum containing antibodies to specific infectious agent in a test tube containing agar. Then allow it to solidify. On to top add the corresponding antigen. The antigen diffuses into the agar and combines with antibody to form a white band (Single diffusion).
   c. Immunoelectrophoresis: At a constant pH, different proteins migrate at different speeds in electrical fields. Based on this immunoelectrophoresis

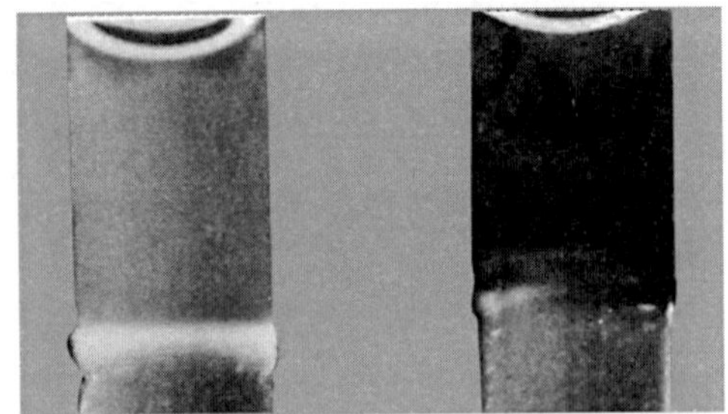

Fig. 13.2: Precipitation reaction. Note the formations of white ring at the junction where antibody and antigen (soluble form) come into contact

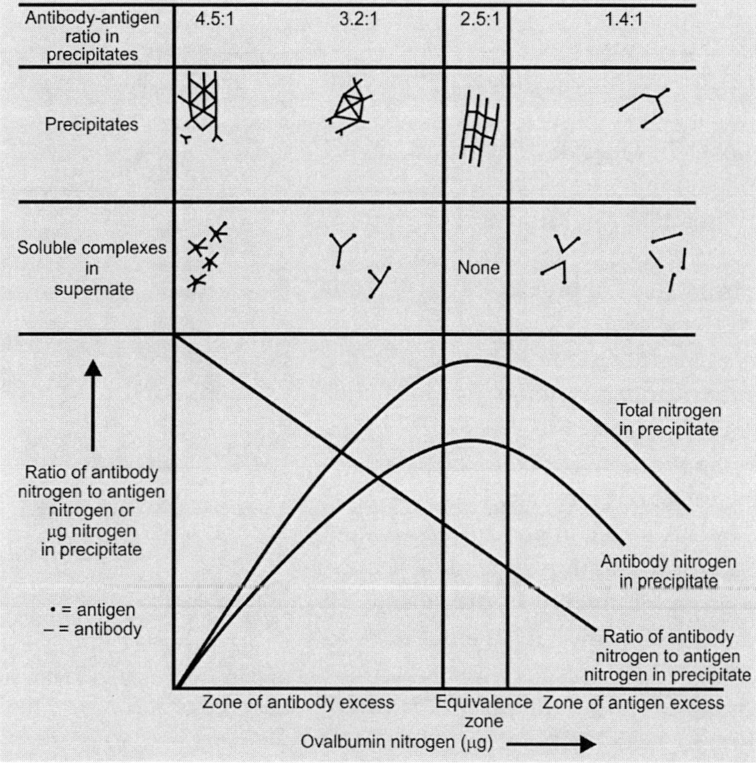

Fig. 13.3: The quantitative precipitin reaction of ovalbumin (valence = 5) with rabbit anti-ovalbumin antibody

is developed on a glass slide with agar gel, first antigen is placed in a well and electricity is applied. If the antigen is a mixture of different proteins, they migrate according to their rate of mobility. Then put the serum in the trough you get different bands. Indicating the numbers of antigens present.

d. Radial diffusion of Mancini: The specific serum is added to molten agar at 50°C and the agar is poured in Petri plates or on glass slides. After solidification, wells are punched in the agar and antigen solution is added to the well. The plates and slides are kept at 4°C for 48–72 hours. If the antigen combines with the antibody present in the agar solution, by diffusion, a white ring around the well is formed, the diameter of which is proportional to the concentration of antigen (Fig. 13.3).

AGGLUTINATION

Agglutination is a type of antigen-antibody reaction in which the antigen is in particulate form and when it is mixed with corresponding antibody clumping of the particulate antigen takes place in the presence of electrolyte like NaCl. That is why agglutination tests are done by suspending the particulate antigen in normal saline (Fig. 13.4). The same principle and mechanism of precipitation is also applicable to agglutination reaction.

Applications

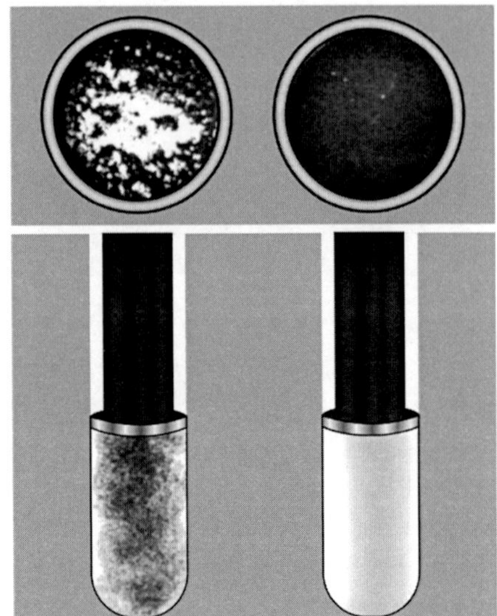

Fig. 13.4: Tube and slide agglutination. Note the clumping of particulate antigen in the presence of antibody specific to antigen (left side) and no clumping in the absence of antibody (right side)

1. To identify an organism, e.g. slide agglutination.
2. To identify the blood group.
3. To diagnose diseases like typhoid fever, atypical pneumonia, etc.
4. Cold agglutination: Agglutination of erythrocytes in the presence of serum from a patient suffering from atypical pneumonia at 4°C but not at 37°C.
5. Paul Bunnel agglutination: Patients suffering from infectious mononucleosis produce antibodies that will agglutinate sheep cells. In the laboratory application of this test helps us in diagnosing infectious mononucleosis.
6. Coombs' test: Another important application of agglutination reaction is to detect anti-Rh blood group antibodies in diagnosing Rh incompatibility or hemolytic anemia in newborn infants.
7. Passive agglutination: Human 'O' or rabbit RBC or inert particles like latex particles can be coated with antigen or antibodies. When these coated particles are treated with serum containing antibodies, one can observe agglutination. Such type of tests are helpful in diagnosing diseases like rheumatoid arthritis or other collagen diseases and bacterial meningitis.

NEUTRALIZATION TEST

Neutralization test is a type of antigen-antibodies reaction in which the toxic effects or the pathogenic effects of an antigen are neutralized by specific antibodies. Organisms of diseases like diphtheria, tetanus, produce powerful toxins and these toxins can be separated and purified. When they are injected in small doses into an experimental animal like rabbit, antitoxins are produced. The potency of such antibodies are measured by their ability to protect an animal from the toxic effects of the particular toxin when both are combined and injected.

1. **International unit of antitoxin:** The amount of antitoxin present in 0.0628 mg of dried serum preserved in State Serum Institute, Copenhagen.
2. **Dose:** Smallest amount of toxin when mixed with 1 unit of antitoxin and injected into guinea pig weighing 250 g causes death of the animal within four days.
3. **Lf dose:** The amount of toxin that forms visible precipitate rapidly with corresponding antibody.

COMPLEMENT AND COMPLEMENT FIXATION

Bordet and Gengou toward the end of 19th century found that, certain types of antibodies can cause lysis of bacteria or cells in the presence of normal serum (without antibodies). The component responsible for such lysis is ultimately found to be a mixture of glycoproteins and they are collectively named as complement.

Complement is defined as a mixture of heat labile glycoproteins that are normally present in serum in low concentration, and it nonspecifically can attach to an antigen-antibody complex and bring down the lysis of the antigen if it is in the form of a cell. The mixture can be separated into 9 components depending upon molecular weight, sedimentation. They are C1 to C9. They are inactivated at 56°C in 30 minutes. Complement fixation, a type of antigen-antibody reaction in which the antibody causes lysis of the cells in combination with complement due to a series of enzymatic reactions resembling the cascade system of blood clotting.

Sheep red blood cells when injected into rabbit, antibodies are produced in the rabbit serum against sheep RBC.

Take a known quantity of sheep cells and add equal amount of antibodies. To this mixture add a known quantity of serum containing complement (usually fresh human or guinea pig sera are rich in all components of complement and the complement level increased by feeding the guinea pigs with carrots). This will result in the lysis of sheep RBC due to a series of enzymatic reactions involving the components of complement C1 to C9. This is known as classical pathway. Whereas in alternate pathway which is usually stimulated by endotoxin or snake venom, separate serum factors called factor B, factor D (called initiating factors) in the presence of Mg^{++} directly cleave the factor 3 to 3a, 3b and from then onward, the rest of the mechanism follows that of classical pathway.

Functions of the Complement

1. Can lyse the gram-negative organisms or red blood cells.
2. Can enhance the phagocytic activity of the white blood cells and also release of enzymes by WBC that can digest bacteria.
3. Can enhance inflammatory reaction by releasing substance, which can increase the permeability of the vessels.
4. In conjunction with specific antibody, can cause immune disease like nephrotoxic nephritis, cutaneous vasculitis, and paroxysmal nocturnal hemoglobinuria.

A low concentration of complement is usually found in diseases like SLE.

The fact that complement attaches nonspecially to any Ag+Ab complex can be used to diagnose various diseases like virus infections, bacterial or fungal or parasitic infection and the test is called complement fixation test.

Let us take an example:

Patients serum containing antibody + antigen → Ag + Ab complex

Ag + Ab complex + complement (by adding in the form of normal guinea pig serum in a known concentration)

- If +ve complement attaches and gets fixed and no more free complement will be available.

To detect whether complement is fixed or not, now add to the Ist system sensitized RBC (i.e., sheep cells coated with its corresponding antibody) incubate whole mixture.

- If 1st test is positive——no lysis of RBC because no complement is available.
- If 1st test is negative——lysis of coated RBC because complement is freely available.

C1 activated at the site of Ag + Ab complex may spread to other sites or it may spread from antibody to antibody. Enable the neighboring bystander cell responsive to lysis by C8 and C9 a process known as reactive lysis.

Aggregated antibody molecule can activate complement (such aggregation can occur in the presence of tannic acid, kaolin particle, uric acid crystals).

Bovine serum contains an unusual component called conglutinin (K), which causes clumping of particles, or cells coated with C1 and the process is called conglutination. Conglutination like activity can be produced by immunization with C1 coated particles. They also occur in autoimmune diseases. High immune conglutinin levels are seen in saliva and interstitial tissue. They are IgA molecules whose significance is not known.

Chapter 14

Immune Response

INTRODUCTION

The immune system mainly consists of reticuloendothelial system, i.e. bone marrow, liver, lymph nodes, spleen and thymus.

The cells involved in immune mechanisms are:

1. Macrophages.
2. Polymorphonuclear cells—neutrophils, basophils, eosinophils.
3. Lymphocytes.
   i. B cells: Derived from bursa Fabricius of birds—the equivalent organ in human is not known. But it may be Payer's patches, tonsils or appendix. Twenty percent of the circulating lymphocytes are B cells. They can function normally even in the absence of thymus. These are the cells, which synthesize immunoglobulins.
   ii. T cells: These are called thymus dependent lymphocytes. They are derived from area vasculosa of embryo therefrom bone marrow and they are circulated through thymus. While traveling through thymus they acquire a new antigen due to the influence of thymic hormones and hence called T cells. Their function is impaired in the absence of thymus. Eighty percent of the circulating lymphocytes are T cells. They do not form immunoglobulins. Depending upon their function they are further divided into:
      - Suppressor cells: Suppress the activity of B cells and inhibit antibody formation.
      - Helper cells: Cooperate with B cells and stimulate them to produce more antibodies.
      - Null cells or killer cells: They are cytotoxic and can kill abnormal cells or aged cells of the body or bacteria.

In the peripheral lymphoid system such as lymph nodes, spleen, contain predominantly T cells and these areas are called thymus dependent areas.

B cells that are stimulated by an antigen, undergo rapid multiplication and produce cells. These cells are capable of producing antibody. They are called plasma cells; the B cells which are sensitized by a specific antigen retain the memory and whenever the same

Table 14.1: Differentiating features of T and B lymphocytes

	T lymphocytes	B lymphocytes
Surface Ig	–	Present
Receptor for	–	Present
IgG	–	+
EAC rosette	–	–
SRBC	+	–
Blast transformation with PHA	+	–
Con A	+	–
Endotoxin	–	+

antigen enters into the body, the B cells immediately proliferate and become plasma cells to produce high concentration of antibodies (Table 14.1).

Immune response is mainly divided into two types humoral or antibody mediated immunity and cell-mediated immunity.

HUMORAL-MEDIATED IMMUNITY

This consists of three steps:

A. Entry of the antigen
B. Processing of the antigen and
C. Secretion of the specific antibody.

1. Entry of the antigen: Once the antigen enters the body, its fate depends upon its physical and chemical nature, its dose, route of entry and whether it is entering the body for the first time or second time.

   Most of the antigen that enter will be excreted after engulfment by macrophages. But a part of it may be transferred to B cells. It stimulates the B cells for the production of antibody. If it is entering for the 1st time, the immune response and thereby the antibody formed is called primary response. During this response small amount of antibodies are formed and they are mostly IgM type. Some antigens can induce formation of a very small quantity of specific IgG. It is the production of IgG that determines duration of immune response. If the antigen entering for the first time stimulates both IgM and IgG, it can give rise to longlasting immunity if not short-lived immunity. Production of IgG induces a sort of memory and the body can repeat response to same antigen.

   If the same antigen enters for the second time, now the immune response is mainly of IgG type and this is called secondary response. The amount of antibody formed during secondary response is directly proportional to the concentration of antigen. At the peak of antibody production if some more antigen is introduced, again the response is increased. This continues upto certain level. Afterwards even the concentration of antigen entering the body is more, the antibody level will be the same.

2. Age: Poor antibody production at the extreme of the age.
3. Nutritional status: Malnutrition decreases antibody production.
4. Route of administration: For particulate antigen IV route gives maximum antibody production. For soluble antigen, IM or SC is useful. Oral or normal route of administration of antibody induces IgA antibody.
5. Multiple antigens: Simultaneous administration of multiple antigen sometimes may have beneficial effect, e.g. DPT.
6. Adjuvant: When antigens are suspended in certain chemical like alum, or water in oil emulsions, the antigens are slowly absorbed and slowly metabolized, giving a prolonged stimulation to the body. Such substances when mixed with antigen, improves the antibody production, are called adjuvants. Adjuvants are two types:

   Adjuvant
   - Complete – Freund's adjuvant (Mycobacteria killed are suspended in oil)
   - Water in oil, aluminum hydroxide, etc. (incomplete adjuvant)
7. Immunosuppressive agents: Corticosteroids, X-rays, antimetabolites, antibodies to lymphocytes and antibody production, cancer therapy.
8. Effect of antibody: Presence of already circulating antibody to a specific antigen, suppresses antibody formation.

CELL-MEDIATED IMMUNITY

In certain diseases like tuberculosis, leprosy or against certain antigens one cannot demonstrate specific antibody. The reason is, such diseases or such antigens do not stimulate the B lymphocytes but they stimulate directly T lymphocytes. Those T lymphocytes, which are stimulated by such antigens or diseases, they become activated and produce a variety of soluble, protein like factors of low molecular weight, which are called lymphokines or cytokines. These lymphokines when they are circulated through the body in turn activate many T lymphocytes or stimulate their multiplication (blastogenesis). These activated lymphocytes now attracted toward the site of antigen or bacteria, which stimulated them and digest or kill it. This type of protective action mediated by proliferation of activated lymphocytes, instead of specific antibody is called cell-mediated immunity.

The best example for cell-mediated immunity is skin test by purified tubercular protein (PPD). When such a protein is injected intracutaneously into a person who is already exposed to tuberculosis infection, after 24 to 48 hours one can observe features of the formation of nodule at the site of injection. If you examine histological nodule, it contains polymorphonuclear cells, lymphocytes and macrophages. If you examine this serum for antibodies, it will be negative. But if you transfer the lymphocytes from this person to another normal healthy person, he will also exhibit (i.e., formation of nodule after injection of PPD) similar response, indicating that such type of immunity is mediated by activated cells but not by antibody.

Chapter 15

Hypersensitivity

INTRODUCTION

Normally the antibodies formed or the cells activated against a particular infecting agent are protective. That means they try to neutralize the effect of pathogenic organisms. Sometimes in doing so, they may also damage the host tissue. Such type of altered reactivity, leading to injury to the host tissue is called hypersensitivity.

It was Portier and Richet who first demonstrated hypersensitivity in dogs. According to Gell and Coombs, hypersensitivity is classified into six types:

- Type I: Anaphylaxis
- Type II: Cytolytic and cytotoxic
- Type III: Immune complex mediated
- Type IV: Delayed hypersensitivity
- Type V: Stimulatory hypersensitivity
- Type VI: Antibody-dependent cell-mediated cytotoxicity.

ANAPHYLAXIS

Anaphylaxis is an immediate type of hypersensitive reaction. Many chemicals like egg albumin, penicillin G, B-complex injections, can cause anaphylaxis. The sequences of events are as follows:

1. **Sensitization:** Adequate dose of antigen, usually smaller dose must be given, preferably subcutaneously to sensitize the given host.
2. **Waiting period:** After initial administration of the antigen wait for 2 or 3 weeks during this period. The antigen injected subcutaneously, stimulates the production of antibodies.
3. **Demonstration of anaphylaxis:** After the waiting period, inject the same antigen, preferably through intravenous route, in higher dosage. Now, immediately after 5 to 10 minutes, the animal starts sneezing, scratches its nose, then feels difficulty in breathing and finally dies off respiratory arrest. If you conduct postmortem and examine, there

will be marked bronchoconstriction and hyperemia of the lungs. Here the target organ is respiratory tract. If such reaction occurs in human beings due to administration of drugs like penicillin, the person will have redness of the face, rash over the body, dyspnea, cyanosis and profound shock due to extreme cutaneous vasodilatation. Here the target organ is circulatory system and the type of anaphylaxis is called generalized anaphylaxis. Instead of injecting the chemical or antigen by IV or IM route if you inject intracutaneously into an already sensitized animal or person, you can observe erythema and wheal formation within 3 to 5 minutes and subsides in an hour. This type of anaphylaxis is called cutaneous anaphylaxis.

If the serum from a sensitized person is removed and if it is injected subcutaneously into a normal person and antigen is given intravenously along with a dye like Evans' blue coloration of the area is seen, where you have previously injected the serum and this is called passive cutaneous anaphylaxis, indicating that anaphylaxis is mediated by antibodies present in the serum. This is also called as Prausnitz and Kustner reaction and local anaphylaxis is another type where the entry of the antigen stimulates such type of reaction. About 10 percent of population shows various types of local anaphylaxis in the form of:

- Bronchial asthma
- Urticaria
- GIT disturbances, etc. due to various antigens present in pollen, food, etc.

4. **Mechanism of anaphylaxis:** When the first dose or sensitizing dose is given a small amount of immunoglobulins are formed. Because the dose is small, it usually stimulates IgE type or low concentration IgG type. Both have the property of getting fixed to the surface of basophils or mast cell. The antibodies are called cytotropic antibodies. When the second dose of antigen is given now, the antigen reacts with the cell fixed antibody to form a complex. During this process due to distortion of the mast cell or basophil, its cell membrane gets digested and releases granules consisting of various vasoactive substances such as histamine, serotonin, SRSA, bradykinin, permeability factors which act on the smooth muscles of the respiratory tract or blood vessels, giving rise to symptoms of anaphylaxis. During the Ag+Ab complex formation on the surface mast cell, there will be decreased cGMP inside the mast cell, which favors the degranulation of the vasoactive substance.
5. **Treatment:** Administration of corticosteroids, adrenaline, antihistamines, drugs like disodium cromoglycate or desensitization therapy.

   There is strong evidence that allergic disorders are largely familial and genetically controlled. Hence, the reason to elicit the history before administering any drug is essential.

CYTOLYTIC OR CYTOTOXIC HYPERSENSITIVITY

Suppose a cell is carrying antigen and when this antigen combines with antibody, the reaction stimulates phagocytosis of the whole cell or the cell may be acted upon by NK cells or the complement gets fixed to the Ag+Ab complex and during this interaction, the cell is lysed.

This type of hypersensitive is seen in cases like:

1. Drug induced hemolytic anemias.
2. Aplastic anemias.
3. In ingestion of parasites or tumor cells.
4. Transfusion of mismatched blood.
5. Rh incompatibility in congenital erythroblastosis or hemolytic jaundice.
6. Organ transplantation procedures
7. Autoimmune diseases.

IMMUNE COMPLEX-MEDIATED HYPERSENSITIVITY

Type III hypersensitivity occurs with soluble antigen. Antigen and antibody complexes are commonly formed in response to a wide range of microbial infection or foreign antigens. These complexes are usually cleared by phagocytic cells without causing any damage to the host. But under certain conditions, the antigen-antibody complex or antibody complexes may lead to localized tissue inflammation depending upon the ability of the complexes to form or deposit at a fixed tissue and then activate complement. This results in tissue damage.

1. **Two types: Arthus reaction**: Occurs in antibody excess. Inject soluble antigen intradermally into rabbit having high concentration of antibodies to the antigen injected. There will be erythema, edema in 3 to 8 hours which subsides. Local infiltration with PMN is seen.
2. **Hay fever:** This type of reaction can be seen in cases like Farmer's lung or hay fever.
3. **Serum sickness:** In certain diseases like diphtheria or tetanus, antitoxin (i.e. horse serum) is administered as a part of treatment. In some cases after 5th day of administration of the serum, the patient starts developing fever, lymphadenitis, rash, abdominal and joint pains and slowly it subsides. The reason for this is formation of antibodies against horse serum and Ag + Ab complex formation leads to hypersensitivity reaction as described earlier.
4. **Arthus reaction:** This occurs when an antigen is injected intradermally into host who is having antibodies against same antigen. The antigen-antibody reaction results in local hypersensitivity.

DELAYED HYPERSENSITIVITY OR CELL-MEDIATED ALLERGY

Delayed hypersensitivity was first demonstrated by Robert Koch in relation to tuberculosis. During his experiments with tubercle bacilli, he injected tubercle bacilli into a normal guinea pig. Then there was a formation of nodule, which later on broke down to a shallow ulcer and ultimately healed off. To this animal which had already injected with tubercle bacilli, he again injected tubercle bacilli, this time the formation of nodule occurred after 24

Table 15.1: Immediate and delayed types of hypersensitivity

Immediate type	*Delayed type*
1. Anaphylaxis, cytolytic or cytotoxic, Arthus reaction, serum sickness, drug reactions.	Tuberculosis, leprosy, fungi, parasitic infections, contact with chemicals dyes
2. Reaction is immediate	Reaction occurs after 24 to 48 hours
3. Histologically, capillary dilatation, PMN infiltration, edema	Induration, lymphocyte, macrophage infiltration.
4. Can be passively transferred to a normal person by administration of serum from the sensitized person	Can be transferred passively by lymphocytes and their extracts

hours and it rapidly broke down to shallow ulcer healed quickly as compared to the time taken for first time. Similar results were obtained when dead tubercle bacilli or protein from it was injected in an already infected animal. Such an enhanced reaction due to previous sensitization, which is mediated through activated cells but not by antibody was called Koch's phenomenon or delayed type of hypersensitivity. Later on such type of delayed hypersensitivity was also demonstrated in many other infections (Table 15.1).

Cell-mediated hypersensitivity can be seen in:

1. Bacteria infections like tuberculosis, leprosy, syphilis, listeriosis.
2. Fungal infections: Candidiasis, histoplasmosis.
3. Parasitic infections: Amebiasis, helminthic infection.
4. Viral infections: Measles, herpes simplex, mumps.
5. Contact dermatitis: Eczema, exposure to chemicals like benzene, metals like nickel, hair dyes.
6. Insect bites and autoimmune diseases.
7. Nonliving antigens like dead bacilli with adjuvant or without adjuvant.

Mechanism is same as CMI: The relationship between CMI and DTH is not fully known although both are dependent on specifically sensitized lymphocytes. Contact hypersensitivity is induced by a process of percutaneous absorption. Most of such antigens are fat-soluble. Hence, they may gain entry by passing through sebaceous glands.

Chapter 16

Transplantation Immunity

INTRODUCTION

Many attempts have been made to transplant fresh organs to replace the diseased organs. These attempts are partly successful and still pose many problems. The problems involved in grafting or transplanting the organs are dealt with under transplantation immunity because they are due to immunological reactions.

DEFINITIONS

Before going to the details some definitions will be useful to understand the basic mechanisms.

1. **Graft:** The transplanted tissue is called a graft, e.g. skin, kidney, heart, liver, pancreas, lung, etc.
2. **Autograft:** The tissue of the same person transplanted to another region, e.g. skin from the thigh region can be grafted on to the face. This type of graft takes perfectly without any complications.
3. **Isograft:** Tissue exchange between two genetically identical persons. Graft takes without complication.
4. **Allograft:** Tissue exchange between two genetically different persons. Graft is sometimes taken and sometimes rejected, e.g. kidney transplantation, blood transfusion.
5. **Xenograft:** Tissue exchange between two different species, e.g. monkey to man—always rejected.

Second and third we are not interested because the grafts take up without complications. The 5th one is still under experimental stage. The most important one concerned in medicine is allograft.

What are the events that taken place in case of allograft? Let us take an experimental example.

Take two different guinea pigs and exchange the skin grafts between them and observe carefully upto 7th day; both grafts appear normal and one can expect that they have been accepted. But after 7th day the grafts become pale, ischemic and there will be violent inflammatory reaction around the graft with infiltration and vasodilatation. By 10th day the graft becomes necrosed and by 12th or 14th day it is rejected. If you once again attempt exchange of skin grafts between these two animals, there will be violent reaction and the grafts are rejected within 4 days (IInd stage).

The events can be explained in the following way during the first 7 days of first stage rejection, blood vessels start communicating with the graft, resulting in circulation of the antigens of the graft into the host immune system. Now the host gets sensitized to these antigens, provokes antibodies and activated cells, which attack the whole graft and reject it during the second stage rejection. The events are accelerated because the animal is already sensitized.

Why this Type of Rejection Occurs?

The rejection of the transplanted tissue between two genetically different person is due to presence of different types of certain specific antigens called histocompatibility antigens or HLA system (human leukocyte antigen system) which are genetically determined on 6th chromosome in humans. There are two types of HLA antigen: (i) major, (ii) minor. If there is an identity in major antigens and small differences are present in minor antigens, the graft usually survives. If there is no identity, the graft is rejected. If the major antigens are similar, but if there are many types of nonidentical minor antigens—graft is rejected. Consequently, the likelihood of compatibility between two genetically different individual is very rare.

In addition the lymphocytes possess different types of antigens that also take part in transplantation rejections.

1. Male donor: Female recipient—graft rejected even in highly inbred strains.
2. Female donor: Male recipient—graft accepted.

The reason is that X chromosome genes are common whereas Y chromosome genes are not. This unilateral sex-linked histocompatibility is called Eichwald-Silmser effect.

Detection of histocompatibility: Before transplantation

1. One has to checkup whether there is any compatibility between donor and recipient just as we do matching of blood groups before transfusion one has to carry the typing of the tissues using antibodies against major and minor HLA antigens.
2. **Normal lymphocyte transfer:** The lymphocytes from the recipient blood are separated and injected intradermally into donor. If there is delayed type of hypersensitivity, it indicates incompatibility that means the donor is not suitable for transplantation. *Disadvantage:* Transmission of infections.
3. **Mixed lymphocyte culture:** The T lymphocytes of the recipient are mixed with killed lymphocytes of donor. If there is an incompatibility, the recipient T cells are activated and they become more basophilic and divide, indicating incompatibility.

Sometimes the lymphocytes present in the graft will attack the host tissue. This is called graft versus host reaction leading to retardation of the growth of the host and other complication like diarrhea, etc.

Prevention of Graft Rejection

1. Tissue matching.
2. Immunosuppressive drugs.
3. Antilymphocyte globulin.

Clinical Experience

Corneal grafts are taken up without any problem because they are avascular. Similarly, grafts of the cartilage are successful because it is not penetrated by lymphocytes and polymorphs. Similarly, areas where lymphatic drainage is absent, the chances of survival of graft is more. Kidney transplants can survive upto more than 6 years if the HLA antigens are carefully matched. Forty to fifty percent of the heart transplants are usually rejected in one year and also it is a problem to get a healthy heart. Liver transplants usually survive 1 year.

Tumor Immunity

Whenever a cell undergoes malignant transformation, it acquires new antigens on its surface. These are called tumor specific transplantation antigens or tumor associated transplantation antigens. They produce antibodies or activated cells against these tumor cells, whereby they are killed. In some cases the malignant cells possess antigens that are normally present in fetus not in the normal adult and their detection helps in early diagnosis of malignancy (e.g. α-fetoprotein). It has been shown that in normal healthy person, malignant cells are continuously formed but they are killed or disposed of by the effective immune system of the body. If the immune system is defective, or if the malignant cells grow beyond the capacity of immune system to tackle then the tumors may become clinically evident. Both HMI, CMI exit against tumor but they are not quite effective, due to some unknown reasons. But in certain cases the immune system can be activated by stimulating it with specific human cell vaccines or nonspecifically with substances like BCG or adjuvant. This sometimes helps to stop the rapid metastasis of the cancer and prolongs the life to certain extent.

Chapter 17

Bacterial Infections

INTRODUCTION

Bacterial infections that are communicable, are very common in developing countries, in spite of availability of specific treatment, these diseases still continue to occur resulting in a number of deaths, or disabilities. In this section, bacterial infections are discussed according to their priority.

TUBERCULOSIS

Tuberculosis is one of the ancient diseases which was even described in Ayurveda. It is a chronic disease which mainly involves respiratory system because the infection is airborne. The disease is caused by a gram-positive bacterium known as *Mycobacterium tuberculosis*. The tubercle bacilli enter the respiratory system through inhalation of dust particles containing the bacilli. Depending upon the individuals resistance the infection subsides without treatment and remains dormant in the body. The infection may get reactivated during anytime. The tubercle bacilli can cause disease in any organ of the body but most of the times lung infection is very common. The disease is characterized by low grade fever (especially evening rise of temperature), cough with expectoration, loss of weight, loss of appetite, night sweats. Infection may spread to kidney resulting in urinary tract infection or to the brain resulting in meningitis. Tuberculous meningitis (brain fever) is a common complication of tuberculosis in children.

The disease is diagnosed by finding the tubercle bacilli in the smears of sputum or other body fluids by Ziehl-Neelsen staining (*see* Fig. 25.4). These are acid-fast bacilli. Culturing of tubercle bacilli in the laboratory on LJ (Lowenstein-Jenson) medium (Fig. 17.1), X-ray examination of the lung, raised erythrocyte sedimentation rate (ESR) and by Mantoux test. The organisms multiply slowly and may take 8–10 weeks to grow on LJ medium. Modified media are available for rapid growth of organisms.

The infection should be treated effectively and the duration of the treatment varies from 6 months to 1 year depending upon the severity of the disease. BCG vaccination given

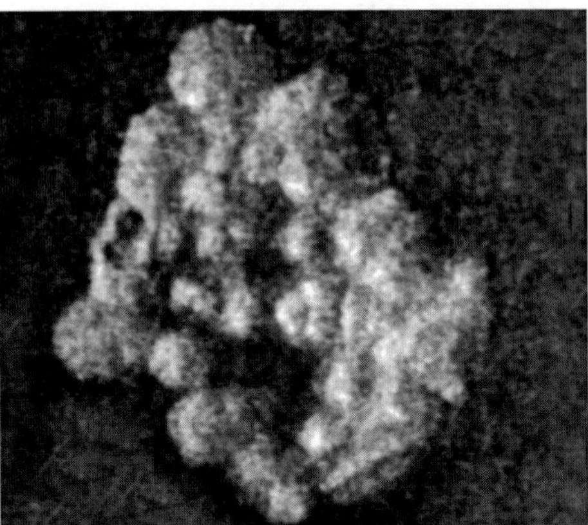

Fig. 17.1: Growth of *M. tuberculosis* on LJ medium. Note the color and shape of the colony (*For color version, see Plate 4*)

to the children offers protection against childhood tuberculosis and its complications but does not offer protection against adult tuberculosis.

LEPROSY

The disease is also known as Hansen's disease named after the person who discovered the disease. There are approximately 12 million people with leprosy throughout the world. The disease is commonly seen in countries like Africa, South and South East Asia, Central and South America, Mexico and Philippines. In India the disease is more prevalent in Tamil Nadu and Andhra Pradesh. Humans appear to be the only natural host for leprosy. Leprosy is caused by *Mycobacterium leprae* (*see* Fig. 25.3). Infection occurs by contact with patients with lepromatous leprosy (one type of leprosy) who excretes large number of bacilli in their nasal secretions and ulcers. But the actual mode of transmission of the disease is not known.

Close contact is necessary for the infection to occur. The major route of entry of these bacteria into the human body is probably through respiratory tract. Biting insects and breast milk may also be an important source of infection. Leprosy is classified as lepromatous leprosy (LL), borderline lepromatous (BL), borderline (B), borderline tuberculoid (BT), and tuberculoid type (TT). Among these types lepromatous leprosy is highly contagious and tuberculoid type is mild and less communicable. The other forms exist in between lepromatous leprosy and tuberculoid leprosy. The incubation period varies from 2 to 5 years but it can be as short as 3 months and as long as 40 years. The early symptom of leprosy is usually asymptomatic, slightly hypopigmented (discolored) skin patches several centimeters in diameter. In tuberculoid type the patches are a few in number. In lepromatous leprosy the patches are more, distributed bilaterally. Because of damage to the nerves, the patches will show less sensation to pain, touch and temperature. Eyebrows and eyelashes are gradually lost and damage to the nerves gradually leads to injury and secondary infection. In untreated cases death occurs due to respiratory obstruction, kidney failure and frequent infections.

Leprosy is diagnosed by the demonstration of lepra bacilli in the smears of skin clippings taken from the patches, in nasal scrapings, earlobes and tissue secretions. The bacilli are numerous in lepromatous leprosy. Study of the biopsy material for characteristic histological response is helpful in tuberculoid leprosy, where the lepra bacilli are often impossible to detect.

Early detection and treatment of infected persons as well as their close contacts help in the prevention of the disease. BCG vaccination offers some protection against leprosy.

DIPHTHERIA

Diphtheria is an acute infection caused by a gram-positive bacteria, *Corynebacterium diphtheriae* (also known as Klebs-Loeffler bacilli or diphtheria bacilli). Diphtheria is worldwide in distribution and in developing countries an estimated 10 lakh deaths occur in a year due to diphtheria. Diphtheria may give rise to epidemics during any period of the year but the number of cases are high in winter season due to overcrowding and close interpersonal contact. Humans are the only natural hosts to diphtheria bacilli. Symptom free carriers and persons who are in the incubation period of the disease are the major source of the infection. The infection is transmitted from person to person through respiratory route. Discharges from extrarespiratory sites such as skin ulcers provide another major source of infection. The infection is characterized by sudden low grade fever, weakness and mild sore throat. The local lymph nodes are enlarged and painful. Spread of the disease from the throat to the larynx and trachea results in airway obstruction resulting in difficulty in breathing, suffocation and death. This is because of the formation of thick greyish pseudomembrane which causes obstruction to the airflow into the lungs. The bacilli multiply at the local site and produce a powerful exotoxin which can cause paralysis and damage of the heart muscle. Primary and secondary lesions may occur in other parts of the body and skin diphtheria is very common in tropical areas. Rarely diphtheria infection of the eye, ear, vagina, secondary to pharyngeal and skin infection can be seen.

Diphtheria is diagnosed by the demonstration of typical bacilli in the smears taken from the tonsillar area or from the skin lesions, culturing of the diphtheria bacilli in the laboratory and demonstration of production of toxin by the diphtheria bacilli by inoculating the experimental animals like rabbits or guinea pigs. Diphtheria can be treated with antibodies and triple antigen comprising diphtheria toxoid pertussis and tetanus toxoid is given as a part of universal immunization program prevents diphtheria. Adults who are not vaccinated in their childhood sometimes develop diphtheria infection. However, such cases are very rare.

MENINGITIS

Infection of the protective layers (mininges) covering the brain is known as meningitis or pyogenic meningitis. The incidence of pyogenic meningitis (also known as bacterial meningitis) is 5 to 10 per 100,000 per year in developed countries and it is more in developing countries. Seventy to ninety percent of meningitis cases are due to one of the following organisms:

a. *Neisseria meningitidis* (Meningococci)
b. *Haemophilus influenzae* type b.
c. *Streptococcus pneumoniae*
d. *Staphylococcus aureus*
e. Group B streptococci
f. *Escherichia coli*

Meningococcal meningitis occurs in epidemics, *H. influenzae* meningitis occurs in children below 5 years age and *Streptococcus pneumoniae* meningitis is seen frequently in adults above 40 years age.

The disease is characterized by headache, fever, neck and back pain and stiffness, vomitings, altered levels of consciousness, fits and photophobia (intolerance to light). In meningococcal meningitis rashes can be seen in 50 percent of the cases.

Meningitis is a serious condition and requires hospitalization and immediate diagnosis and treatment. The diagnosis is made by examination of cerebrospinal fluid (Fig. 17.2) obtained by lumbar puncture. The cerebrospinal fluid is analyzed for the presence of increased protein, decreased sugar and chloride, presence of plenty of white cells and smear may show typical bacteria on staining (Fig. 17.3). Other tests like detection of C-reactive protein, lactic acid and bacterial specific products may be useful in rapid diagnosis and treatment. The persons who are in close contact with the patient should be given appropriate antibiotics to prevent the development of disease in them. Counter immunoelectrophoresis is a rapid method for the detection of antigen of meningococci in the spinal fluid.

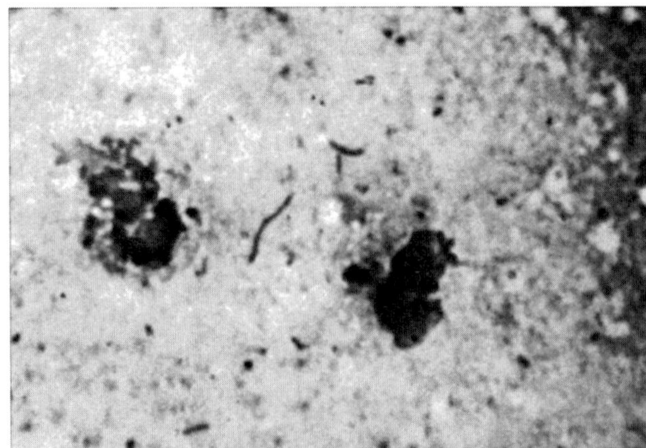

Fig. 17.2: Gram-stained film of the CSF from a patient of *Haemophilus influenzae* meningitis (*For color version, see Plate 4*)

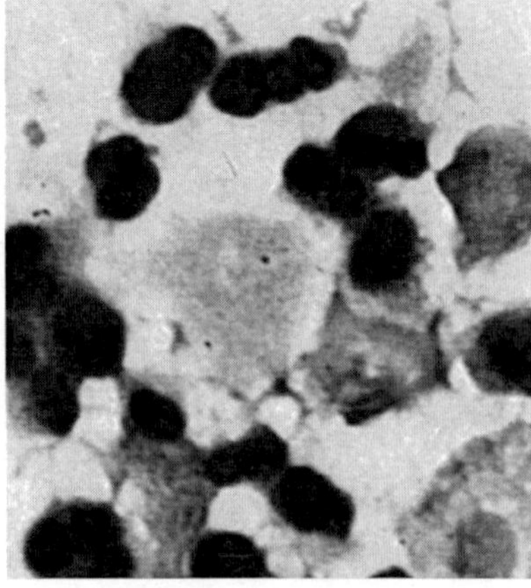

Fig. 17.3: Gram-stained film showing Gram-negative diplococci within the cells (meningococci) (×100) (*For color version, see Plate 4*)

TYPHOID AND PARATYPHOID FEVERS

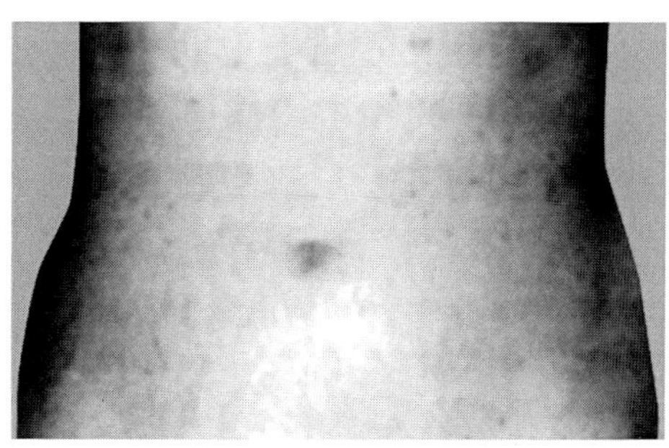

Fig. 17.4: Rose spots in a patient with typhoid fever (*For color version, see Plate 4*)

Typhoid fever is also known as enteric fever. It is mainly caused by a gram-negative motile bacterium called *Salmonella typhi,* other organisms like *Salmonella paratyphi* also can cause typhoid fever. The disease is endemic in India, South East Asia, Middle East (Gulf countries), Africa and Central as well as South America. The infection occurs through food and water contaminated by feces (stools) or urine of a sufferer or carrier. The incubation period is about 2 weeks. The infected person will have persistent continuous high fever and headache, weakness, anorexia (loss of appetite) dry cough and constipation. There may be altered consciousness in the second week of infection, abdominal distention and yellowish green colored diarrhea may occur in third week. In patient with fair skin one can see spots (rash) on lower chest and upper abdomen (Fig. 17.4). The liver and spleen may be enlarged. Pulse rate may be low. Altered consciousness, distended abdomen, perforation of intestine and shock may be seen as complications during the third week of infection. Other complications like intestinal bleeding, jaundice, abscess formation are rarely seen.

The disease is diagnosed by culturing the blood, bone marrow bile or urine for the specific organism. Antibodies against *Salmonella* organisms may be raised which can be detected by "Widal test" but this is not reliable. Every attempt should be made to culture the organism in the laboratory for the confirmation of the diagnosis. Patients should be treated promptly with antibiotics, rest and easily digestible diet. Patient should be given adequate fluids to avoid dehydration and shock. In cases of complications like bleeding or perforation of intestine, blood transfusion and surgery are indicated.

ENTERIC FEVER—CHANGING TRENDS

Systemic reactions with bacterimia as a consequence of infection with *Salmonella,* and other members of the family Enterobacteriaceae constitute a spectrum of syndromes involving differences in pathogenesis from the most common clinical manifestation of acute diarrheal diseases. Included representatives of such entities are "Typhoid fever," other enteric fevers, enteropathogenic *E. coli* infection and septicemia due to *Salmonella choleraesuis.* The exact incidence of typhoid fever in developing countries is not clear. In India, it has been estimated that 1 million people are affected every year. Another study indicates that the isolation of *Salmonella* is approximately 0.5/1000 cultures.

General Considerations

The *Salmonella typhi*-serotype is uniquely adopted humans, and human carriers represent the sole source of these organisms. Carriers can be convalescent carriers who excrete these organisms for a short period of time or chronic carriers who shed these organisms for longer than an year. Approximately three percent of the typhoid patients become carriers. The majority of these chronic carriers are older women with gallbladder disease. The organism resides in the gall stones or scars in the biliary tree. Typhoid fever occurs through ingestion of contaminated water and food. In developing countries without adequate control measures typhoid fever remains a major health problem involving thousands of people.

Pathogenesis

Approximately 25% of the people get infected on ingestion of 10 organisms and with 10^9 organisms nearly 95% people can be infected. During the first week of infection nonspecific symptoms like lethargy, fever, malaise, body pains are very prominent. Constipation rather than diarrhea is the rule. The organism penetrates the intestinal bloodstream, and also the other parts of reticuloendothelial system. The organisms are ingested by monocytes but they are not killed. Following the multiplication in monocytes the organisms invade bloodstream once again resulting in bacterimia, invasion of the Peyer's patches of intestine. Complications like intestinal perforation, bleeding, thrombophlebitis, cholecystitis and pneumonia, localized infections such as abscess formation in thyroid gland, secondary infection of a hydatid cyst may occur occasionally. The death rate is between 2 and 10 percent and lowest when the supportive therapy is available. Relapse may occur in approximately 20% of the infected persons. *Salmonella* septicemia is prolonged and comprises of fever, chills, anorexia and anemia. Focal lesions like osteomyelitis (especially common in persons with sickle-cell trait), pneumonia, pulmonary abscess meningitis or endocarditis. In patients with schistosomiasis, chronic bacterimia due to *Salmonella typhi* has been described because the parasite carriers these organisms. However, this distinctive textbook picture of a patient of typhoid fever is now not seen in more than 50% of patients and change is being observed in clinical presentation and complications.

Salmonella group of organisms produce a variety of virulence factors including surface antigens, adhesions, endotoxins, and cytotoxins. The role of these virulence factors varies with individual serotype and the immunocompetency of the host. The surface antigens like 'O', Vi help the organism to attach to complement-mediated lysis by normal serum. The uptake of the organism by macrophages is also affected by the deposition of complement on the surface of the organism. For some strains the 'O' antigen is more important for the survival of the organism within the intestine. The role of 'Vi' antigen in the pathogenesis is not very clear. However, it has been shown that Vi strains are more resistant to phagocytosis. Fimbrial strains are slightly more virulent than nonfimbriate strains. Whether plasmids encode for the changes in the surface properties of *Salmonella* facilitate the spread of the organism is not known.

Syntheses of new bacterial proteins are required when grown in the presence of mammalian cells. Under low oxygen concentration, the adherence is more pronounced and strains are more invasive. Endotoxin also plays an important role, especially during the bacterimic phase. Presumably, it is responsible for fever. Endotoxin may activate complement system and may localize the leukocytes. *Salmonella typhi* produces least amount of cytotoxins and they inhibit protein synthesis.

Changing Clinical Spectrum

As mentioned earlier, a number of new facts of typhoid fever have been noticed and attention has been drawn to the various known and unknown complications which were not encountered earlier or did not noticed with more attention. Typhoid affects almost every system of the body. The disease can lead to a variety of complications such as neuropsychiatric complications like encephalopathy, delirium, convulsions, meningism, acute brain syndrome, psychosis, peripheral circulatory failure myocarditis, shock, intestinal hemorrhages, perforation, arthropathy, hepatitis, nephritis, typhoid spine, and rarely orchitis, perinephritic abscess, etc.

Because of the several odd presentations, and atypical signs and symptoms, the initial clinical diagnosis mainly depends upon high degree of suspicion. Bizarre symptoms with prolonged fever, gastroenteritis, acute bronchitis mimicking like acute bronchopneumonia should alert the physician. Toxic manifestations like headache, dry coated furred tongue, cough, abdominal symptoms, bradycardia, malaise may be observed only in 50% of cases.

All age groups are susceptible and men are affected more commonly than women. However, there are no supportive studies to postulate whether the immunity is sex-linked. Though a genetic factors seem to be implicated in determining the severity of the disease, the classical step ladder pattern of the fever, bradycardia may not be seen in many patients. On the other hand continuous, remittent fever with or without chills and rigors may be seen. This is important to bear in mind because in tropical countries malaria may also present with similar symptoms. Among Indian patients rose spots are not seen, very frequently because of skin complexion. Epistaxis and hepatosplenomegaly are seen very frequently. Presence of 'gurgling' cecum is an important sign especially during 1st and 2nd weeks, and this clinical sign should alert the physician.

A high incidence of neuropsychiatric manifestations has been observed, which may present as acute delirium and convulsions and involvement of organic reflexes such as urinary in continence, or patients may present with fever, toxemia and may develop semicoma or coma with gradual involvement of organic reflexes. It is to be noted that the extent of neuropsychitric manifestations is not related to the degree of temperature. Anemia and malnutrition are responsible for higher incidence of psychiatric disturbances in typhoid fever. Rarely pseudo- bulbar palsy, encephalomyelitis can occur. Parkinsonian type of rigidity has been noticed in typhoid patients which is reversible and it is a good prognostic index. This may be due to the action of endotoxins interfering with cholinergic dopaminergic control of the basal ganglia. True typhoid meningitis is uncommon. The biochemical basis of neuropsychiatric disturbances points toward the alterations in the serum, and CSF calcium and magnesium levels.

Approximately 10% of the patients may show ECG abnormalities which may be slight or severe in the form of myocarditis and rhythm alterations. Significant changes in the serum levels of SGOT and SGPT enzymes were observed in patients with myocarditis.

Persistence of various abnormalities in ECG and development of arrhythmias carry a poor prognosis.

Intestinal perforation is another important complication of typhoid fever. The incidence of which varies from 1.9 to 11.2 percent. Patients with typhoid fever if develop pain around umbilicus, physician should suspect impending perforation. Very high or low leukocyte count, fall in the body temperature, delay in the diagnosis, poor nutritional status are some of the factors that influence the outcome of the perforation. Presence of air under the diaphragm radiologically is a late sign. Classical signs of intestinal perforation in a typhoid patient are an exception than the rule.

The incidence of hepatosplenomegaly in these patients varies from 13 to 65 percent. Hepatic encephalopathy as a manifestation of typhoid hepatitis is rare. The jaundice in typhoid patient may be confused with viral hepatitis. Typhoid hepatitis if associated with other complications carrying a poor prognosis. Severe infection reduces gastric acidity making the person more prone to infection. Intestinal hemorrhage is seen as a complication along with intestinal perforation and hepatitis.

Functional or pathological changes can occur in the kidney during the course of typhoid fever. Transient glomerular disease or acute renal failure due to hemolysis may be seen direct involvement of kidneys in typhoid fever is more frequent in patients with concurrent existence of renal disease. The development of toxic nephritis depends on the immune status. The approximate incidence of typhoid associated nephritis is about two percent and it carries poor prognosis. Depositions of *S. typhi* Vi antigen has been demonstrated in the glomerulitis due to typhoid fever. Circulating immune complexes have been demonstrated following a renal injury due to typhoid and subsequently they disappear following the recovery. Hence, their detection has some prognostic role and needs further evaluation. Histological studies in typhoid nephritis showed no glomerular or tubular abnormality. However, irreversible damage occurs in toxic and moribund patients, and they may progressively pass on to renal failure.

Peripheral circulatory failure, arthropathy, typhoid spine, perinephritic abscess, bronchopneumonia, orchitis, ottitis media osteomyelitis, pericarditis have been documented as some of the rare complications following typhoid fever.

Current Knowledge on Laboratory Findings

Blood picture shows leukopenia, absence of eosinophilia and relative predominance of mononuclear cells. Acute hemorrhage, hemolytic uremic syndrome, disseminated intravascular coagulation (DIC), consumptive coagulopathy have been documented. The cause for DIC in typhoid is not known but seems to be associated with clinical shock which is usually seen in gram-negative sepsis. Depression of reticuloendothelial system may play a role in the development of DIC in these patients. Thrombocytopenia was another common finding in acute typhoid infection. The decreased number of platelets is (a) due to decreased production, (b) increased destruction, and (c) subclinical DIC, (d) drugs. Bone marrow is essentially normocellular. An increase in plasma cells has been observed in most patients and they may play a nonspecific role in humoral immune response. Both cell-mediated immunity (CMI) and humoral response develop regularly independent of each other. Specific

CMI response, which usually appears in the second week-influences the outcome of the patient. Clinical recovery of patients with complications correlates with the specific CMI and this is depressed in patients with complications. Studies on T and B lymphocytes in typhoid fever patients showed that the difference in both early and late rosette forming T lymphocytes was found to be significantly high.

Humoral immune response is unrelated to complications. The age old Widal test for determining the 'O' and H antibody titers is routinely done in all laboratories. It is one of the commonly prescribed tests for all kinds of fevers and many a time treatment is given based on the positive report. However, Widal test has its own limitations and one has to consider many criteria, such as (a) previous exposure, (b) vaccination, (c) anamnestic reaction for careful interpretation. It is a well-known fact that sera of a portion of persons in any country contain antibodies capable of reacting to a variable titer in the Widal test. Even in the developed countries where enteric fever is uncommon one to two percent of normal population may show agglutinin titers ranging from 1:20 to 1:320. In countries where enteric fever is endemic, 25% of population may show "H" antibodies. Similarly antibodies against "O" antigens are also seen very frequently because these antigens are widely distributed in not only among the Serotypes of salmonella but also in other enterobacteria. Though some 'O' antibodies may result from the experience of Salmonella infection others may well not.

Extensive studies conducted by Brodie in 1977 and during the Aberdeen typhoid outbreak in 1964 revealed that Widal test is of limited value. The study was conducted on 10,000 serum samples and 11, 043 cultures were done to isolate *Salmonella typhi.*

The popular belief that 'O' antibodies appear early and disappear early and 'H' antibodies appear late and persists longer is not absolutely true. On the contrary, 'H' agglutinins appear towards the end of the 1st week and reach maximum by 3rd week and persists for months or years afterwards. 'O' agglutinins in excess of 1: 80 are usual at some stage of the disease but they may appear quite late during the early stages of the disease hampers the antibody formation has been found to be erroneous by Robertson et al. (1970). The diagnostic significance of estimation of agglutinins in single serum sample is controversial. While high titers may be useful in the diagnosis of enteric fever where the disease is uncommon it seems likely that many patients in the endemic areas who give rapid and strong antibody response have had the endemic areas who give rapid and strong antibody response have had earlier exposure to typhoid bacilli. Substantial rise in titers during the course of disease may be misleading because this often occurs as an anamnestic reaction during the course of unrelated fevers. Rise in 'O' agglutinins is suggestive of active infection not necessarily due to *Salmonella* infection and by no means diagnostic.

A variety of serological tests are under active consideration to replace the Widal test. Tests like counter immunoelectrophoresis (CIEP), passive endotoxins, latex agglutination, ELISA have been tried using different antibodies, or antigens like lipopolysaccharide or porins, but they are not completely reliable. Antibodies to yet unidentified antigens probably play an important role in protection.

Treated patients will have a positive culture of blood during the first week of illness. The incidence of culture positivity drops down to 40% in the face of prolonged antecedent microbial therapy. However, cultures of bone marrow are still positive. Ninety percent of the times cultures can be positive even after one or two doses of antibiotic administration. Recently, a new medium called Ranbach agar has been developed which shows red colonies of *Salmonella* in contrast to blue and pale colonies of other coli forms.

Interestingly, it has been observed that during the acute phase of typhoid fever serum cholesterol and triglycerides are increased which comes to normal level during convalescence. However, serum triglycerides remain high for a prolonged period as compared to other bacterial infections. These changes by and large reflect the catabolic status lipase activity and enzymatic effects of *S. typhi* infection. High density lipoproteins are also decreased in typhoid fever depending upon the severity of the infection, nature of infecting organism and the energy sources that are available. Changes in the lipid profile are transitory and not related to the severity or impending complications of the infections.

Management and Problems

Chloramphenicol, amoxycillin + clavulenic acid, cotrimoxazole is the antibiotics of choice for treating the typhoid fever. Chloramphenicol is contraindicated in the presence severe anemia and bone marrow depression should be kept in mind as a complication of treatment which is of course not very common.

The second problem is development of resistance to chloramphenicol by some strains of *S. typhi*. Chloramphenicol resistant typhoid fevers have severe toxemia and a prolonged course. The acquisition of chloramphenicol resistance is either by mutation or by plasmid mediated. Plasmid-mediated chloramphenicol resistance is usually seen in endemic area or due to indiscriminate use of the antibiotic. As a result of increased resistance to chloramphenicol and ampicillin in tropics, quinolones and cephalosporins are now emerging as promising therapeutic agents. Presently even quinolones are also not very useful for the treatment because of high acquired resistance. Severe infections may require corticosteroids. However, the serum cortisol level was found to be high in acute phase of infection. Low dose of cortisone for a short period is indicated in all seriously moribund patients. Possibly steroids decrease the toxic macrophage products released during the interaction between macrophage and endotoxins of *S. typhi.*

In conclusion the spectrum of typhoid is thus definitely different in the tropics and a more serious profile is now being reported. Though the mortality has definitely come down with the advent of chloramphenicol. Nevertheless, due to various factors like late diagnosis, malnutrition, alterations in immune response, emergence of drug resistant strains an upward trend in mortality upto 18% has been observed especially in hospitalized patients. The changing pattern of clinical, and laboratory findings of typhoid fever should be kept in mind to initiate prompt treatment whenever there is a high degree of suspicion.

CHOLERA

Cholera is highly communicable disease caused by a motile gram-negative comma shaped bacterium known as "*Vibrio cholerae*" which exists in two forms classical and 'Eltor' type. Cholera is endemic in Bengal region of India and Bangladesh. Since 1817 there were seven pandemics of cholera spreading all over the world. The infection is transmitted by contaminated food and water. Until recently there has been a high mortality associated with the disease. In 1947, in Egypt 20,000 deaths occurred due to cholera. In United States in 1866, 50,000 people died of cholera infection. Humans are the carriers of the disease and are below the age of 50 years and they excrete the bacilli in feces intermittently.

The incubation period for cholera is few hours to 2 or 3 days. There is an abrupt onset of diarrhea (which is typically looks like rice water without any fecal matter) and vomiting. Fluid loss in the form of diarrhea may be 15 to 20 liters/day. This results in shock with sunken eyes and cheeks. The skin turgor is diminished. The diarrhea is watery, odorless and without any normal bacteria of intestine.

The diagnosis of cholera should be done as rapidly as possible, examination of the watery diarrhea under the microscope shows plenty of rapidly motile bacilli. The motility can be inhibited by adding antiserum or distilled water. The cholera organisms can be isolated in the laboratory using various nutrient media.

The patient should be given large amounts of fluid and electrolytes. Intravenous infusion of saline may require in severe cases. Cholera is self-limiting disease and does not need any antibiotic therapy. Cholera vaccine is not very useful. A completely new type of cholera bacilli had emerged in India in 1992 in Madras. It is named as *Vibrio cholerae* 0139 (serotype) Bengal. It produces clinical picture similar to vibrio cholera but the severity is more and the organism is more susceptible to some antibiotics. It has spread throughout India and went to Bangladesh in 1993 and then to China, Thailand and South East Asia.

DYSENTERY

The gram-negative non-motile bacilli belonging to the genus *Shigella* (named after the discoverer) are the major causes of bacillary dysentery. Among the species *Shigella dysenteriae* and *Shigella sonnei* are responsible for majority of infections. The other species are *Sh. boydii* and *Sh. flexneri.*

The infection spreads from person to person through contaminated water and food. The reservoir is the carrier who sheds the organism in the feces. Chronic carriers have been described. From the carriers, the organisms can spread by flies, fingers food or feces. *Shigella* organisms can be isolated from clothing and toilet seats. The infection is common in children between age group 1 to 10 years and it is characterized by severe abdominal cramps, and frequent painful passage of small amounts of stools containing blood and mucus. In severe cases the patient may have high grade fever, chills convulsions along with frequent loose motions containing blood and mucus. The deaths are usually due to dehydration and fluid electrolytes replacement is necessary for recovery along with antibiotics. Breastfeeding throughout the first year is effective in reducing dysentery in children. *Shigella dysenteriae* can produce powerful toxin called Shiga toxin, which can cause paralysis.

GASTROENTERITIS

Acute gastroenteritis is the most common problem infants and children with which the clinician is frequently faced. In it is one among the ten leading causes of death in the childhood. It has been estimated in India the death rate due to diarrheal diseases in children is about 20.6/1000 children/year. The etiology of the acute gastroenteritis is multifactorial. In 25 percent of cases we have bacterial agents such as *Escherichia coli, Salmonella, Shigella, Vibrio cholerae, Yersinia enterocolitica, Campylobacter jejuni,* etc. and in other 25 to 50 percent cases we have the viral agents such as rotavirus, adenovirus, enteroviruses, etc. but in 25% cases the etiology is obscure. Acute infectious diarrhea exacerbates nutritional deficiencies so caloric requirements are increased. In addition, catabolic steroids, glucagons and adrenergic amines increase the breakdown of structural proteins adding to the disease picture. Repeated episodes of infectious diarrhea amplify the ill-nourished state. Malnourished individuals are more susceptible to infectious diarrhea, and are susceptible to an increasing number of episodes.

As mentioned earlier viruses, bacteria, parasites are the most frequent cause of diarrhea; fungi are involved only rarely most often in immunosuppressed persons. Older asymptomatic persons presumably serve as the reservoir for the various pathogens responsible for diarrheas. Several factors affect the occurrence of the disease such as age, seasonal variation, individual hygienic habits, socio-economic status, the dose of the causative agent, gastric acidity, health of the mucous membranes, intestinal motility, normal flora of the gut, humoral and cellular immunity possibly associated with coproantibodies, nonspecific resistance factors, intestinal epitopes or receptor sites of the attachment of the microorganisms, the adherence mechanism of the microbes and their toxic moieties.

In the tropics peak incidence of diarrhea is seen in the summer while in temperate areas diarrhea occurs more often in winter season.

Microorganisms produce diarrhea by a variety of mechanisms such as neurotoxins, enterotoxins or cytotoxins. Among the bacterial agents *Escherichia coli* needs special attention because its mechanism of pathogenicity is still poorly understood. In recent years there are four recognized classes of *Escherichia coli* that cause diarrheal disease in humans, namely (a) enterotoxigenic *E. coli,* (b) enteroinvasive *E. coli,* (c) enteropathogenic *E. coli* and the recently recognized enterohemorrhagic *E.coli.* Each of clinical syndrome and epidemiology and each falls within a different set of "O" antigen serogroups.

Enterotoxigenic *E. coli* (ETEC) causes diarrhea in infants, in less developed countries and in travelers from industrialized areas who visit developing countries. ETEC strains produce a heat labile enterotoxin that resembles cholera toxin, polypeptide heat stable enterotoxins or both. Genes encoding production of these heat labile (LT) and heat stable (ST) occur in transmissible plasmids. Studies have been conducted to determine the other determinants associated with ent^+ plasmid such as antibiotic resistance, metallic salt resistance, fermentation or utilization of organic or inorganic substrates. It is not clear whether a single strain of *Escherichia coli* possesses single virulence factor or multiple virulence factors for expressing its mechanism of pathogenicity and also whether all of them are mediated by a single plasmid or multiple plasmids. Among the most common serogroups of human ETEC are 06, 08, 015, 020, 025, 027, 063, 078, 080, 085, 0115, 0128, 0148 and 0159. The most frequent clinical syndrome of an ETEC infection includes watery diarrhea, abdominal cramps, low-grade fever, nausea and malaise. Michael et al. (1980) used antisera of "O" serogroups to identify ETEC strains in stools of 618 patients with diarrhea. Compared with standard enterotoxin testing using rabbit ileal loop model or infant mouse model, testing with antisera had a sensitivity of 64%, specificity of 96% and a predictive accuracy of 89%. Serological grouping may have to be standardized according to the prevalence of ETEC strains with respect to a given geographical area.

Enteroinvasive *E. coli* (ETEC) resembles *Shigella* in many ways. They are often nonmotile, nonlactose fermenting, and they possess a large circular 140 MDa plasmid genes that confer the ability containing to invade epithelial cells. The "O" serogroups in which enteroinvasive *E. coli* are found include 028, 0112, 0124, 0136, 0143, 0144, 0147, 0152 and 0164. The clinical syndrome due to ETEC is identical to bacillary dysentery and includes high grade fever, malaise, toxemia, severe abdominal cramps, diarrhea followed by dysentery and tenesmus.

Enteropathogenic *E. coli* (EPEC) represent the first recognized diarrheagenic class of *E. coli,* having come to light between 1940–1950 as the main cause of outbreaks in infant nurseries and as a cause of sporadic infant diarrhea. The term EPEC was coined by Neter et al. for a collection of "O" serogroups, 026, 055, 086, 0111, 0125, 0126, 0127, and 0128 which occurred more frequently in diarrheal patients than healthy controls. Further studies in 1970 revealed that these strains were negative for virulence markers such as enterotoxins, enteroinvasiveness, leading to a debate that the classic EPEC, including volunteer studies, identification of novel virulence properties and partial elucidation of pathogenesis, recognition of typical histopathological lesion in the affected intestine and modern epidemiological studies. Since 1978 EPEC have come to be appreciated as a new separate class of diarrheagenic *E. coli* that cause diarrhea by distinct pathogenic mechanisms. The pathogenesis of these strains appears to involve both enteroadhesiveness and production of toxin identical to Shiga toxin. The adhesiveness is plasmid mediated. The lesions involve dissolution of micro villi by bacteria, effacement of the enterocytes outer membrane and formation of pedestal around the bacterium at the point of contact. EPEC are the important cause of infant diarrhea. Reservoirs of infection include (a) infants and young children with either clinical or asymptomatic infection, (b) asymptomatic adult carriers or animals. The association of infection with bottle-fed infants and sparing the breastfed infants raises the possibility that (a) breast milk is not subjected to contamination, (b) there is little opportunity for the bacteria for multiplication, (c) breast milk lowers the pH of the intestine, (d) breast milk has bacteriostatic effect due to iron binding protein notably lactoferrin and finally (e) passively acquired specific immunoglobulin A through the breast milk.

More recently outbreaks and sporadic cases of bloody diarrhea and colitis have been reported that are due to *Escherichia coli* 0157:47. The clinical syndrome is somewhat distinct from bacillary dysentery since fever is not prominent and the bloody discharges are copious rather than scanty. These strains possess a 60 to 70 MDa plasmid and are relatively potent producers of a cytotoxin (verotoxin) that appears to be identical to Shiga toxin and is believed to be important in the pathogenesis of diarrhea seen in infection due to enterohemorrhagic *E. coli.* These strains are further responsible for hemolytic uremic syndrome.

Among the various pathogenic mechanisms, production of toxin is the most important mechanism responsible for diarrhea. Enterotoxins are produced by organisms like *Vibrio cholerae,* certain strains of *E. coli* and many of the non-cholera *Vibrio* species. Enterotoxin increases the cyclic AMP in luminal epithelia, resulting in copious fluid secretion. The most widely studied example is cholera toxin which induced the formation of adenylate cyclase resulting in an increase of cyclic AMP concentration. The enterotoxins produced by other vibrios and certain of the *E. coli* toxins act in a similar fashion and are antigenically related to the cholera toxin. While immunoassays and molecular testing for the presence of enterotoxins depends on the use of ligated small bowel segments of animals such as rabbits or infant mice, cell culture systems. An increase in secreted fluid volume after the introduction of enterotoxins into the bowel segments indicates the presence of enterotoxin or cytopathic effect in cell cultures. The enterotoxins of *Shigella dysenteriae* and *Bacillus cereus* have also been studied. It is suspected that *Salmonella, Klebsiella, Citrobacter* and *Enterobacter* may possess heat stable, labile toxins but they do not display these particular attributes with great frequency.

The second type the cytotoxins act by destroying the intestinal mucosa leading to an inflammatory colitis. Cytotoxicity is particularly a property of *Shigella, Clostridium perfringens,* and *Vibrio parahaemolyticus.* The delta toxin of *Staphylococcus aureus* is also cytotoxic. *Clostridium difficile* apparently produces a cytotoxin in addition to its enterotoxin. *Escherichia coli* cytotoxic activity is present in a number of serogroups and leads to production of Vero and or Shiga toxin like moieties, especially with *E. coli* 0157:H7.

The other types of neurotoxins are produced by bacteria in food prior to ingestion. These are elaborated by bacteria like *Clostridium botulinum, Staphylococcus aureus* and *Bacillus cereus.* The neurotoxin of *Staphylococcus aureus* resembles the enterotoxin the enterotoxin in its action, but instead of acting on the intestinal epithelium its acts on the automatic nervous system. Another toxin elaborated by *Staphylococcus* aureus results in hyperperistalsis. Certain of the neurotoxins of *B. cereus* have an emetic effect. The various toxins produced by *C. botulinum* act on neuromuscular juncture preventing the release of acetylcholine from presynaptic vesicles.

The mere presence of these pathogens in the intestinal lumen is not sufficient to produce symptoms. Most microorganisms prefer attachment to a substrate and in the intestinal tract. Attachment is significant for the overt clinical manifestations of disease. The mechanism of attachment has been studied with a variety of bacteria particularly with *E. coli.* These bacteria produce fimbriae, protein organelles, for attachment specifically and nonspecifically to a variety of mammalian cells. They are identified as colonizing factors like CFA I and CFA II.

The ability to invade and destroy luminal epithelial cells of colon is characteristic of many *Shigella* strains and of invasive *Escherichia coli.* They cause an inflammatory or dysenteric type of diarrhea. This capacity to invade and destroy may be related to the 'O' antigen. Chemical alterations and thus it is concluded that they are involved in invasiveness.

Other organisms related to disease severity exist. For example, it is believed that the ability of *Salmonella typhi* to elicit pathology is in part related to the 'Vi' antigen in combination with specific 'O' polysaccharide and parts of the outer membrane of the organism (Table 17.1).

Table 17.1: Clinical diseases induced by *Salmonellae*

Symptoms	*Enteric*	*Septicemia*	*Gastroenteritis*
Incubation	7–20 days	Variable	8–84 hours
Onset	Insidious	Abrupt	Abrupt
Fever	Gradual	Rapid spikes	Low grade
Duration	Several weeks	Variable	2–5 days
GI symptoms	Early constipation	Often none	Nausea, vomiting, diarrhea
Blood culture	Positive	Positive during high fever	Negative
Stool culture	Positive during 2nd or 3rd week	Infrequently positive	Positive soon after the onset

Another important pathogen commonly responsible for diarrhea is *Campylobacter jejuni*. These curved, gram-negative motile organisms were originally placed in genus '*Vibrio*'. The infection has long incubation period. Stool cultures may be positive in 2 to 5 weeks in patients who have not received specific therapy. Males under the age of 14 are commonly affected. The incidence is apparently high in children, but this may be due to over sampling. The infection is more prevalent in warmer months but its significance is obscure. The infection is prevalent in tropical countries. Symptomatic patients act as reservoirs. The exact incidence of infections in humans caused by animal sources is not known. The infective rate is very low probably due to poor survival of the organism. Mothers suffering from *Campylobacter* infection towards the end of confinement may transmit the disease to the newborns. Milk food that is handled improperly is likely major sources of infection.

The organisms are present in less than 1 percent population and are truly pathogens and not merely opportunists as they can infect. High degree of specific antibody is developed during infection. *Campylobacter* spp are pathogenic mainly by the virtue of a direct invasiveness and that LT-like enterotoxins may be responsible in some cases. The principal site of infection is jejunum, and it is hemorrhagic and congested. Passage of bright blood in stools suggests the involvement of colon. *Yersinia enterocolitica* another notable intestinal pathogen may cause infection due to LT-like enterotoxins.

Among the viruses the Rota and Norwalk viruses produce their effect by the destruction of villus tip cells of the small intestine, but they spare the secretory crypt cells. This action produces changes in the absorptive fluid balance and reduces the enzyme secretion of intestinal brush border. Some variation of this type of microbial attachment involved in the bacterial over growth syndrome and may be used in part by EPEC, and parasites like *Giardia lamblia, Strongyloides* and *Cryptosporidium.*

The host parasite equilibrium is an important factor in enteric infectious disease. Micro-organisms alter the normal physiological equilibrium by disturbing the water and electrolyte balance in the small intestine or by the destruction of ideal or colonic mucosa or by penetration of the mucosa and infection of the reticuloendothelial system. Water and electrolyte imbalances result in watery diarrhea in which no fecal leukocytes are demonstrated. Pathogens that produce this type of diarrhea are *Vibrio cholerae*, ETEC, some *Salmonella* species, possibly *V. parahaemolyticus Giardia lamblia*, Rotavirus, Norwalk agent and related viruses as well as cryptosporidium.

The three types of disease manifestations can be distinguished by: (a) absence of leucocytes indicate a noninflammatory process. The diarrhea produced is a result of upper small intestine intoxication or the presence of *G. lamblia* or any one of the forementioned viruses. Noninfectious causes are non-beta cell islet tumor, medullary tumor, and medullary carcinoma of thyroid, carcinoid tumor, benign or malignant neoplasms, tropical sprue, enzyme deficiencies, and ulcerative colitis. (b) Presence of polymorphonuclear cells in feces is encountered when there is inflammatory and invasive process in the colon or distal small bowel. Amebic dysentery involving the colon, however, demonstrates few if any polymorphs. If they are present the nuclei are usually picnotic. (c) The ability to penetrate intact mucosa frequently in the distal small intestine, with consequent multiplication in lymphatic or reticuloendothelial cells results in a systemic febrile illness. Diarrheal stools accompanying these conditions reveal at times mononuclear leukocytes.

Rapid stool examination for the presence of leukocytes, demonstration of drop in pH may be useful in the early initiation of treatment. Preservation of stool samples in buffered glycerol saline is necessary to ensure the survival of pathogenic bacteria. Selective media micro-aerophilic atmosphere are necessary for the isolation of the fastidious organisms. If pseudo-membranous colitis is suspected examination of feces for toxins is required. The isolation of *Clostridium difficile* is not required but toxin should be demonstrated in the fecal samples. For *Yersinia enterocolitica* cold enrichment of the specimen in buffered saline for 1 to 3 weeks can be helpful.

It is very difficult to establish the role of *Escherichia coli* in inflammatory diarrhea, bloody diarrhea, diarrheal outbreaks in nurseries and in individuals with diarrhea. Cluster outbreaks or epidemic studies require assistance of a reference laboratory.

Persistent diarrhea, especially with blood and weight loss suggests that the infection may be due to *Entamoeba histolytica, Giardia or Strongyloides.* Cryptosporidiosis may be responsible for diarrhea in immunocompromised patients.

Indications for antimicrobial therapy in diarrheal diseases:

a. Severe *Shigella* infection
b. Systemic salmonellosis
c. Typhoid and paratyphoid fevers
d. Compylobacter infection when severe and prolonged
e. Cholera
f. Yersiniosis
g. Diagnostic doubt between septicemia and gastroenteritis
h. Amebic dysentery
i. Giardiasis
j. Enterohemorrhagic or invasive *E. coli* infection.

Schematic Approach to the Diagnosis of Diarrheal Diseases

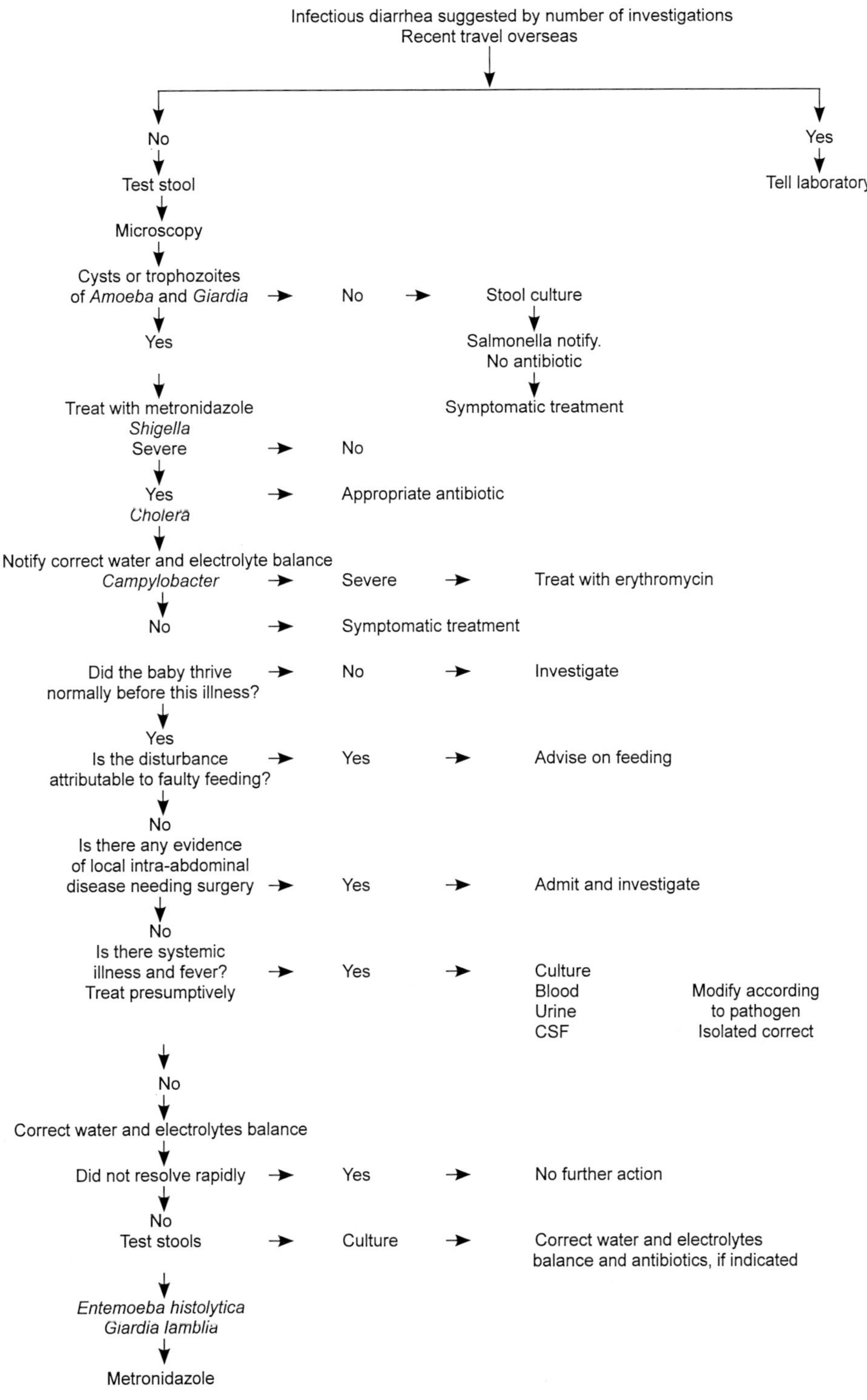

Carrier Status of Intestinal Pathogens

Generally symptomless excretion does not last more than a few weeks. Carrier rate is more in *S. dysenteriae*, compared to other species of *Shigella*. But in India *S. flexeneri* is more common and carrier rate with this is very much less prolonged. In an endemic area carrier rate is approximately 3.8 percent. In one of the large series of study in England 0.4 percent carrier rate was detected. Not more than two percent of the convalescents carried the bacilli for over 3 months, and the carrier stage may extend upto 10 weeks. About two to three percent of patients may have the symptoms of chronic colitis after recovery.

Infection is derived as a rule from cases particularly mild, ambulant cases of the disease from healthy convalescents from usually temporary carriers and probably far less often from chronic carriers. The experience of most workers, however, shows that chronic carriers, i.e. who excrete the organisms more than one year are very infrequent. In mental institutions it is not the relapse but reinfection is more common.

One of the largest series of carrier study of *Salmonella* wherein 14,500 normal persons were investigated the carrier rate was 0.14 percent.

The incidence of contact carriers in cholera is about 4 to 20 percent for household carriers and 1.5 percent among the community carriers.

Since dehydration is the cause health in all types of watery diarrhea, including cholera, the key to management is adequate rehydration either through oral or parenteral routes. The discovery of oral dehydration salt (ORS) has revolutionized the treatment of diarrheal diseases. Further home available fluids (HAF) can be substituted for ORS. However, oral rehydration therapy implementation programs in various developing countries, including India still need to accelerate to a considerable extent in order to achieve a substantial reduction in the diarrhea related mortality.

Laboratories should establish a protocol for the examination of stool specimens which reflect the most likely causative organisms in their area, the various stages of severity and duration of diarrhea. Suspected organisms repeatedly isolates from stool specimens should be regarded as potential disease causing agents.

GONORRHEA

Gonorrhea is a sexually transmitted disease caused by a gram-negative intracellular, kidney shaped diplococci known as *Neisseria gonorrhoeae* (Fig. 17.5). Gonorrhea is the most common of the classic sexually transmitted disease. The increase and decrease in incidence have been associated with seasonal peaks, major social changes, and desruptions caused by wars. When compared to many other infectious diseases gonorrhea is not highly contagious. The incubation period is 2 to 8 days; with the onset of infection patient feels burning sensation on micturition and yellowish discharge from the urethra. There may be associated fever and increased white cell counts in the blood. In 10% of cases there are no symptoms but the person can transmit the disease to others through sexual contact. The complications of untreated cases include stricture urethra (narrowing of urethral canal), swelling and pain of the testes, spermatic cord and prostate gland. Rarely meningitis,

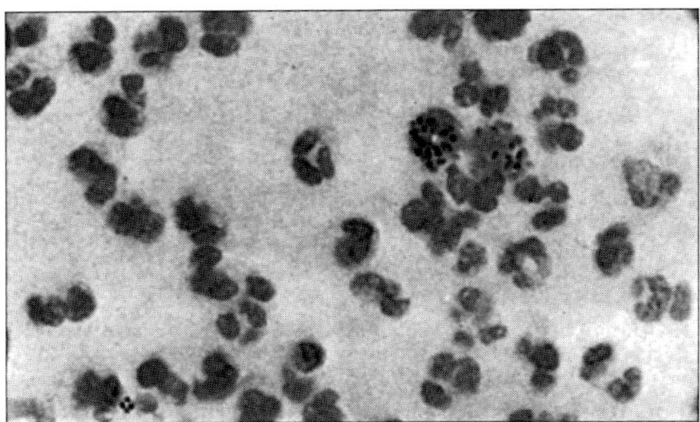

Fig. 17.5: Intracellular gram-negative cocci in pairs. Gonococci (×100) *(For color version, see Plate 4)*

septicemia may occur. In women also burning sensation on urination, vaginal discharge and abdominal pain are the main symptoms. Many women are nonsymptomatic and they do not have any complaints. Complications like infection of fallopian tubes of the uterus, sterility, secondary infections may occur. When the infection spreads throughout the body typical skin lesions, joint pains, fluid accumulation in the joints, is seen. The diagnosis of gonococcal infections is done by the examination of stained smears of the urethral discharge. Culturing of the discharge for the isolation of the organism in the laboratory. Significant number of cases also occur in infants and children. In infants the infection occurs during birth and the most common complication is infection of the eye. Earlier this infection was the cause of blindness in majority of infected children. Presently this disease is rare because routine application of 1 percent silver nitrate into the eyes of newborn. This sometimes may not prevent infection of the eye especially in premature babies. Pharyngitis can occur due to gonococcal infection in adults who are habituated to abnormal sexual practices. Gonococcal vulvovaginitis can occur in girls 2 to 8 years age due to child abuse. Gonococcal conjunctivitis in newborn is called ophthalmia neonatorum.

SYPHILIS

Syphilis is a sexually transmitted disease caused by a spiral shaped bacteria known as *Treponema pallidum*. During the 15th century syphilis was recognized in Europe and rapidly reached epidemic proportions at that time. The course of the disease was first described by John Hunter in 1767. Syphilis is not a highly contagious disease. It is transmitted by sexual contact and the disease has relatively long incubation period. The groups that are frequently affected are the drug users; prostitution for drugs or for money to purchase drugs represents the central epidemiological aspects of the problem. The infections occur on the genital organs of both males and females. The disease has 3 stages. In the primary stage the genital organs are affected and there will be a formation of painless ulcer on the genital organs which is known as 'chancre'. The regional lymph nodes are enlarged but not painful. After 2 to 10 weeks the patient may develop secondary stage of syphilis which is characterized by fever, sore throat, enlarged lymph nodes, headache and rash. The rash is very prominent on palms and soles. Ulcer may be seen in the mouth. The secondary stage is highly infectious. During this stage joints, kidney may be affected. The secondary stage is followed by latent stage during which period the patient is asymptomatic except that his blood examination shows the evidence of exposure to syphilis infection. The latent period may vary from 4 years to many years. If the patient does not receive proper treatment he will develop third stage disease which involves nervous system or heart resulting in complications like meningitis, blindness, loss of memory, heart failure and death.

Infants get infected with syphilis during birth and may develop congenital syphilis.

The disease is diagnosed by demonstration of organisms from the serous fluids obtained from the ulcers. It is not possible to culture the organism in the laboratory but rabbits can be infected and the organisms can be maintained by inoculating the organisms into the testes of the rabbit. The other methods of diagnosis include VDRL test or *Treponema pallidum* hemagglutination test (TPHA) and fluorescent treponemal antibody absorption test (FTA-ABS), *Treponema pallidum* immobilization test, etc. These tests are carried out on serum obtained from the infected person and the tests are performed in a reference laboratory.

RELAPSING FEVER

According to Bergey's Manual of Systemic Bacteriology, spirochetes of the genus *Borrelia* belong to the family *Spirochaetaceae* in the bacterial order Spirochaetales. The spirochetes of the genus *Borrelia* are responsible for the disease in humans known as relapsing fever. Relapsing fever has been known to Western sphere of the world since the time of Hippocrates. The infection has been associated with poverty, overcrowding and warfare. Detailed clinical description of relapsing fever was presented by Bryceson et al. Otto Obermeir discovered spirochetes in the blood of the infected person in 1868 while working in Berlin. Motshukoffsky in 1876 inoculated the blood from the infected person to healthy volunteers and reproduced the disease in them, thus, confirming the association between the spirochetes and the relapsing fever. Mackie in India confirmed the earlier suggestions of Munch and Fliggie that the disease is transmitted by human body louse. Dutton and Todd reported the mechanism of infection of tick, *Ornithodoros moubata* and the transovarial passage of spirochaetes to succeeding generations of ticks.

After the First World War louse-borne relapsing fever spread to countries of Europe and dislocated the civilians, soldiers and the prisoners. Large epidemics occurred throughout Europe, Africa, Asia and South America during World War II. As many as one million reported cases and nine million unreported cases, with a case fatality rate of five percent said to have occurred during the war time. Epidemics of relapsing fever and typhus fever occurred simultaneously in many parts of the world. The spirochetes of the genus *Borrelia* got separated from other spirochetes based on their ultrastructural morphology as seen under the electron microscope. The speciation of the members of the genus *Borrelia* is primarily based on the arthropod vector responsible for the transmission.

Much of our knowledge and experience in understanding the clinical manifestations of human borreliosis owes to the experimental induction of fever with *Borrelia* species in patients infected with syphilis. The symptom and severity of the disease depends upon immune status of the host, geographic location, and the strains of the *Borrelia* species and the phase of the epidemic. The differences between tick-borne and louse-borne relapsing fevers are mentioned in the Table 17.2.

The incubation period is about 6 days, ranging from 2 to 14 days. In the late stage of incubation period, the patient develops sudden onset of chills, fever, headache, tachycardia and myalgia. The primary attack lasts for 3 to 7 days (may be longer for louse-borne type) and ends by crisis. The fever is usually continuous type. Variable number of patients may show macular rash that appears generally near the end of the first attack. The symptoms like jaundice, hepatosplenomegaly and vomiting are common. Respiratory tract involvement may result in bronchitis or bronchopneumonia. Meningismus without encephalitis may be seen in about 30% of the some patient groups. The crisis coincides with immune response. Rarely crisis may result in shock. The temperature usually returns to normal and the patients are free till the subsequent attack. The interval between primary attack and the relapse is shorter in louse borne relapsing fever. The number of relapses may vary from nil to four or more and the percentage of patients with single or multiple relapses varies from 16 to 27 percent.The relapses are usually shorter in duration with less severe and shorter duration of pyrexia. Majority of cases go unrecognized until one or more relapses have occurred.

Diagnosis of borreliosis is based mainly on the detection of spirochetes in the peripheral blood of febrile persons and animals or in the hemolymph or the tissues of arthropod vectors. During the febrile period most spirochetes circulate in the blood and can be detected by either light microscopy of wet preparations made from a drop

Table 17.2: The clinical manifestations of relapsing fevers

Clinical findings	*Tick-borne relapsing fever*	*Louse-borne relapsing fever*
Incubation period	7 days	—
Duration of primary infection	3.1 days	5.5 days
Duration of a febrile interval	6.8 days	9.25 days
Duration of relapse	2.5 days	1.9 days
Number of relapses	> 3	1
Body temperature	40.5°C	—
Splenomegaly	41%	77%
Hepatomegaly	18%	66%
Jaundice	07%	36%
Rash	16%	34%
Respiratory symptoms	16%	34%
CNS involvement	8.9%	30%

of the blood mixed with a small drop of sodium citrate and covered with a cover slip. Any one or combinations of Romanowsky stains can be used to stain both thick and thin smears of the blood to demonstrate the spirochetes. For initial diagnosis thick films are ideal because spirochetemia may be mild and always tend to become milder with each succeeding relapse. Thick films should be of one centimeter in diameter and they may be dehemoglobinized and air dried before staining to make the smears more transparent. This is useful to detect the blue stained spirochetes. A microhematocrit concentration technique detects spirochetes more rapidly in the blood specimen of mildly infected person.

In the arthropod vectors like body louse, the spirochetes are limited to the hemolymph which can be obtained by the amputation of one or more legs of the distal end of the vector. The hemolymph test can also be conducted on the large ticks. However, the test is not sensitive because the *Borrelia* are not always abundant in the body fluids of the infected ticks that have been without a blood meal for a long period. The feeding of infected ticks on experimental animals may not always lead to the transmission of the spirochetes. Hence, this method is not recommended for routine diagnosis unless feeding experiments are carried out repeatedly. Spirochetes in the arthropod vectors are more reliably detected by direct immunofluorescent technique using species-specific antibodies labeled with fluorescent dyes like FITC or careful examination of the tissues under dark-field microscopy and by inoculating the susceptible animals with tick triturates. Polymerase chain reaction has been used to detect the DNA of the *Borrelia* species.

Borreliae can easily be cultivated in their arthropod vectors or in a large variety of vertebrate animals particularly small rodents. Embryonated eggs can be used for successful isolation of these organisms. Kelly medium has been developed for the *in vitro* cultivation of *B. hermisii, B. parkeri, B. turicatae, B. hispanica* and *B. recurrentis.* However, spirochetes cultured for even relatively short periods of time may be quite different from the naturally occurring ancestral strains due to changes in the protein profiles, migration of lipopolysaccharide material in the polyacrylamide gels and the reduction in the numbers of detectable plasmids.

During late relapses of relapsing fever the spirochetes in the blood of the infected person or animal may be very low in numbers and may not be detected by microscopy. In such circumstances one should call for the inoculation of susceptible laboratory animals with whole blood or triturated blood clots. Suckling Swiss mice and suckling rats are the animals of choice for both louse-borne *B. recurrentis* and tick-borne borreliosis. Other animals like monkeys, rabbits, guinea pigs or chicken are useful depending on the species involved. About 0.05 to 0.2 mL of 1:1 dilution of blood in sodium citrate is injected intramuscularly or intraperitoneally in the selected laboratory animals. Spirochetes in the infected laboratory animals can be detected within three days of inoculation. Blood films are examined daily for 14 days before the animal is considered negative for spirochetemia.

Because of the spontaneous changes in the antigenic composition of the spirochetes serodiagnosis of borreliosis is difficult. Indirect-immunofluorescent antibody technique appears promising in detecting the specific antibodies against the cultured spirochetes as antigens. The test can be used for the characterization of antigenic types of *Borrelia* and for detecting the mixed population and serotypes of spirochetes.

Borrelia are susceptible to many antibiotics but for treatment tetracyclines are the drugs of choice. They reduce the relapse rates and rid central nervous system of spirochetes. Rapid destruction of the organisms may produce Jarisch-Herxheimer reaction. Although the dosage and the route of administration of antibiotics are debatable, good results have been obtained with 500 mg 6th hourly for 4 to 5 days. Single dose of 100 mg doxycycline is also as good as tetracycline therapy. To avoid Jarisch-Herxheimer reaction, a combination of procaine penicillin 4 lakh and tetracyclines can be used.

LEPTOSPIRA

Leptospirosis is now identified as one of the emerging infectious diseases, exemplified by recent large outbreaks in Nicaragua, Brazil, India, Southeast Asia, and the United States and most recently in several countries as a result of the Eco Challenge Sabah 2000 competition in Malaysia. In the landmark Institute of Medicine report "Emerging Infections: Microbial Threats to Health in the United States," leptospirosis was used as an example of an infection which had in the past caused significant morbidity in military personnel deployed in tropical areas.

Leptospirosis is a zoonosis of ubiquitous distribution, caused by infection with pathogenic *Leptospira* species. The spectrum of human disease caused by Leptospira is extremely wide, ranging from subclinical infection to a severe syndrome of multi-organ infection with high mortality. This syndrome, icteric leptospirosis with renal failure, was first reported over 100 years ago by Adolf Weil in Heidelberg.

The importance of occupation as a risk factor was recognized early. The role of the rat as a source of human infection was discovered in 1917, while the potential for leptospiral disease in dogs was recognized, but clear distinction between canine infection with *L. interrogans serovars icterohaemorrhagiae* and *canicola* took several years. Leptospirosis in livestock was recognized some years later.

Leptospirosis has been described as a zoonosis of protean manifestations.

Clinical presentation of leptospirosis is biphasic with the acute or septicemic phase lasting about a week, followed by the immune phase, characterized by antibody production and excretion of leptospiras in the urine. Most of the complications of leptospirosis are associated with localization of leptospiras within the tissues during the immune phase and thus occur during the second week of the illness (Fig. 17.6).

The great majority of infections caused by Leptospira are either subclinical or of very mild severity, and patients will probably not seek medical attention. A smaller proportion of infections, but the overwhelming majority of the recognized cases, present with a febrile illness of sudden onset. Other symptoms include chills, headache, myalgia, abdominal pain, conjunctival suffusion, and less often a skin rash. If present, the rash is often transient, lasting less than 24 hours. This anicteric syndrome usually lasts for about a week, and its resolution coincides with the appearance of antibodies. The fever may be biphasic and may recur after a remission of 3 to 4 days. The headache is often severe, resembling that occurring in dengue, with retro-orbital pain and photophobia. Myalgia affecting the lower back, thighs, and calves is often intense.

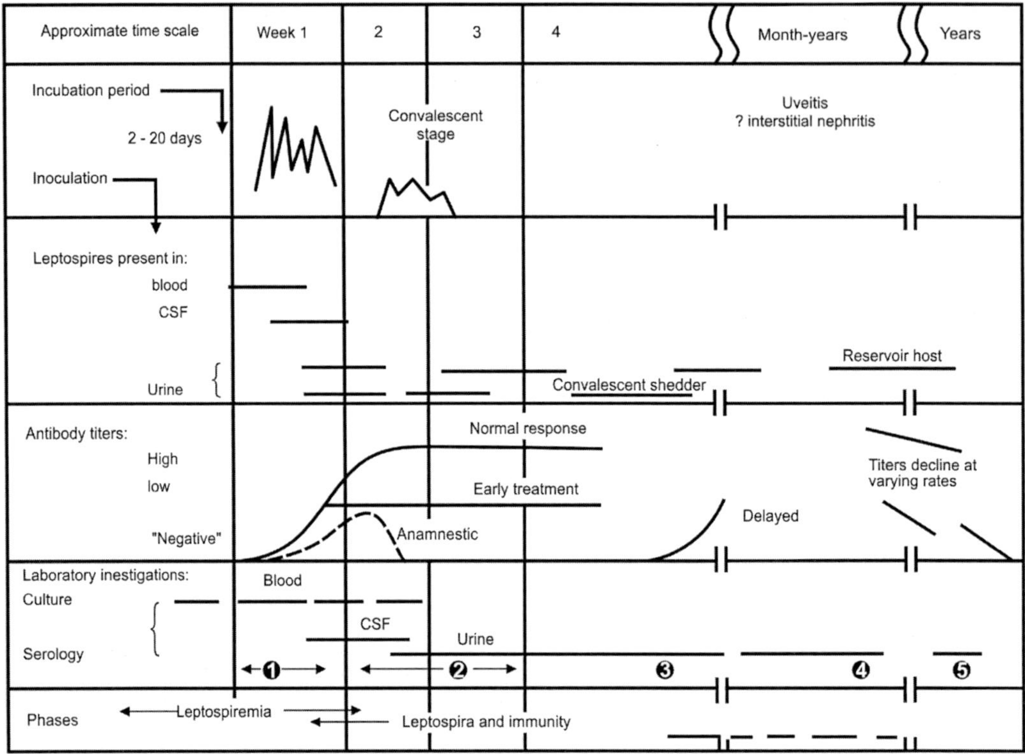

Figure 17.6: Biphasic nature of leptospirosis and relevant investigations at different stages of disease

Aseptic meningitis may be found in ≤25% of all leptospirosis cases and may account for a significant minority of all causes of aseptic meningitis. Patients with aseptic meningitis have tended to be younger than those with icteric leptospirosis. Mortality is almost nil in anicteric leptospirosis, but death resulting from massive pulmonary hemorrhage occurred in 2.4% of the anicteric patients in a Chinese outbreak.

Icteric leptospirosis is a much more severe disease in which the clinical course is often very rapidly progressive. Severe cases often present late in the course of the disease, and this contributes to the high mortality rate, which ranges between 5 and 15%. Between 5 and 10% of all patients with leptospirosis have the icteric form of infection.

The complications of severe leptospirosis emphasize the multi-systemic nature of the disease. Leptospirosis is a common cause of acute renal failure (ARF), which occurs in 16 to 40 percent of cases. A distinction may be made between patients with pre-renal azotemia (non-ARF) and those with ARF. Thrombocytopenia occurs in ≥ 50% of cases and is a significant predictor for the development of ARF. The occurrence of pulmonary symptoms in cases leptospirosis ranges from cough, dyspnea, and hemoptysis to adult respiratory distress syndrome. Intra-alveolar hemorrhage was detected in the majority of patients, even in the absence of overt pulmonary symptoms. Pulmonary hemorrhage may be severe enough to cause death. Cardiac involvement in leptospirosis is common but may be underestimated.

Ocular manifestations of severe leptospirosis were noted in early reports. Conjunctival suffusion in the presence of sclera icterus is said to be pathognomonic of Weil's disease. Anterior uveitis, either unilateral or bilateral, occurs after recovery from the acute illness in a minority of cases. Uveitis may present weeks, months, or occasionally years after the acute stage. Acute infection in pregnancy has been reported to cause abortion and fetal death but not invariably so.

Rare complications include cerebrovascular accidents, rhabdomyolysis, thrombotic thrombocytopenic purpura, and Guillian-Barre syndrome. Anecdotal reports suggest that leptospirosis may include chronic symptoms analogous to those produced by other spirochetal infections such as Lyme disease.

Treatment of leptospirosis differs depending on the severity and duration of symptoms at the time of presentation. Patients with mild, flu-like symptoms require only symptomatic treatment but should be cautioned to seek further medical help if they develop jaundice. Patients who present with more severe anicteric leptospirosis will require hospital admission and close observation. If the headache is particularly severe, a lumbar puncture usually produces a dramatic improvement.

The management of icteric leptospirosis requires admission of the patients to the intensive care unit initially. Specific antibiotic treatment was reported soon after penicillin became available, with mixed results. Oxytetracycline was also used. Doxycycline (100 mg twice a day for 7 days) was shown to reduce the duration and severity of illness in anicteric leptospirosis by an average of 2 days. Doxycycline (200 mg orally, once weekly) has been shown to be effective for short-term prophylaxis in high-risk environments. Anecdotal evidence suggests that doxycycline but not penicillin may be used successfully after exposure in laboratory accidents.

Leptospiras may be visualized in clinical material by dark-field microscopy or by immunofluorescence or light microscopy after appropriate staining. Dark-field microscopic examination of body fluids such as blood, urine, CSF, and dialysate fluid has been used but is both insensitive and lacking specificity.

Staining methods have been applied to increase the sensitivity of direct microscopic examination. These have included immunofluorescence staining and immunoperoxidase staining of blood and urine. A variety of histopathological stains have been applied to the detection of leptospiras in tissues. Leptospiras were first visualized by silver staining, and the Warthin-Starry stain is widely used for histological examination. More recently, immunohistochemical methods have been applied. Leptospiras are tightly coiled spirochetes; usually 0.1 μm by 6 to 0.1 by 20 μm. Leptospiras may be stained using carbol fuchsin counter stain.

Leptospiras are obligate aerobes with an optimum growth temperature of 28 to 30°C. They produce both catalase and oxidase. They grow in simple media enriched with vitamins (vitamins B2 and B12 are growth factors), long-chain fatty acids, and ammonium salts. Long-chain fatty acids are utilized by as the sole carbon source and are metabolized by β-oxidation.

Detection of leptospiral antigens is clinical material would offer greater specificity than dark-field microscopy while having the potential for greater sensitivity. An evaluation of several methods concluded that radioimmunoassay (RIA) could detect 10^4 to 10^5 leptospiras/mL and an enzyme-linked immunosorbent assay (ELISA) method could detect 10^5 leptospiras/mL. A chemiluminescent immunoassay was applied to human blood and urine but was no more sensitive than earlier ELISA. More recently, immunomagnetic antigen capture was combined with fluoroimmunoassay to detect as few numbers as 10^2 leptospiras/mL of urine of cattle infected with serovar hardjo. Inhibitory substances have been reported in urine, indicating the need for treatment of urine prior to testing.

Growth of leptospiras in media containing serum or albumin plus polysorbate and in protein-free synthetic media has been described. Several liquid media containing rabbit serum were described by Fletcher, Korthoff, Noguchi, and Stuart. The most widely used medium is Ellinghausen-McCullough-Johnson-Harris (EMJH). Leptospiras are more fastidious and require the addition of either pyruvate or rabbit serum for initial isolation. Growth of contaminants from clinical specimens can be inhibited by the addition of 5-fluorouracil.

Leptospiramia occurs during the first stage of the disease, beginning before the onset of symptoms, and has usually finished by the end of the first week of the acute illness. Therefore, blood cultures should be taken as soon as possible after the patient's presentation. One or two drops of blood are inoculated into 10 mL of semisolid medium containing 5-fluorouracil at the patients beside.

Other samples that may be cultured during the first week of illness include CSF and dialysate. Urine can be cultured from the beginning of the second week of symptomatic illness. Cultures are incubated at 28 to 30°C and examined weekly by dark-field microscopy for upto 13 weeks before being discarded. Contaminated cultures may be passed through a 0.2 µm or 0.45-µm filter before subculture into fresh medium.

Identification of leptospiral isolates. Isolated leptospiras are identified either by serological methods, or more recently, by molecular techniques. Traditional methods relied on cross-agglutinin absorption.

Most cases of leptospirosis are diagnosed by serology. Antibodies are detectible in the blood approximately 5 to 7 days after the onset of symptoms. Serological methods can be divided into two groups: those which are genus specific and those which are serogroup specific. The use of agglutination test was described soon after the first isolation of the organism. Many other methodologies have since been applied to serological diagnosis, but the definitive serological investigation in leptospirosis remains the microscopic agglutination test (MAT).

Microscopic Agglutination Test

The reference method for serological diagnosis of leptospirosis is the MAT, in which patient sera are reacted with live antigen suspensions of leptospiral serovar. After incubation, the serum-antigen mixtures are examined microscopically for agglutination, and the titers are determined. Formerly, the method was known as the agglutination-lysis test because of the formation of lysis balls or lysis globules of cellular debris in the presence of high-tittered antiserum. However, these are tightly agglutinated clumps of leptospiras containing live cells and not debris.

Several modifications of earlier methods led to an MAT method which can be performed and read in microtiter trays. Protocols for performing the MAT have been described in detail. Live cultures of serovars required for use as antigens must be maintained. This applies equally whether the test is performed with live or formalin-killed antigens. The repeated weekly subculture of large numbers of strains presents hazards for laboratory workers, and laboratory-acquired infections have been reported. Other drawbacks include the continuous risk of cross-contamination of the antigen cultures, necessitating periodic verification of each serovar. MAT titers are affected by the culture medium in which the antigens are grown.

The range of antigens used should include serovars representative of all serogroups and all locally common serovars. Antibody titers to local isolates are often higher than titers to laboratory stock strains of serovars within the same serogroup. It is usual to include one of the serovars of the nonpathogenic species *L. biflexa*. Such a wide range of antigens is used in order to detect infections with uncommon or previously undetected serovars. Contrary to a widely held belief, the MAT is a serogroup-specific assay. The MAT is also the most appropriate test to employ in epidemiological serosurveys, since it can be applied to sera from any animal species and the range of antigens used can be expanded or decreased as required. It is usual to use a titer of ≥100 as evidence of past exposure. However, conclusions about infecting serovars cannot be drawn without isolates; at best the MAT data can give a general impression about which serogroups are present within a population.

IgM antibodies have been detected by ELISA in CSF from patients with icteric leptospirosis. In patients with meningitis without a proven etiology, IgM was detected in the CSF in 15% cases. IgM has been detected in saliva. ELISA methods have been applied in a number of modifications. An IgM–specific dot-ELISA was developed in which polyvalent leptospiral antigen was dotted onto nitrocellulose filter disks in microtiter tray wells, allowing the use of smaller volumes of reagents. Further modifications of this approach have been used to detect IgG and IgA in addition to IgM and have employed an immunodominant antigen and a polyester fabric-resin support in place of nitrocellulose. A commercial IgM dot-ELISA dipstick has been shown to be as sensitive as a microtiter plate IgM-ELISA. Another dipstick assay has been extensively evaluated in several populations. A dot immunoblot assay using colloidal gold conjugate allowed completion of the assay within 30 minutes. The indirect hemagglutination assay (IHA) developed at CDC was shown to have a sensitivity of 92% and specificity of 95% compared with the MAT.

TETANUS

Tetanus is still a common uncontrolled infectious disease in the developing countries. The infection occurs due to the entry of *Clostridium tetani* a gram-positive, obligate anaerobic (grows in the absence of oxygen) motile bacteria and its spores through injuries. The bacilli multiply in the deeper tissue under anaerobic condition and secrete a powerful exotoxin which produces typical symptoms. The tetanus bacilli and their spores are present in large number in feces of animals like cattle, horses, goats and sheep. The spores of tetanus bacilli can survive for years and under favorable conditions they become bacilli. The spores are resistant to heat, disinfectants like phenol, cresol but destroyed by autoclaving. Tetanus follows an abortion. Otogenic tetanus occur due to infections of the ear. Umbilical cord which is cut with contaminated blades or scissors, may result in neonatal tetanus.

The infection is characterized by frequent painful spasms of muscles especially the muscles of the mouth (lock-jaw), face, muscle of the back and neck, lower limbs, and abdomen. Even slight stimulus like light may trigger spasms.

The tetanus can be prevented by cleaning the wound thoroughly with disinfectant and water, antibiotics and immunization with tetanus toxoid.

In India tetanus is an important endemic infection. The average annual incidence is about 100 per 100,000 population. It is also an important cause of infant mortality.

WHOOPING COUGH (PERTUSSIS)

This infectious disease occurs all over the world. With the introduction of vaccine against this disease the incidence has fallen remarkably but still the disease is prevalent in many parts of the world. It occurs endemically and epidemically in tropical countries. Though the reports are inadequate, it is estimated that in India about 58 cases occur per 1,00,000 population with 5 to 15 percent mortality.

Infection is caused by a gram-negative bacteria *Bordetella pertussis* which is responsible for majority of cases. About five percent cases occur due to *Bordetella parapertussis. Bordetella pertussis* infects only man. The infection occurs through inhalation of bacilli which are present in undiagnosed cases. The incubation period is 3 weeks and the infection is common in children below 5 years age. Though the infection can occur at anytime, it is more common in winter season.

The disease is characterized by onset of mild fever irritating cough gradually becoming paroxysmal with characteristic 'whoop' (a loud crowing inspiration). The complications include pneumonia, hemoptysis and subconjunctival hemorrhages, and bleeding from the nose.

PLAGUE

Plague is essentially a disease prevalent in rats and transmitted by insects known as rat fleas. Man is accidentally exposed to infection when a rat flea containing plague bacilli bites a man. Plague is caused by a gram-negative nonmotile bacteria, which has typical safety pin appearance. It is called *Yersinia pestis*. Plague was very prevalent in India until 1940 and thereafter declined speedily and became free of the disease in 1960. There has been no laboratory confirmed human plague since 1966. However, these were two reported outbreaks in Himachal Pradesh, Tamil Nadu and Andhra Pradesh in 1984. Similarly, an unconfirmed outbreak of plague occurred in 1993 in Latur district of Maharashtra.

Wild rodents like rats, small animals are the natural reservoirs of the infection. The infection occurs by the bite of 'rat flea', an insect belonging to arthropod. The infection can also be transmitted from man to man due to inhalation of bacilli.

The disease is characterized by swelling of the lymph nodes (Bubos) pneumonia, fever. Hence, it is classified as bubonic plague, pneumonic plague and septicemic plague.

STAPHYLOCOCCAL INFECTIONS

Staphylococci are gram-positive spherical or oval shaped organisms arranged in clusters that look like 'bunches of grapes'. They measure about 0.8 to 1 μm in size. They are nonmotile, nonsporing, grow aerobically on simple media like nutrient agar, peptone water. Some of them produce golden yellow or lemon yellow colored pigment. They grow at a pH of 7.2 to 7.4. They can also grow under anaerobic conditions. The cell wall contains peptidoglycan, techoic acid and protein A. Many species are present under the genus *Staphylococcus*. Important species are: (i) *Staphylococcus aureus*, (ii) *Staphylococcus epidermidis*, (iii) *Staphylococcus saprophyticus, Staphylococcus haemolyticus*, etc. Among the species *Staphylococcus aureus* is an important pathogen. It produces enzymes like coagulase, staphylokinase, lipases and hyaluranidase. It also produces toxins like α-hemolysin, β-toxin, δ-toxin, γ-toxin, leucocidin enterotoxins, exfoliative toxin and toxic shock syndrome toxin I. All these enzymes and toxins are responsible for the virulence of the organism.

Staphylococci are part of the normal flora of the human body. The source of infection is either a patient or a carrier who is usually one of the members of hospital staff. Patients with infection are dangerous as they may spread the infection to others. Direct contact through hands is the single most important route of transmission.

Staphylococci are responsible for abscesses, skin infections like carbuncles and furuncles. Initially the hair follicle is infected and from there the infection extends subcutaneously resulting in pus forming lesion, the boil or furuncle. Carbuncle is similar to furuncle but the infection spreads into the deeper layers of the fibrous tissue. Most of these lesions heal by spontaneous drainage of pus within 3 to 5 days. Impetigo is characterized by the formation of encrusted pustules. When the crusts are removed, one can see red area oozing with pus. The disease is highly contagious and can spread in an epidemic manner in nurseries or in neonatal units.

Staphylococci also cause scalded skin syndrome, which comprises of three distinct but related clinical diseases. They are: (a) generalized exfoliative dermatitis which is characterized by painful erythema and desquamation of large area of the skin, (b) bullous impetigo, and (c) staphylococcal scarlet fever which is a mild generalized form (Fig. 17.7).

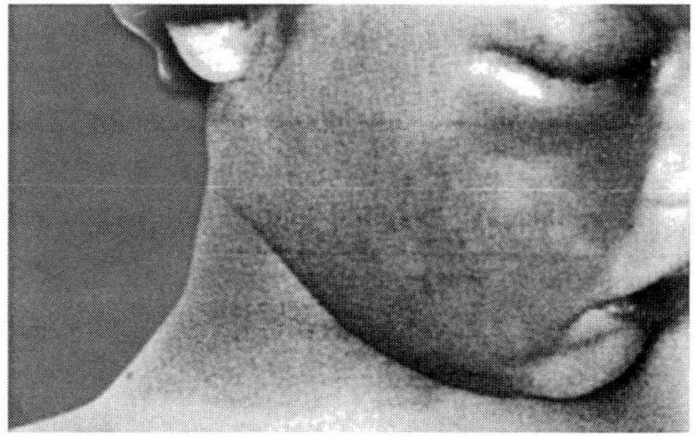

Fig. 17.7: Staphylococcal infection
(For color version, see Plate 4)

The other clinical manifestations of staphylococcal infections include pneumonia, osteomyelitis, septic arthritis, septicemia, bacterial endocarditis and food poisoning. Toxic shock syndrome (TSS) is another important disease caused by staphylococci.

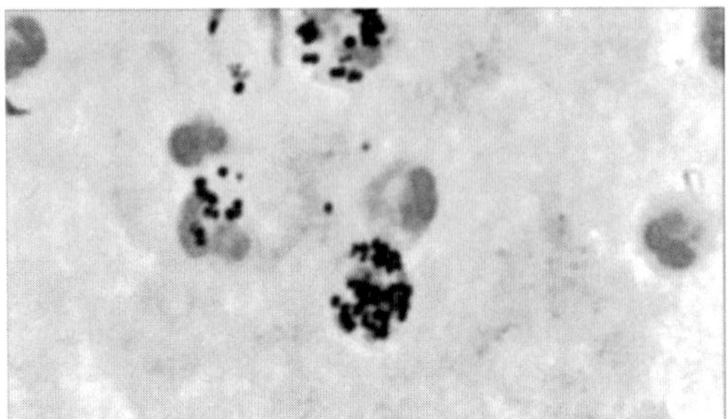

Fig. 17.8: Gram-positive cocci in clusters. Note many of them are intracellular staphylococci (×100) (*For color version, see Plate 5*)

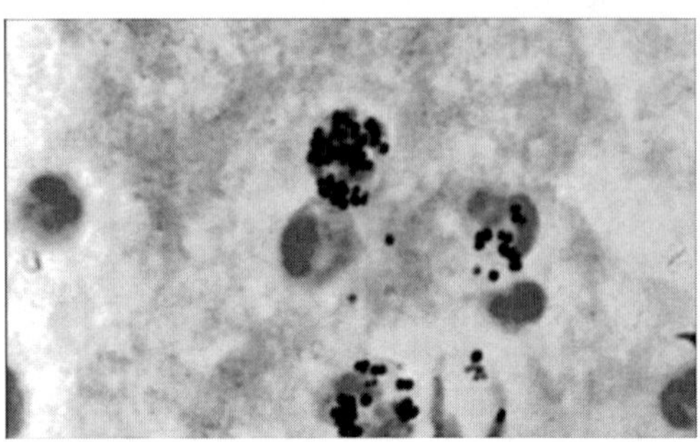

Fig. 17.9: Gram-positive cocci in clusters along with pus cells. Staphylococci (×100) (*For color version, see Plate 5*)

This is usually seen among young women during their menstrual cycle but others also may be affected. The clincial features include fever, marked hypotension, diarrhea, conjunctivitis, myalgias.

Laboratory diagnosis of staphylococcal infection comprises collection of pus from the pustules or carbuncles, postoperative wounds. Blood, urine or sputum samples are collected aseptically. Gram smear of the specimens show gram-positive cocci in clusters (Figs 17.8, and 17.9). The specimens are inoculated onto blood agar or mannitol salt agar. The identification of the growth on these media is done by Gram's smear, coagulase test and mannitol fermentation and phosphatase production.

The staphylococci initially were quite sensitive to penicillin during early 1950s. Later on they developed resistance to penicillin. Subsequently they also acquired resistance to many antibiotics like tetracyclines, etc. Presently methicillin resistant *Staphylococcus aureus* (MRSA) strains are widely distributed all over the world and are responsible hospital infections. They are also resistant to many commonly used antibiotics like aminoglycosides, cephalosporins and quinolones. They can be treated either by vancomycin or teicoplanin or linzolid. Monotherapy with rifampicin is not recommended as the bacteria acquire resistance to refampicin a very rapidly.

STREPTOCOCCAL INFECTIONS

Streptococci are gram-positive arranged in short or long chains typically resembling 'chain of pearls'. They are spherical or oval in shape measuring 1 to 2 μm in size, nonmotile, nonsporing can grow under aerobic as well as anaerobic conditions. Streptococci when grown on culture medium containing blood may produce either greenish discoloration (α-hemolysis) or clear zone of hemolysis around the colonies (β-hemolysis) (Figs 17.10 and 17.11). Some streptococci are nonhemolytic (γ-hemolytic). Several species of streptococci are present as commensals, parasites or saprophytes in the environment. Based on the cell wall carbohydrate composition, Lancefield in 1933 grouped them into different groups like Groups A, B, C, D, E, F, G,- - - upto P, Q, R, S except I, J. Among these groups streptococci belonging to Groups A, B, C, D, G cause infections in humans although other groups may rarely cause infections.

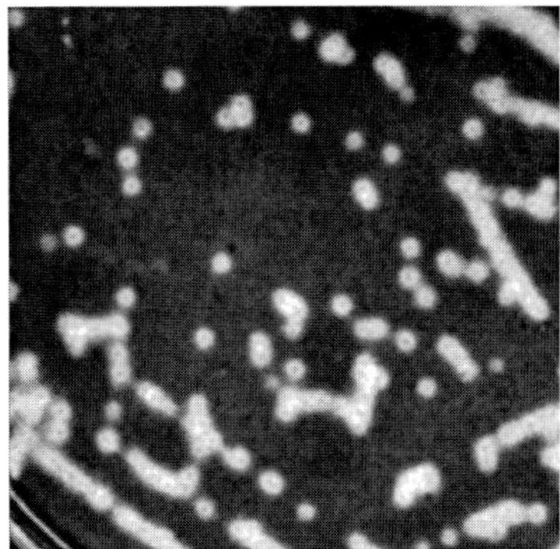

Fig. 17.10: Colonies of β-hemolytic streptococci. Note the clear zone of hemolysis on sheep blood agar (*For color version, see Plate 5*)

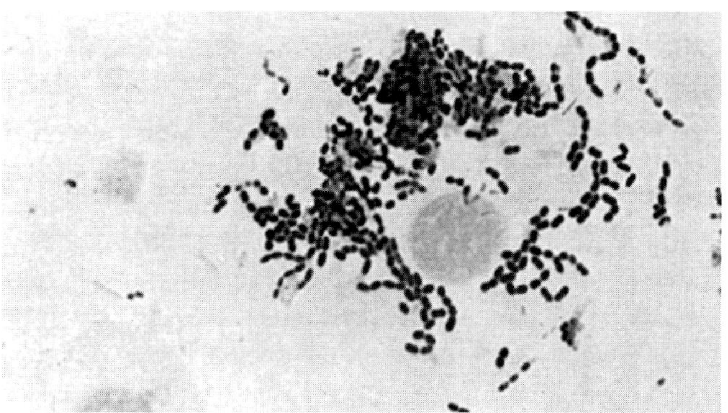

Fig. 17.11: Gram-positive cocci arranged in chains streptococci. Gram stain (×100) (*For color version, see Plate 5*)

Group A streptococci comprises of an important species *Streptococcus pyogenes*. These are gram-positive, produce β-hemolysis on blood agar medium. It can grow at 37°C under aerobic as well as anaerobic conditions or under CO_2 tension. Group A streptococci are sensitive to bacitracin. Apart from the group specific carbohydrate, *Streptococcus pyogenes* has M and T proteins, capsular polysaccharides. When cultured, *Streptococcus pyogenes* produce two types of hemolysins, namely streptolysin 'O' and streptolysin S. These are responsible for clear zones of β-hemolysis around the colonies on blood agar. Streptolysin 'O' is oxygen labile and is antigenic following infection due to *Streptococcus pyogenes;* antistreptolysin antibodies are formed which are of diagnostic significance. But these antibodies are formed in high concentrations following pharyngeal or systemic infection but it is low following skin infections, other virulence markers produced by this organism are erythrogenic toxin, deoxyribonuclease, hyaluronidase, streptokinase and neuraminidase and a cardiohepatic toxin. *Streptococcus pyogenes* causes acute pharyngitis, tonsillitis, and scarlet fever. Following a streptococcal pharyngitis some patients develop acute rheumatic fever, which is characterized by arthritis (bilateral, symmetrical fleeting type) carditis, chorea (a neurological complication characterized by involuntary movements) and erythema marginatum or subcutaneous nodules. In untreated cases of acute rheumatic fever leads to rheumatic heart disease. Acute glomerulonephritis occurs especially in children and most of times recovery is complete in children but in adults it may be associated with poor prognosis (Fig. 17.12).

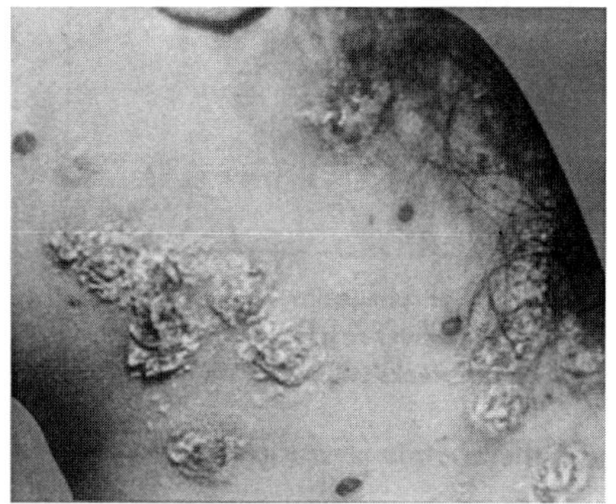

Fig. 17.12: Streptococcal infection (*For color version, see Plate 5*)

Group B streptococci are similar to that of *Streptococcus pyogenes* in morphology and cultural characters. They may produce yellow, red or orange pigments when grow anaerobically. These are normally found in the throat, gastrointestinal tract, and vagina. Group B streptococci cause endocarditis, puerperal infection, skin infections in adults, septicemia, meningitis in newborn infants. Group D streptococci are also known as enterococci. These are either hemolytic or nonhemolytic, can grow in media containing 6.5 percent sodium chloride or 40 percent bile. They can withstand heat upto 60°C for 1 hour. Enterococci are important causative agents of urinary tract infections, septicemia, and endocarditis, wound infections respiratory tract infections.

Viridians group of streptococci produce α-hemolysis on blood agar. They ferment a number of carbohydrates based on which the species are characterized. These viridians groups of streptococci are responsible for infections like cellulitis, sinusitis, intra-abdominal infection, subacute bacterial endocarditis, brain abscess and dental caries. Laboratory diagnosis of streptococcal infections depends upon type of infection. Specimens like throat swabs, wound swabs, pus, blood and urine are cultured on blood agar, on which they show typical pinpointed colonies with or without hemolysis. Further characterization is done on serological grouping bacitracin sensitivity, ability to grow in medium containing 6.5 percent sodium chloride (especially enterococci) type of hemolysis produced on blood agar and ability to resist in activation by heat at 60°C for 1 hour. Group A streptococci are sensitive to penicillin, erythromycin and tetracycline whereas other streptococci are sensitive to broad spectrum antibiotics like cephalosporins, aminoglycosides and quinolones. Antibody titers against streptolysin 'O' and anti-DNase, B antibodies are useful in the diagnosis of streptococcal infections.

PNEUMOCOCCAL INFECTIONS

Streptococcus pneumoniae is a gram-positive 0.5 to 1.0 μm in size, lanceolate in shape, arranged in pairs (Fig. 17.13) capsulated organism. It grows on blood agar at a pH 7.2 to 7.4 and requires 10% CO_2 for growth on blood agar; it shows greenish colored hemolysis around the colonies on blood agar or small and shows 'poached egg' appearance with central depression. Pneumococci are capsulated organism. Capsular polysaccharide is antigenic and it resists phagocytosis. Pneumococci are bile soluble, optochin sensitive ferments inulin. They produce a variety of enzymes like neuraminidase; proteases and toxins like pneumolysin 'O' (similar to streptolysin 'O') and purpose producing principle, which causes damage to the capsular polysaccharide as many as 84 serotypes have been identified. In the presence of specific antiserum against the capsular polysaccharide, the capsule swells and become more prominent. This is known as 'Quellung' reaction. Healthy persons carry pneumococci in the nasopharynx and form major source of infection.

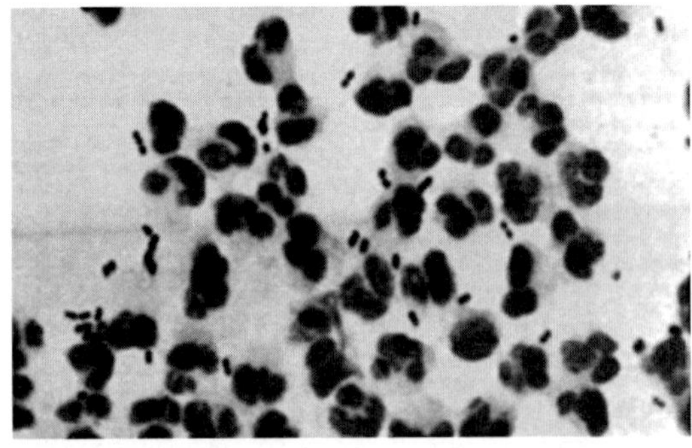

Fig. 17.13: Pus cells with gram-positive cocci in pairs. Pneumococci Gram stain (×100) *(For color version, see Plate 5)*

Pneumococci causes lobar pneumonia, upper respiratory tract infections, ear infections and meningitis. Laboratory diagnosis include sputum examination by Gram's smear, culture of sputum, cerebrospinal fluid or blood depending upon the clinical presentation. Diagnosis can also be made by the detection of capsular polysaccharide by special techniques. Pneumococcal infections are treated with penicillin, cephalosporins, aminoglycosides, tetracycline and chloramphenicol. Pneumococcal vaccine is available and it is given to patients who are immunocompromised (e.g., children, elderly patients, patients who had transplantation and patients with HIV infection).

GAS GANGRENE

Gas gangrene is caused by gram-positive thick bacilli, measuring 2 to 4 μm in size, capsulated spore forming bacteria, that grow under anaerobic conditions (absence of oxygen). The most common organisms responsible for gas gangrene are *Clostridium perfringens, Clostridium sordellii.* Except *Clostridium perfringens* others are motile. These organisms are also known as histotoxic bacteria and cause severe infection of the muscle, clostridial myonecrosis or otherwise known as gas gangrene or clostridial myositis (Fig. 17.14).

Gas gangrene used to be a major disease during World War II. The clostridial group of organisms responsible for gas gangrene can be cultured on blood agar, nutrient agar or serum agar. The organisms grow well in Robertson's cooked meat medium. Production of hemolysis on blood agar, opalescence in serum or egg yolk media, inhibition of opalescence in the presence of specific antiserum (Nagler reaction) fermentation of milk agar with stormy clot appearance (medium is cracked due to excessive gas formation) are some of the important characters which identify these organisms.

These organisms cause skin and soft tissue infection, where presence of anaerobic conditions due to ischemia or vascular damage, favor the growth of these organisms. Wounds contaminated with soil, cloth or metal may lead to the growth of clostridial species. Road traffic accidents, septic abortions, compound fractures, surgical complications lead to clostridial infection. A number of toxins produced by these organisms attack the healthy

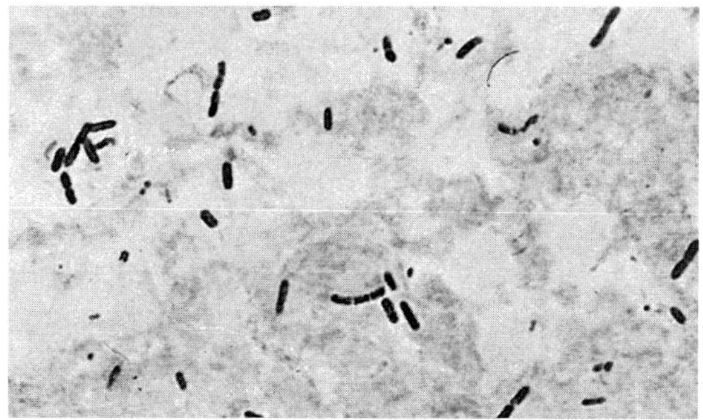

Fig. 17.14: Gram-positive thick bacilli from a gangrene patient. *Clostridium* species (×100) *(For color version, see Plate 5)*

muscles and surrounding tissue and help the survival of the organisms under anaerobic conditions. Further infection leads to anaerobic cellulitis, gas gangrene and septicemia. Necrosis of large muscles and resulting edema may cause severe shock and renal failure.

Treatment consists of clearing of the wounds, surgical removal of dead tissue administration of antibiotics like penicillin and administration of anti-gas gangrene serum.

MYCOPLASMA INFECTIONS

The genus *Mycoplasma* belongs to the class 'Mollicutes'. The species that causes human infection is *Mycoplasma pneumoniae*. This was first isolated in hamsters and was named as Eaton agent or pleuropneumonia like organism. It is a part of normal flora of human respiratory tract or genitourinary tract but can cause infection like atypical pneumonia, otitis media (middle ear infection), meningoencephalitis, etc.

These are small pleomorphic organisms measuring about 0.2 to 0.8 μm. They lack cell wall. Hence the organisms are resistant to penicillin and cephalosporin group of antibiotics. They multiply by binary fission. These organisms require cholesterol and other related sterols for the synthesis of cell membrane. They require complex culture media enriched with horse serum, yeast extract and nucleic acids. They grow aerobically at 37°C. The growth is very slow and it may take 7 days to 3 weeks for the culture to grow in the laboratory. The colonies appear like fried egg or poached egg. The colonies are stained by a special stain called 'Diene's' stain. *Mycoplasma* produces infection by means of adhesion to the cell surface. Some species of *Mycoplasma* produce neurotoxin. Due to infection by *Mycoplasma*, the antibodies are produced which can agglutinate human 'O' red blood cells at 4°C. These are called cold agglutinins.

The infections due to *Mycoplasma* are worldwide, epidemics occur every 4 to 6 years interval especially among school going children, army personnels. Spread of infection requires close contact.

The organisms can be isolated from sputum, throat swabs and body fluids. Liquid media can be used initially and from them the subcultures are made on complex solid media.

The diagnosis can also be made by immunofluorescent antibody detection or by cold agglutination test. Passive hemagglutination or ELISA tests are available for serological diagnosis. Drugs like erythromycin and tetracycline are the drugs of choice. No vaccine is available to prevent this disease. Use of tetracycline prophylactically are helpful to some extent.

The other species like *Ureaplasma urealyticum*, *Mycoplasma hominis* can cause puerperal fever, septic abortion, and infection of the urogenital tract. These are normally present in the female genital tract and cause opportunistic infections including arthritis.

RICKETTSIAL INFECTIONS

Rickettsial infections played a very significant role in the history of western civilization. In both World Wars rickettsial infections killed thousands of people. The name Rickettsia was coined in the honor of Sir Howard Ricketts who first discovered the organism, cultivated in the laboratory and died of rickettsial infection.

The family *Rickettsiaceae* comprises 6 genera are given in Table 17.3.

Rickettsiae are small pleomorphic gram-negative intracellular organisms. They are poorly stained by Gram's stain but stained easily by Giemsa or Macchiavello stain. The morphology and structure is similar to gram-negative bacteria. Except *R. quintana,* all other species require living cells for growth such as tissue culture or embryonated eggs. They remain viable for long periods at – 70°C. Some species are resistant to heat and drying. Apart from culture diagnosis can be made by detecting specific antibodies in patients who suffer from these infections. Earlier proteus species antigens were used to detect antibodies

Table 17.3: Six genera of *Rickettsiaceae*

Genera	*Species*
1. *Rickettsia*	• *Rickettsia rickettsii*
	• *Rickettsia akari*
	• *Rickettsia prowazekii*
	• *Rickettsia tsutsugamushi*
2. *Rochalimaea*	• *Rochalimaea quintana*
3. *Coxiella*	• *Coxiella burnetii*
4. *Ehrlichia*	• *E. sennetsu, E. canis, E. ewangi*
5. *Bartonella*	• *B. basilliformis*
6. *Chlamydia*	• *C. trachomatis, C. psittaci*

Table 17.4: Types of infections by *Rickettsiaceae*

Diseases	*Agents*	*Arthropod vectors*	*Animal reservoirs*
Spotted fevers			
1. Rocky Mountain spotted fever	*R. rickettsii*	Tick	Dogs, wild rodents
2. Rickettsial pox	*R. akari*	Mite	Mouse
3. Queensland tick fever	*R. australi*	Tick	Wild rodents
Typhus fevers			
4. Epidemic typhus	*R. prowazekii*	Body louse	Humans
5. Brill-Zinsser disease	*R. prowazekii*	None	Humans
6. Murine typhus	*R. typhi*	Rat flea	Small rodents
7. Scrub typhus	*R. tsutsugamushi*	Mite	Wild rodents
Other fevers			
8. Q fever	*C. burnetii*	Tick	Cattle, sheep, goats
9. Trench fever	*R. quintana*	Body louse	Humans
10. Sennetsu fever	*E. sennetsu*	Unknown	Humans

against rickettsia due to cross-reaction. This test is known as Weil-Felix agglutination test. Because of unreliability of the results currently this test is not usually carried out.

The infection occurs due to bite of the arthropods like ticks, lice and mites. Types of infections include as in Table 17.4.

Most of these fevers start abruptly with headache, fever and chills. Myalgias are very common. Usually rash appears and it first appears on the ankles and wrists then spreads all-over the body. Sometimes people suffer from gastroenteritis and appendicitis.

Laboratory diagnosis include demonstrative of organisms in the smears using special staining techniques, immunofluorescence, culture and detection of specific antibodies. Chloramphenicol and tetracyclines are the drugs of choice. Prevention includes using protective wear, control of ticks, mites and lice. No vaccine is available at present.

Chapter 18

Microbial Food Poisoning

INTRODUCTION

The anabolic and catabolic process occurring in living cells is energy dependent and this energy is derived from the various components of food that is being taken by every living organism. The heterotrophs take already available from animal or plant products which they break into simpler substances such as amino acids, sugars, fatty acids which are used as building blocks by the living organism for growth, cell division and reproduction. Human beings consume food both in the raw form (such as fruits, pulses, cereals, leafy vegetables, roots) as well as cooked food both vegetarian and nonvegetarian. The present technology in the processing of food is well advanced and many readymade foods such as bread, butter, jams, fruit juices, instant mixes, icecreams, and cheese are all available ready to consume with attractive colors, flavors and tastes. While such availability ready to use food made the life easy, nevertheless it is associated with risks of *contamination*, spoilage leading to a specific disease entity known as *food poisoning*.

Bacterial food poisoning is the term applied to acute gastroenteritis which follows the ingestion of bacteria or their products. The disease follows as a result of ingestion of performed toxins, the classical examples being staphylococcal food poisoning and botulism. Acute gastroenteritis is due to *Salmonella* species, enterotoxin producing *Escherichia coli*, *Vibrio parahaemolyticus*, *Bacillus cereus*, and *Clostridium perfringens* develops following the multiplication of ingested bacteria within the intestinal tract.

There has been an approximately three-fold increase in bacterial food poisoning in each 5-year interval over the past 30 years. In the United States alone an estimated one million cases occur every year. Of these staphylococci assumed to be responsible for 60 to 70 percent, Salmonellae for 15 to 20 percent. In United Kingdom 95% of the food poisoning outbreaks have been associated with *Salmonellae*, three percent with staphylococci, 2 percent with *Clostridia*.

In our country the true incidence of food poisoning is not clear. It has been stated that in each outbreak the number of persons affected varies from 20 to 600 and 5 or 6 such outbreaks are being noticed in Andhra Pradesh state only in each year. Most of the outbreaks are seen among children and are mainly due to either *Salmonella* or enterotoxigenic or enteropathogenic *Escherichia coli*. Fule and Kaundinya (1986) studied 196 strains of enterotoxigenic strains from infantile diarrhea case and concluded that detection of permeability factor has a good relationship with the enterotoxin production by the *Escherichia coli* strains responsible for infantile diarrhea. They also described in the same year the isolation of *Salmonella cerro* (18:z4,z23-), a rare serotype from infants with acute diarrhea.

Talwar *et al.* (1986) studied the enterotoxin production among 115 *Staphylococcus aureus* strains isolated from routine nonfecal clinical specimens and found that 33% of the strains are enterotoxigenic. Among the enterotoxigenic strains 78.9% produced single type of enterotoxin and the rest produced more than one type. Enterotoxin C_2 was found to be very common in their series. No correlation with phage group was observed.

Borle and Gupta (1987) studied the incidence of fungal contamination of areca nut contaminated with *Aspergillus flavus, Aspergillus niger* and *Rhizopus*. Samples of areca nut positive for fungus growth were subjected to aflatoxin estimation. It was shown that contaminated areca nut showed the presence of B_1 and G_1 aflatoxins. The pathogenesis of aflatoxins will be discussed later.

These are few recent studies show that the incidence of poisoning and the causative agents are widely prevalent in our tropical country and capable of causing epidemic or sporadic outbreaks from time to time although the exact incidence is difficult to assess.

Among the various microbial agents responsible for food poisoning, the following deserves special mention in view of their frequent occurrence.

STAPHYLOCOCCAL FOOD POISONING

Strains of *Staphylococcus aureus* belonging to the phage groups III and IV have the ability to produce enterotoxin and consequently staphylococcal food poisoning. These particular strains of *Staph. aureus* have been isolated from healthy carriers, and from noses as well as hands of food handlers who contaminate food. The organism grows well above 18°C and capable for producing, enterotoxin both under aerobic and anaerobic conditions. Milk and meat products provide excellent media for the synthesis of enterotoxins. The initial number of staphylococci in the food influences the extent of enterotoxin production but the more important determining factor is length of storage of food at temperatures, congenial for the multiplication of the organism and subsequent synthesis of enterotoxin. Among the enterotoxins which are distinct antigenitically, type A is the most common and it is produced by 90% of the strains of staphylococci isolated from outbreaks of food poisoning. Approximately eight percent strains produce type B enterotoxin and two percent strains produce both the types. About 80% of strains isolated from the noses of healthy persons are capable of producing type A enterotoxin. This is due to the fact that 42D phage type strains of staphylococci are lysogenized by temparate phage carrying the gene responsible for the type A enterotoxin production.

Chemically enterotoxins are basic proteins of molecular weight about 24,000. They are resistant to acid, heat and proteolytic enzymes and can withstand boiling for more than 100°C for 30 minutes.

Man is uniquely sensitive to staphylococcal enterotoxin. In most outbreaks the incidence approaches 100%. The incubation period is usually averages to 3 hours with a range of 1 to 6 hours after ingestion. The severity of the disease is proportional to the amount of toxin ingested. Symptoms like salivation, nausea, vomiting, retching, abdominal pain, and diarrhea occur in varying intensity and persists for 6 hours. Recovery is usually complete within 24 hours. But occasionally death may occur in infants and debilitated adults. Ingestion of one microgram enterotoxin is sufficient to cause symptoms. Enterotoxins act as mitogens and induce the release of mediators such as interleukin-1 from lymphocytes and trigger systemic effects. Staphylococcal enterotoxin produces its effects by its action on the nervous system but not on the intestinal epithelium. No convenient laboratory animal is susceptible to the action of enterotoxin. Enterotoxins can be detected by agar gel diffusion technique. Sensitive precipitation assays are available which can detect 0.02 μg toxin/g food.

Staphylococcal food poisoning occurs worldwide especially with a peak incidence in summer. Prevention is by personal hygiene of the food handlers and proper preservation of food under refrigerated conditions especially the milk and milk products as well as meat products. There is no specific treatment. Affected persons should be treated symptomatically taking care to correct water and electrolyte balance to prevent shock. Patients recover well within 24 hours. There is little evidence that significant levels of immunity accompanies recovery from the disease.

OTHER ORGANISMS

Ananthan *et al.* (1989) isolated *Escherichia coli* as a predominant pathogen in 70.54% of diarrheal cases. Two hundred eighty four in the age group of 1 to 6 months showed *Escherichia coli* as the predominant organism. Classical enteropathogenic *Escherichia coli* (EPEC) were detected in 311 cases among them 277 did not produce either heat stable or heat labile toxin. Ten percent strains produced these enterotoxins. Two strains belonging to serotypes 086:K61; 0142:K86; 0128:K67; 0126:K71; 0125:K58; 055:K59 showed both localized and diffuse adherence to Hela cell lines. The study concludes that EPEC strains are capable of causing diarrhea in infants and children and warrant that these strains should be subjected for their enteropathogenic, enterotoxigenic, enteroadherent properties in addition to serotyping in epidemic as well as sporadic occurrences. Rai *et al.* (1990) studied 150 fresh samples of locally prepared bread collected from small canteens and bakeries and cultures them for isolating the fungi. Twenty samples showed that the presence of various species of fungi like *Aspergillus flavus, A. niger, A. fumigatus, Rhizopus, Trichoderma* spp, *Trichothecium* spp, etc. Among these *A. fumigatus* and *A. niger* were commonly isolated which are known to cause toxicity in human beings. Rout *et al.* (1989) conducted studies on a rice contaminating fungus '*Curvularia lunata*' which produces curvularin a potent mycotoxin. Experimental pheohypomycosis and mycotoxicosis were observed in albino rats. Spore suspension produced localized lesion, with simultaneous steroid therapy, lesions could be seen in distant organs. The mycotoxin curvularin produced hepatic necrosis. However, authors could not say whether human liver is susceptible to this toxin or not.

BOTULISM

Botulism is an intoxication due to ingestion of minute amounts of the most potent toxin produced by the organism *Clostridium botulinum* which is a gram-positive, spore forming, rod-shaped organism, growing under anaerobic conditions. The spores are highly resistant to heat and survive in improperly canned or preserved food. The spores germinate and the vegetative forms elaborate the toxin. The toxins are antigenitically distinct and have been designated as types A, B, C, D, E and F. Type A, B and E are primarily involved in human disease. Only few human cases have been due to types C and D. Botulinum toxins are inactive protoxins which are converted to active toxins by proteolytic enzymes. These toxins have a varying molecular weight between 70,000 to 1,00,000. Type A toxin in the crystalline form has a molecular weight of 70,000, with a sedimentation constant of 15.5S. It is highly resistant to proteolysis by pepsin. At pH 9.2 the toxin is irreversibly dissociated into a principal component with a sedimentation rate of 7S and molecular weight of 1,58,000. The dissociated fragment can be extensively degraded by pepsin but it retains the property of toxicity. The molecular sizes of these degraded fragment is not known but may be around 3,800. Similar findings were also seen with type E toxin.

After ingestion type A botulinum toxin is present as 7S toxin or in a form that is susceptible to pepsin or trypsin digestion into 4.4S to 11.4S fragments. Type A toxin is 50,000 times more lethal by oral route than other routes. Crystalline type A toxin has a minimal lethal dose of 45 million/mg. The liquid cultures of *Clostridium botulinum* can yield 200 million MLD/mL. All types of botulinum toxins have similar pharmacological properties but differ greatly in relative lethality to animals. The lethal dose of type A toxin to man is less than 1 μg.

The preformed botulinum toxin is highly acid resistant and can traverse the stomach unchanged. In the intestine the protoxin is activated by proteolytic enzymes. The toxin circulates in the bloodstream and finally reaches peripheral nervous system and acts antagonistically to acetylcholine and causes reduction of the miniature end plate potentials without changing their amplitude. The rate of paralysis induced by botulinum toxin is influenced by the factors governing the metabolism of acetylcholine.

The incubation period is usually ranges between 12 to 36 hours but it may be as short as 6 hours and as long as 8 days. The incubation period is inversely proportional to the amount of protoxin ingested and the case fatality rate is directly proportional to the incubation period. The toxin produces mild intestinal symptoms, fatigue, diplopia, difficulty in swallowing and speech. Death occurs due to respiratory failure. The mortality rate is higher with type A toxin then type B or type E toxin.

Laboratory diagnosis comprises of mouse protection test. The suspected items of food are prepared in the form of suspension and inoculated into both untreated as well as mice protected with antitoxin. Occasionally, the test may be positive when 1 mL of blood of the patient is used as the source of toxin.

The incidence of botulinum food poisoning varies widely with the distribution of organisms in the soil, the potency of toxin, and the eating habits of the people. Outbreaks due to type A toxin are more frequent. In Europe type A and type B toxin outbreaks are common and are associated with consumption of preserved meat products. Type E toxin is associated with eating of raw fish as seen in British Columbia, Alaska, Japan and Baltic Africa.

Annual number of cases reported are very low. From 1899 to 1972, 1,731 cases have been documented of which 86 percent were associated with home prepared food and 14 percent with commercial food products. Outbreaks due to contaminated commercial products were due to type E toxin whereas type A toxin outbreaks were associated with home-made foods.

Proper cooking of the food prevents botulinum food poisoning. Treatment for established cases is of little value. However, polyvalent antitoxin should be given to all persons who consumed contaminated food. Affected persons should be given symptomatic support. Active immunity in man can be produced by injecting 3 doses mixed toxin at 2 months interval. But it is not generally recommended, because of low incidence of the disease.

Rare cases of wound infections with *C. botulinum* resulting in characteristic signs and symptoms of botulinism have been recorded.

The 'floppy child syndrome' describes a young child usually less than 6 months old with flaccid paralysis that is ascribed to the growth of *C. botulinum* in the intestine at a state in development when colonization resistance of the gut is poor. There are various grades of the syndrome. Some of the cases recorded in the literature have been attributed to the presence of *C. botulinum* spores in honey.

SALMONELLA FOOD POISONING

Acute gastroenteritis characterized by nausea, vomitings diarrhea and abdominal pain as well as fever. It can be caused by the ingestion of a wide variety of bacteria or their products, several viruses, and a number of vegetable toxins and inorganic chemicals. The 'bacterial food poisoning' is conveniently restricted to cases and epidemics of acute gastroenteritis that are caused by the ingestion of food contaminated by bacteria or their toxins. It is an important feature to remember that in bacterial food poisoning, the bacteria need the opportunity to multiply in the food to reach infective concentration before being eaten. Infections like hepatitis A, bacillary dysentery, cholera in which food may be incidental vector, are not usually considered to be examples of food poisoning. *Salmonellae* are common causes of food poisoning worldwide.

Salmonella food poisoning usually occurs in the form of diarrhea, malaise, headache, nausea and vomiting after 8 to 48 hours incubation. The onset is usually abrupt with a low grade fever. The symptoms may persist for 2 to 5 days. Blood cultures are usually negative but stool cultures may be positive soon after the onset. Severe cases may have hypotension, dehydration, cramps and renal failure. Most often infection occurs in very young and elderly. Mild and subclinical infections are also quite common. Persistent or high fever suggests bacteremia possibly with metastatic infection. Common food poisoning serotypes are *S. typhimurium, S. enteritidis*. Strains isolated from patients and contaminated food should be phage typed if possible to match source. The examination of vomit is rarely of value.

The zoonotic salmanellosis is very complex in its epidemiology. The cooked meats, eggs, milk and milk products are the most common sources of food poisoning infection.

Salmonella serotypes causing human infection cause only mild or in apparent infection in animals. Thus, it becomes difficult to recognize the infected animal and mixing up of infected animal during slaughtering is more important hazard. Poultry, ducks, turkeys are the most significant sources of reservoir of infection responsible for food poisoning. Rats and mice are commonly infected with food poisoning salmonellae and may contaminate human food with their excreta. Food poisoning may occasionally be caused by food handled by a carrier. The more sophisticated the manipulation of food, the greater the chance of contamination. Contamination of meat products can occur during chilling, or by instruments or during transportation. Infection in pigs is due to feeding of swill containing infected animal matter. Improper cooking may fail to destroy the vegetative bacteria.

Food poisoning incidences occur suddenly among members of a community sharing a common meal, as in factories, hospitals, schools or at some celebratory feast. However, sporadic incidences affecting a single family or a person are more common.

As in most other efforts to control the spread of infection, human element plays the pivotal role so that proper health education; personal hygiene of food handlers is the most important and continuing requirement.

OTHER TYPES OF FOOD POISONING

Spores of *Bacillus cereus* are particularly heat resistant and most strains produce toxins. The organisms are ubiquitous and found in raw food materials, especially cereals. The food poisoning due to *B. cereus* is by preformed toxin often found in lightly cooked Chinese dishes. The incubation period is usually 6 hours and vomitings is the main symptom. The toxins are low molecular weight peptides which are heat and acid resistant and can withstand the proteolytic effect of intestinal enzymes. *B. cereus* can also produce enterotoxin which is heat labile. This can cause diarrhea similar to that caused by *Escherichia coli* or *Salmonella*. Presence of high number of *B. cereus* organisms in food material and absence of other pathogens clinches the laboratory diagnosis.

Food poisoning associated with *Clostridium perfringens* is an infection rather than intoxication. The gastroenteritis starts usually after 8 to 18 hours of incubation period after eating contaminated food. Diarrhea and abdominal cramps are the predominant symptoms. Vomiting is a rare symptom. The organisms produce enterotoxin like that of *Escherichia coli*. Readily perishable foods are hazardous and should be thoroughly cooked to destroy the spores. Food should be kept either hot or cold. Many outbreaks are known to have occurred when the food was allowed to cool slowly before it was refrigerated and was subsequently eaten without adequate reheating.

Vibrio parahemolyticus is the most common cause of food poisoning in Japan and has been responsible for numerous outbreaks during summer due to ingestion of contaminated shell fish, crabs and shrimps. The organism is halophillic requiring three to seven percent salt concentration. Patients infected with *Vibrio parahaemolyticus* experience an acute exudative diarrheal disease, presumably the result of the ability of the microorganism to penetrate epithelial cells lining intestinal mucosa.

AFLATOXINS

Aflatoxins are one of the well studied group of toxins of fungal origin. In 1960, in England, a localized outbreak of an undiagnosed Turkey disease characterized by anorexia, lethargy, weakness leading to death with head extended and legs drawn backward. Autopsy revealed liver necrosis, hemorrhage and congested kidneys. Soon similar outbreak occurred in ducks in same area and an epidemic of hepatomas in Rainbow trouts of USA. Investigations revealed that these were associated with a feed made from Brazilian peanut meal. A methanol chloroform extract of the same feed resulted in same toxicity in experimental animals. It was also noted that the feed contained large numbers of *Aspergillus flavus* hyphae. Studies with chemical extraction and chromatography showed that the fungus yielded the toxic substance responsible for clinical manifestations. This was named as aflatoxin. Children eating fermented soyabeans developed hepatic necrosis and excreted aflatoxins in urine. Fodder containing aflatoxins reduced the milk yield in cows and also offsprings got affected.

Aflatoxins are mycotoxins which are complex substances of fatty acids and quinone derivatives. *Aspergillus* species are the most common source for aflatoxins. This mycotoxicosis is common in tropical and subtropical countries with high humidity and a mean temperature of 12 to 40°C.

Aflatoxins are the secondary metabolites. These are formed during the stationary phase of fungal growth. There are 17 naturally occurring types of aflatoxins. Important types are B_1, B_2 and G_1, G_2 according to fluorescence (Blue or green). Aflatoxin M derived from Cow's milk is further subdivided into M_1 and M_2. Other aflatoxins are P_1P_3, T_2B_{2a}, G_{2a}. Among the types B_1 is the most potent. Aflatoxins are soluble in chloroform, stable at high temperature. They can be absorbed through gut, respiratory tract and skin. Maximum concentration is seen in liver within 48 hours after ingestion of which 60 percent is excreted through bile. Toxicity can be studied experimentally in one day old ducklings, embryonated duck eggs. In tissue culture there is inhibition of mitosis and gaint cell formation. Chemical studies include 'thin layer chromatography', radioimmunoassay or ELISA.

Acute toxicity comprises of hepatic necrosis, bleeding, nephritis and congestion of lungs. Chronic toxicity includes cell damage, carcinogenicity, mutagenicity, teratogenicity, sublethal doses use proliferation of bile ducts, and hepatocellular carcinoma. These are one of the most potent carcinogenic agents.

Biochemically they combine with DNA and suppress DNA and RNA synthesis. Affects both mitochondria and the nucleus. Pregnant rats showed retardation of fetal growth and central nervous system abnormalities have been shown in Hamsters. The toxins have mutagenic effect on human leukocyte cultures.

Table 18.1: Types of toxin, organisms, their sources and actions

Types of toxin	*Fungi*	*Sources*	*Actions*
Aflatoxin	*Aspergillus flavus*	Peanut, grains	Toxic to liver and carcinogenic
Sterigmatocystin	*A. nidulans*	Cereals	Toxic and carcinogenic to liver
	A. versicolor		
Ochratoxin	*A. ochraceus*	Cereals	Toxic to kidney
Leukocidin	*Penicillium* spp	Peas	Toxic
Fallulan	*Penicillium* spp	Apple	Produces edema and toxic to kidney
Zearalenone	Gibberellazea	Corn	Hyperestrogenic
Patulin	*P. miticae*		Produces sarcomas
Sporidesmin	Pithomyces		Causes facial eczema

All food grains particularly groundnuts contaminated with *Aspergillus* contain these toxins. The bitter taste of groundnuts is due to aflatoxins. Such groundnuts are yellow in color and fungus can be seen. Milk and fresh meat contain less amounts of aflatoxins whereas dried meat has high concentration of aflatoxins. Overriped fruits may contain toxins. Safety limits of aflatoxins as per WHO recommendations are 30 parts/billion. Treating the food with ammonia vapors or autoclaving removes aflatoxins. Aflatoxins are sensitive to sunlight, UV rays and alkaline pH.

Zinc is essential for the synthesis of aflatoxin. The lowest concentration of aflatoxins at which no response is observed in noninfected people or the lowest concentration at which minimum cross-reaction observed is considered as diagnostic titer. One day old duckling is sensitive to aflatoxin at a concentration of 0.335 mg/kg body weight. Aflatoxins affect protein synthesis, interfere with electron transport, lysosomes, acid hydrolysis and endoplasmic reticulum. Initially stimulates glycogenolysis and interferes with conversion of amino acids into proteins.

The optimum pH range for aflatoxin production is 6.2. Ions like copper, iron, calcium inhibit their synthesis whereas zinc, manganese, cadmium favor the synthesis. Increased lipid content in the medium lowers the synthesis of aflatoxins. Coenzyme NADPH is essential for the synthesis of aflatoxins.

To summarize bacterial/toxic food poisoning is a community problem. Outbreaks can occur explosively or sporadically. Diagnosis is usually made by history of consumption of contaminated food and clinical symptoms. Majority of cases do not require any specific treatment and many times recovery is seen within 48 hours. Among the toxins botulinum toxin and B_1 aflatoxins are the most potent ones. Prevention of food poisoning consists of avoiding of raw food, proper storage and handling of food, personal hygiene and proper processing of meat, and milk products (Table 18.1).

Chapter 19

Wound Infections

INTRODUCTION

Skin is the largest organ of the human body which protects all the internal organs by controlling the microbial populations, living on the surface of the skin from entering under layers or organs. It also plays a crucial role in sustaining the life through regulation of water and electrolyte balance, thermoregulation and resistance against mechanical, thermal, and chemical aggression. The skin is composed of three layers—epidermis, dermis and hypodermis. The epidermis which mainly comprises of dead cells with PA protein called keratin is responsible for protection against the environment and it is waterproof. The cells on the surface of the skin are constantly being replaced by regeneration from below with top layers sloughing off. The repair of an epithelial wound is merely a scaling up of this normal process.

Exposure of a subcutaneous tissue with wound provides a moist and warm environment suitable for the multiplication of microorganisms. However, wound type, depth, location, quality, level of perfusion and antimicrobial efficacy or resistance are the governing factors for examining the microbial effects on wounds. When the skin barrier is disrupted due to any cause such as ulcers, burns, neoplasm or trauma it cannot function adequately. A wound is defined as a break in the epithelial integrity of the skin. However, the disruption could be much deeper, extending to the dermis, subcutaneous fat, fascia, muscle and the bone. Wounds are generally classified as (a) wounds without tissue loss, (b) wounds with tissue loss as in cases of burns, (c) wounds due to trauma, abrasions or as secondary complications due to venous stasis, diabetic ulcers or pressure sores, and (d) iatrogenic wounds such as skin graft donor sites and dermabrasions. Wounds are also classified by the layers involved, like superficial wounds involving only epidermis and dermis, full thickness wounds involving subcutaneous fat or deeper tissue. Wounds are also classified as acute (post-traumatic wounds, burns, skin ulcers, etc.) and chronic wounds (leg ulcers, pressure sores and diabetic foot ulcers, etc.)

Table 19.1: Types of surgical and traumatic wounds

Type of wound	*Cause*	*Result*
Incision	Surgical (Rarely trauma)	Penetrating
Laceration	Usually trauma	Torn tissue
Contusion	Usually trauma, skin may be intact	Extensive tissue damage
Abrasion	Usually trauma	Superficial epithelial
Combination	Usually severe trauma	Life threatening

ACUTE WOUNDS

These are due to external damage of the intact skin and include surgical wounds, bites, burns, minor cuts and abrasions, and more severe traumatic wounds such as lacerations or gunshot wounds. Acute wounds are classified as surgical and traumatic wounds. Surgical wounds are skin incisions that cause minimal tissue damage. They are made with precision in an aseptic environment where aseptic and antiseptic techniques reduce the risk of infection. Penetrating trauma may cause minimal damage to the skin and the connective tissue but the deeper damage to vessels, nerves and internal organs may be significant. The traumatic wounds are contused wounds with characteristic torn and irregular edges and may contain devitalized tissue and foreign materials Table 19.1.

CHRONIC WOUNDS

A chronic wound is due to the loss of cutaneous substance as a result of ongoing pathological process, which progresses over an indeterminate time period. The normal process of healing is disrupted at one or more points in the phases of hemostasis, inflammation, proliferation and repair. Chronic wounds occur due to chronic venous leg ulcers, arterial, neuropathic, pressure, vasculitis and burns. The most commonly involved site is the lower limbs although chronic ulceration can affect any anatomical region. Nearly 70% of all leg ulcers are due to venous hypertension or venous insufficiency. Diabetes and arterial diseases contribute to the rest. Chronic wounds are more common in elderly age group.

Restoration of tissue continuity after injury is a natural phenomenon. Infection, quality of healing, speed of healing, fluid loss and other complications may enhance the healing time and represents a major challenge in clinical setting. Chronic wounds disrupt normal healing process and are not sufficient to effect uneventful repair. Delayed healing is generally a result of compromised wound physiology. Second major challenge is the prevention of scarring, keloid formation or contractures and a cosmetically acceptable healing. Normal wound healing involves a complex and dynamic but well orchestrated series of events leading to the repair of the injured tissues. Wound healing process comprises of hemostasis, inflammation, proliferation, maturation or remodeling and epithelization. The platelets present in the exposed blood aggregates to form temporary plug to reduce bleeding. The phagocytes at the site of injury clear debris and destroy the ingested substances and degraded products. New vessels proliferate from the fresh granulation tissue and carry oxygenated blood to the wound bed. The fibroblasts lay down a net work of collagen fibers and they are remodeled and finally the process of laying down new skin or epithelial cells takes place.

Acute wounds are expected to heal within the stipulated time frame and with minimal intervention. On the other hand, the chronic wounds are caused by endogenous mechanisms that ultimately compromise the integrity of the dermal and epidermal tissues.

WOUND MANAGEMENT

Wound management is a challenging job and needs the determination of underlying etiology followed by local wound care. All wounds are treated differently depending upon the underlying etiology and severity of the wounds. An important part of wound management is realizing the potential dangers of wound infection. Surgery itself carries a risk of 1 to 5 percent of wound infection and if proper care is not taken, there is a 27% chance of endogenous contamination. Wound infection and presence of pathogen in the skin and the body is primarily responsible for delayed wound healing although host immune response and local environmental factors such as tissue necrosis, hypoxia and ischemia impair immune cell activity. Antiseptics, antibiotics, vacuum assisted wound closure, enzymatic and surgical wound debridement, pressure reduction in the wounds, complementary and alternative therapies are the common techniques of wound management.

The incidence of surgical wound infections depends upon surgical technique, type of surgery, extent of endogenous contamination, duration of operation, underlying disease status such as diabetes, coronary artery disease, chronic liver or kidney disease, operating room environment, organisms shed by the operating room team

WOUND CARE

Diluted liquid antiseptics in a concentration of two to three percent (Cetrimide 15%, Chlorhexidine 7.5%) are used to remove old dried blood/dirt/grease/discharge from the wound. Alcohol should not be used inside the wound as it causes irritation and burning and kills the living tissue. It can be applied around the wound edges to harden the skin and disinfect it. Ether should not be used because it dries up the skin and makes it more susceptible to breaking. Hydrogen peroxide acts by removing the debris from the wound and is less painful. It also increases tissue oxygenation locally for some time. Betadine solution acts only for ten minutes where as the cream acts for six hours.

Wounds should not be touched dirty hands and hands should be thoroughly washed with soap and water and if they are not very much soiled, hands should be cleaned with 70% isopropyl alcohol. One can get the help from the colleague and the dressing tray should be made available. The patient should be explained the procedure that intended. The old dressing must be removed. The wound is examined after wearing gloves, for any swelling, color, tenderness and any oozing from the wound. If necessary, discharge from the wound or the scab should be collected under aseptic conditions and sent for the culture. The edges of the wound are cleaned with 10% betadine, and betadine cream is applied to the wound before the wound is covered with sterile gauze. The old dressing is discarded into the yellow bag for disposal. Unless there is an indication, do not use dynaplast. Only micro pore tape is used to fix the gauze.

Despite the advances in surgical techniques, surgical infections continue to be the major cause of more postoperative mortality and morbidity than any other single cause. Control of wound sepsis requires sound knowledge on the biological and clinical basis of infection and of the host-defense mechanisms. Host resistance to infection virulence of the invading organisms and the hospital environment *per se* are among the main determinants of the pathogenesis of wound infection. Consequently wound infections require a systematic approach.

Bacterial activity of any surgical wound can vary from normal cent percent to 'zero' from 1 mm^2 to the next. A random distribution of bacteria containing particles enters the wound throughout the surgical procedure, and the number of bacteria arriving at any locus in the wound is sufficient when coupled with substantial reduction in local host resistance to cause a suppurative bacterial lesion. Any effort therefore aimed further reducing the wound sepsis rate must concentrate on the host responses while holding down bacterial contamination.

Despite the many advances in careful aseptic surgical techniques available data suggest that 3 to 11 percent of incised wounds become infected. The use of antibiotics prophylactically prior to surgery to prevent infection that do not exist is without redeeming value and may be facilitating colonization of the patient with antibiotic resistant organisms.

Infection of the wound generally occurs during the operation with most of the times patient serving as the source of infection (endogenous). With the exception of group A streptococcal infections which become apparent within 48 hours, the first sign of infection usually develops 5 days after the operation, when there is increased pulse rate and temperature. By 7th day swelling, tenderness, edema and erythema of the wound are apparent. Prompt drainage and antibiotic usage according to the culture and sensitivity are usually effective. Table 19.2 shows the principal agents responsible for etiological surgical wound sepsis in various types of surgery. Among the various microorganisms, staphylococci are the principal causative agents accounting for 30 to 50 percent of wound infections, followed by other organisms.

Table 19.2: Causative agents in wound infections

General surgery	*Gynecologic and obstetric surgery*	*Tracheostomy*
Staphylococcus aureus	Anaerobic streptococci	*Pseudomonas aeruginosa*
Escherichia coli	Nonhemolytic streptococci	*Enterobacter-Klebsiella* species
Enterobacter-Klebsiella species	*Escherichia coli*	*Proteus* species
Proteus species	Peptococci	*Staphylococcus aureus*
Bacteroides species	Viridans streptococci	Fungi

Adequate disinfection of the surgical site before incision, avoiding the shaving off the surgical area one day before the surgery, gentle handling of the tissue and strict aseptic precautions during surgery and restriction of antibiotic prophylaxis only to intraoperative period are some of the methods which are useful in curtailing the incidence of postoperative wound sepsis.

General wounds, and bedsores are cleaned thoroughly with antiseptic soaps and water. The surroundings area of the wound should be cleaned with 70 percent alcohol or betadine. The wound itself can be cleaned with three percent hydrogen peroxide and wound should be free of dead tissue. Any slough present should be removed till healthy granulation tissue is seen. Topical use of antibiotics and sterile wound dressings will help in healing of the wounds which are nonsurgical. The underlying causes like diabetes, immunosuppression if any should be controlled.

Chapter 20

Urinary Tract Infections

INTRODUCTION

Urinary tract infection is a complex situation and it is not a specific entity. Normally the surface of the urinary tract, the ureter, bladder, and urethra has its protective barrier, the simple flow of urine. Instillation into the bladder of organisms capable of causing urinary tract infections is followed by their prompt excretion in urine, with no untoward effects. Except for a few organisms normally found in the lower urethra, urinary tract is free from bacteria and urethral contaminants in urine rarely exceed 1000 colony forming units (CFU)/mL. In symptomatic or asymptomatic urinary infections, however, bacteria ordinarily are present in concentrations more than 10^5/mL. Thus, quantitative studies are of critical importance in distinguishing infection from contamination.

Infection of the urinary tract ranges from asymptomatic bacteriuria through cystitis, urethritis to pyelonephritis. Even in asymptomatic bacteriuria, the bacterial counts may exceed more than 10^5/mL. Pyuria is commonly seen in urinary tract infection; the number of pus cells seen under the microscope depends upon the way the specimen is obtained, the urine flow rate, the intensity of tissue reaction, the volume of urine, time and speed of centrifugation, the volume of the resuspension. Pyuria with no bacteriuria can be seen in: (a) bacterial urethritis, (b) glomerulonephritis, (c) nephrosis, (d) foreign body, (e) tumors, and (f) injury. In 94% of patients with bacteriuria excrete more than 400,000 WBC/hour.

Urinary tract infection are extremely common in women, the incidence being in the range of 10 to 20 percent. The most common mode of infection is ascending type wherein microorganisms present in the host's own intestinal tract produce surface contamination of the urethra and migrate upward through the urinary passages from the urethra, bladder, and ureters to the kidneys. Rarely infection can spread hematogenously as a consequence of systemic infection. Screening of asymptomatic population, recognition of the causes for persistent urinary tract infection (UTI), such as vesicoureteric reflux, intrarenal reflux, immunological and host factors have increased our present knowledge of UTI. Neurologic or structural or obstructive lesions, or instrumentation of female urethra may lead to asymptomatic bacteriuria and chronic pyelonephritis. Lower urinary tract infection may lead to acute pyelonephritis and rarely bacteremia. Most of the infections are asymptomatic appear to be limited to the urethra and bladder and are accompanied by persistent bacteriuria. Urethritis and cystitis are usually mild diseases that subside in a week or less but bacteriuria persists. Finally a significant but variable proportion of untreated patients with symptomatic or asymptomatic bacteriuria develop renal damage or acute pyelonephritis. Although most of the episodes of acute pyelonephritis usually subside in a week to 10 days, the bacteriuria persists and the disease tends to recur due to relapse or reinfection. Chronic pyelonephritis resulting due to persistent infection is a progressive disease and is one of the common and important kind of renal parenchymal diseases.

Among the main predisposing factors, age and sex play an important role in UTI. Urinary infections are 10 times more common in females than in males. However, newborn males may have an higher incidence of bacteriuria due to anatomical abnormalities. Long-term studies have shown that about five percent of the schools going girls have experienced bacteriuria or overt disease. Among the boys the incidence is less than 0.5 percent. During the childbearing age women are 10 times more prone to develop acute pyelonephritis than males. The frequency of bacteriuria among pregnant women is 4 to 10 percent. It is to be noted that 13 to 40 percent of women with asymptomatic bacteriuria in early pregnancy develop overt infection including acute pyelonephritis is about 1 to 1.5 percent. The prevalence of bacteriuria among the females continues to increase with age and 10 to 15 percent of women of 60 years age may have bacteriuria. In the absence of prostatism and genitourinary instrumentation the incidence of bacteriuria in males is less than 0.5 percent. In males over the age of 40 the incidence is 3.5 percent and selected population such as hospitalized patients it may be around 15% or more. Urinary tract infections are more common in patients with anatomical defects associated with an inadequate lumen, diseases of the wall, or functional inadequacy. Instrumentation hospitalization increases the risk of UTI. Urinary tract infections are more common in diabetics especially in females. Persons with sickle-cell anemia are more prone to urinary infection because of obstruction associated with sickling and thrombus formation in the renal medulla.

Microorganisms responsible for UTI are:

1. Aerobic gram-negative bacilli such as *Escherichia coli, Klebsiella, Enterobacter, Proteus, Citrobacter, Pseudomonas, Serratia* and *Chlamydia.*
2. Gram-positive organisms like *Staphylococcus aureus*, coagulase negative staphylococci, enterococci.
3. Yeast like *Candida* species.

   Anaerobic organism is usually rare to find.

Most important organisms for nongonococcal urethritis are *Chlamydia, T-strain Mycoplasma*. All combinations such as bacteriuria can be seen in urinary tract infections.

PATHOLOGY

Cystitis occurring in the presence of obstruction persists and frequently leads to progressive renal damage. In acute pyelonephritis, the lining of the renal pelvis and calyces is inflamed and the infection is usually confined to one or more wedge shaped areas with spikes in the medulla. Upon healing a linear scar remains. In chronic pyelonephritis there are numerous scars scattered over the renal surface with mononuclear infiltration. Renal medullary necrosis usually involves ischemic necrosis of the renal papilla and adjacent portions of the renal medulla together with lesions of acute and chronic pyelonephritis. Gram-negative bacteremia is very common in UTI patients and is associated with endotoxin shock. The exact mechanism by which shock is induced is not very clear. One of the intriguing possibilities is that endotoxin triggers the release of lysosomal enzymes thus initiating the process of circulatory collapse.

LABORATORY DIAGNOSIS OF URINARY TRACT INFECTION

Similar to the epidemiology and pathogenesis, the diagnosis of urinary tract infection is also complex. Pyuria is a nonspecific indicator. Since the counting of bacteria per mL is important, colony counts are very important in the diagnosis of urinary infection. Two consecutive, properly collected, clean voided specimens containing more than 10^5 bacilli/mL of single type correctly establish the diagnosis in 95 percent of the times. Polymicrobial infections are rare but can occur in catheterized patients. Direct examination of wet films under phase contrast microscopy or by Gram stain is a good laboratory indicator. Two organisms per field of Gram's stained smear of an unspun specimen of urine is 90% suggestive of infection. Pyuria is defined as more than 10 WBC/HPF in a centrifuged specimen. Bacterial counts may sometimes be less than 10^5/mL in patients with dysuria. With gram-positive organisms or fungal infections counts may be 10^4/mL. Eighty-five percent of the urine cultures performed will be either hightly or heavily infected with *E. coli* and 95% of the UTI are caused by single pathogen. Thus, identification of a mixed infection it is better to treat the predominant pathogen. Ninety nine percent of the UTI are caused by less than 10 major different type of bacteria.

METHODS FOR URINE CULTURE

A. Filter paper method
B. Dipslide method
C. Cup method
D. Pad culture method
E. Pipette method
F. Pour plate method
G. Miles and Misra method
H. Roller tube method
I. Streak plate method by calibrated loop.

Medical microbiologist should be consulted for selecting the appropriate method for diagnosing the urinary tract infection.

Localization of Urinary Tract Infection: The following methods are available for localizing the infection in the urinary tract infection.

a. Ureteric catheterization
b. Fairley's technique
c. Serum antibodies
d. Urine concentration technique
e. Analysis of *E. coli* serotype
f. Renal biopsy.

These laboratory techniques facilitate the diagnosis of upper and lower urinary tract infections. This differentiation is necessary in certain situations like chronic nephritis, chronic pyelonephritis, before transplantation, etc.

Although culture is the mainstay of diagnosis of UTI it is not without its drawbacks. It is therefore, important to the aware of the limitations to the accuracy of culture when making comparisons between it and other techniques used to diagnose UTI—predicting UTI is not same as predicting a positive culture result. There are several reasons why cultures do not always give is true indication of infection. The number of bacteria in urine is influenced by various factors like level of fluid intake, the frequency of voiding, and organisms may only become apparent on prolonged incubation of the culture. All these factors indicate that cultures must be interpreted in the light of other laboratory findings and clinical condition.

Majority of bacterial culture causes UTI or respiratory tract infection (RTI) or surgical wound reports the gram-negative bacilli that belongs to formally called Enterobacteriaceae. These group of organism are generally resistant to many antibiotics, including cephalosporin, because of their ability to produce extended spectrum of β-lactamase (ESBL), a group of enzymes that are capable to inactivate penicillin, a cephalosporin group of antibiotics. However, these bacteria are susceptible to a combination of penicillin derivative, a cephalosporin when combined with a β-lactamase inhibit or like clavulenic acid, sulbactam and tazobactam. These β-lactam inhibit combination of carbapenems like meropenem imipenem are in severe infection or in situation where culture sensitive is not available.

Chapter 21

Respiratory Tract Infections

Respiratory infections account both for the majority of all human illnesses and bulk of human infections. This has been well supported by clinical, epidemiological, microbiological and serological data obtained by carefully controlled studies. Viruses are the causative agents in more than 90% respiratory infections while bacteria are responsible for the balance. Further there are significant differences between upper and lower respiratory tract infections also between children and adults which can be noticed from Table 21.1.

INCIDENCE

About 30% morbidity (27 to 40%) was accounted for upper respiratory tract infections and 20 to 24 percent of deaths in children are due to lower respiratory tract infections. Attack rates varying from 0.26 to 4.1 per person per year have been reported in children below the age of 5 years. The incidence decreases with advancing age. In the age group of 0 to 5 years the incidence is high in males whereas in the age group of 41 to 50 years females showed an higher incidence. The incidence is influenced by climatic conditions, seasonal variation, more number of cases being seen in winter. In tropical countries, the incidence is 3 times more common in cold weather. The respiratory tract infections are common in temperature and wet seasons. Laryngeal infections are common in dry-hot season. Overcrowding, malnutrition, age and sex are some of the influencing factors. About 2.2 million deaths occur due to acute respiratory disease every year. If all causes of respiratory disease are taken into account, 61% of deaths due to respiratory illness result with acute respiratory disease.

Among the etiological agents 90 percent of the infections are due to viruses, which have been mentioned already. There was no correlation with the type of organism and the disease except *Bordetella pertussis* and *C. diphtheriae*, which are more or less specific. *Streptococcus pneumoniae*, *Staphylococcus aureus*, hemolytic streptococci, *Klebsiella pneumoniae* and *Pseudomonas aeruginosa* are the most common bacteria, responsible for lower respiratory tract infection especially in pneumonias. Any of the above-mentioned bacteria could be secondary invader following an acute viral infection.

Table 21.1: Differences in respiratory tract infections of children and adults

Clinical syndromes	*Causative agents*
A. Common cold	Rhinoviruses, influenza viruses, Respiratory syncytial virus, Corona viruses, Adenoviruses, Coxsackieviruses A and B, Echoviruses, *Mycoplasma*
B. Sinusitis	Pneumococci, Staphylococci, Streptococci secondary to viral infection, fungi like *Aspergillus*
C. Acute respiratory disease and febrile pharyngitis	Mostly viral, Streptococci, *Mycoplasma*
Lower respiratory tract	
A. Bronchitis infants and children	Respiratory syncytial virus. Parainfluenza viruses, *Mycoplasma,* and rhinoviruses. *Haemophillus influenzae*
Adults	Influenza virus
B. Chronic bronchitis, bronchietasis Emphysema in adults	Aggravated by acute bronchitis due to *H. influenzae*, Pneumococci secondary to a viral infection
C. Bronchiolitis	
Infants and children	Mostly viruses, *Mycoplasma*
Adults	Influenza virus
D. Epiglottitis,	
Laryngitis, laryngotracheobronchitis in children	Viruses, *Mycoplasma, H. influenzae*
Tracheobronchitis in children	Influenza, Pertussis
In adults	Influenza
E. Bronchopneumonia:	
Infants	Viruses
Children	*Mycoplasma*
Adults	Influenza viruses, Adenoviruses, *Mycoplasma*

The isolation of parainfluenza virus reported in India studies varied from 14.3 to 24.2 percent in acute respiratory infections (ARI) compared to 1.04 to 1.4 percent incidence in normal individuals, serological evidence was found in 6.4 to 44 percent of cases studied. Respiratory syncytial virus isolation from ARI cases varied from 22.6 to 63 percent of cases of ARI.

Because of its antigenic liability influenza virus A affects all ages and recovery is usually uncomplicated. Influenza A causes febrile convulsions, pneumonia and death in children. The isolation of virus similar to A/England/1/51 (HINI) between 1950 and 1957 from Coonoor area in southern India was reported. In 1957 virus A/Singapore/1/57 was introduced in the country and attacked 4.5 million persons resulting in 1100 deaths. Epidemics of influenza caused by strains similar to A/England/42/72 have been reported from Ahmed Nagar, Maharashtra and Andhra Pradesh. During 1978 epidemics have been recorded in Pune and Madras due to A/USSR/77 strains.

Influenza B predominantly occurs in younger age. Symptoms consist of abdominal pain and respiratory tract infection. Significant epidemics occur in every few years with irregular periodicity. Both A and B types circulate concurrently in the same outbreak. Influenza C causes mild and infrequent infection.

Among the 4 immune types of parainfluenza, the first 3 types are common. Types I and II are responsible for croup. Type III causes pneumonia and bronchiolitis. Type II can occur in epidemic form and type I occurs in epidemic form of an interval of several years. Type III is endemic. Infection with type I and type II does not occur in infancy because of the presence of maternal antibodies. As the immunity wanes off overt illness appear.

Respiratory syncitial virus causes epidemics of bronchitis and pneumonia in every season except during summer. The incidence is high at 2 months age and frequent reinfections are common. Passive immunity due to transfer of maternal antibodies are not protective and no laboratory animal is susceptible to infection.

Adenovirus types of 1, 2, 5 are endemic and are isolated continuously. Epidemic serotypes 3, 4, 7 occur with irregular periodicity. Rhinovirus infection is very frequent with multiple serotypes especially in winter and spring. Respiratory infections due to enteroviruses are more common in summer.

Mycoplasma pneumoniae, which is an important organism responsible for primary atypical pneumonia, was first identified in 1962. *Mycoplasma pneumoniae* infections occurred in epidemics at intervals of 3 to 5 years specially in the age group of 5 to 14 years and showed seasonal and geographic variations with a wide range of incidence of 6 to 67 percent of all pneumonias in western world. Apart from lung infection, a number of serious complications and sequelae like meningoencephalitis, pericarditis, Guillain-Barré syndrome, acute pancreatitis have been described with *M. pneumoniae* infection.

Acute fungal infections of human respiratory tract are clinically indistinguishable from bacterial or viral respiratory disorders. Respiratory mycoses differed from bacterial and viral diseases in one important aspect, i.e. they are not transmissible from man to man or from animal to man. The most common fungi responsible for respiratory disorders are *Aspergillus* species, *Candida*, *Histoplasma* and *Cryptococcus*. Bronchopulmonary allergic aspergillosis is fairly common in India.

LABORATORY DIAGNOSIS

The laboratory diagnosis of respiratory tract infection is intended for three purposes, namely:

1. Identification of etiological agent in an already clinically established cases of pneumonia or lower respiratory tract infection.
2. In the differential diagnosis of acute pulmonary conditions such as pulmonary embolism.
3. As a part of routine investigation of a pyrexia of unknown origin where a smear or sputum may show acid-fast bacilli by Ziehl-Neelsen's stain.

By and large the most common specimen subjected for microbiology is sputum. Since it is always mixed with normal flora of the upper respiratory tract, it requires careful interpretation of the cultures. The specimen should represent the infection and hence a well-expectorated mucoid, or mucopurulent or purulent specimens are only to be collected under the supervision of a trained staff. Sometimes postural drainage with the help of a physiotherapist will enable us to get a proper sample of the pathological specimen. *If there is no production of sputum it is futile to perform culture and in such situations one has to depend upon other investigations like chest X-ray, serology, etc.*

Once proper specimen is collected from the patient it is mandatory to perform a Gram's smear, which gives us a lot of useful information. Presence of epithelial cells in large numbers in Gram's smear indicates the specimen is of superficial nature, contaminated largely with saliva and is not suitable for culture. The ratio between inflammatory cells particularly polymorphs and the epithelial cells should be 10:1 and such specimens are considered to be suitable for further processing. Gram smear also helps in studying the type of further processing of staphylococci, gram-negative bacilli, anaerobes and fungus so that appropriate medium can be used for the recovery of the organisms in the laboratory.

Examination of smear either wet mount or Gram's smear helps in:

a. Rejection of specimen.
b. Capsular swelling reaction in case of pneumococci or *Klebsiella.*
c. Smear for AFB.
d. Decision regarding culture on routine media and on additional media.

Once the culture of the sample is justified, the sputum requires homogenization either by physical methods using sterile glass beads or by chemical methods such as treatment with N-acetyl-L-cysteine, sputolysin or one percent buffered pancreatin. The treated samples are inoculated on the blood agar, one percent phenyl ethyl blood agar, MacConkey and chocolate agar. Additional media like Thayer-Martin medium or Sabouraud's agar with and without antibiotics may be included if the smear shows fungal elements. The most common organisms encountered in respiratory infections of bacterial nature are: (a) staphylococci, (b) streptococci, (c) pneumococci, (d) *H. influenzae,* (e) gram-negative bacilli and rarely *Neisseria* spp, *Branhamella* and fungi. To summarize see Figure 21.1.

Once the organism is cultured and identified, antibiograms are performed which form the guideline for a specific antibiotic therapy wherever it is required.

If facilities are available, the best and most rapid method of establishing a laboratory diagnosis of localized respiratory tract infection would be to demonstrate a positive fluorescent antibody reaction on exfoliated epithelial cells. In the hands of experts, this procedure is practical especially for viral infections. However, the multiplicity of antigenic types, the expertise required, and its cost involved generally makes this technique unadaptable for routine work.

Serology plays an important role in establishing the etiological role of viruses, wherein usually a four-fold rise in the antibody titer between acute and convalescent serum confirms the diagnosis. Isolation of specific virus from the respiratory secretions is useful for epidemiological studies but may not contribute much to the management of the patient.

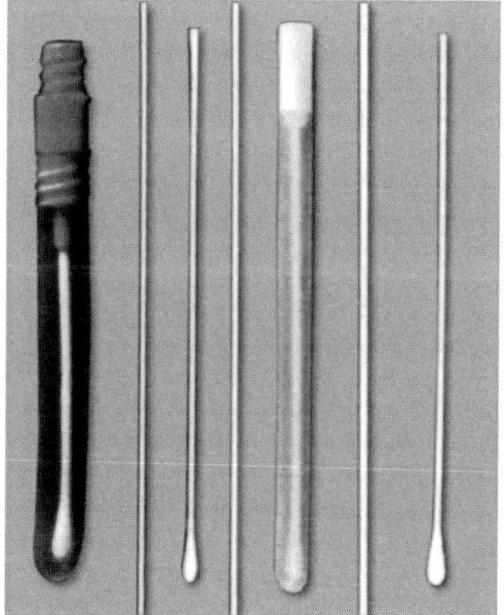

Fig. 21.1: Swabs for the collection of specimens like pus or throat swab, nasal swab, wound swab, etc. (*For color version, see Plate 6*)

For isolation of virus, throat swabs or nasal swabs (Fig. 21.1) or nasopharyngeal secretions are to be collected in Hank's balanced salt solution with 0.22 percent bovine serum albumin and transported at 4°C. The specimens are to be inoculated as early as possible in either fertile hen's eggs (10 to 12 days old), or tissue culture tubes containing monolayer cells of monkey kidney or tissue culture tubes of HELA or HEP2 or HELU cell lines. The inoculated eggs or tissue cultures should be examined after specific virus identification is done either by hemagglutination inhibition or by virus neutralization tests.

Sputum specimens are centrifuged to remove mucus and cells and smears are prepared from the supernatant fluid. The slides are air dried and subjected to indirect immunofluorescence studies for the diagnosis of viral infections.

MANAGEMENT

Respiratory infections of viral origin should be managed symptomatically because most of them are self-limiting. Depending upon the severity of the disease, patient should be under careful observation so as to any complications that may develop subsequently can be handled at an early stage. Where there is a suspicion of influenza viral infections, antibiotics may be prescribed to prevent secondary bacterial invasion and in other viral infections secondary bacterial invasion is rare.

Chapter 22

Viral Infections

HEPATITIS VIRUSES

Viral hepatitis is a systemic infection with hepatic cell necrosis and hepatic inflammation resulting in characteristic constellation of clinical, biochemical, immunological and morphological features. At least five and possibly six viruses with distinctive immunological and epidemiological features are responsible for this clinical entity. The diseases are known as hepatitis A, hepatitis B, hepatitis C, hepatitis D and hepatitis E and they indicate that the infection by hepatitis A virus (HAV), hepatitis B virus (HBV), hepatitis C virus (HCV), hepatitis D virus (HDV) and hepatitis E virus (HEV). The other viruses that are under investigation are hepatitis G virus, hepatitis F virus and transfusion transmitted virus (TTV). Although viruses like cytomegalovirus, Herpes virus may also cause liver cell injury, they differ from hepatitis viruses in that the clinical manifestations due to involvement of other organs are more prominent and more common than evidence of only liver damage.

Hepatitis A and E

As early as 5th century BC outbreaks of jaundice compatible with hepatitis A and E were described in Babylonia, and Hippocrates mentioned about epidemic jaundice in his writings. Recorded history and circumstantial evidence supports the notion that hepatitis A has been a regular concomitant of warfare. However, the virological etiology of epidemic jaundice was recognized only during the early decade of 29th century. Experiments on human transmission during World War II established the existence of distinct agents with characteristic incubation period, routes of transmission and infectivity and provided firm basis for understanding hepatitis A infection. The central role of hepatic cell necrosis and inflammation in all forms of viral hepatitis was recognized with the development of percutaneous needle biopsy introduced in 1930s. In 1947, MacCallum suggested that the virus of infectious hepatitis be named as virus A. Hepatitis A virus was first demonstrated by immunoelectron microscopy in 1973. It is now recognized as RNA virus classified under Picorna virus.

The existence of a second enterically transmitted form of viral hepatitis came into light in the early 1980s and the experimental studies confirmed the presence of HEV, the responsible agent for epidemic jaundice apart from HAV in 1990. The virus was cloned and partially characterized and shown to be an RNA virus and possibly belongs to Calicivirus family or to the subgroup of positive stranded RNA viruses.

Fig. 22.1: Schematic diagram of hepatitis B virus (*For color version, see Plate 6*)

Hepatitis B, D, and C

These three viruses share many historical, epidemiological and clinical characteristics. A type of viral hepatitis that was transmitted by inoculation of human blood was recognized in 1883.In the year 1941, there was an epidemic of jaundice that infected more than 30,000 US army people due to administration of yellow fever vaccine that was contaminated with pooled human serum. Convalescent pooled human serum used for treating infectious diseases caused several epidemics of jaundice. In 1947, MacCallum suggested that the infectious agent that causes hepatitis due to inoculation of serum should be called virus B (Fig. 22.1). The epidemiology of serum hepatitis was extensively studied between 1950 and 1960, and a number of important human transmission studies were performed. Blumberg discovered Australia antigen in 1963 which was subsequently found to be the hepatitis B surface antigen (HBsAg). This discovery resulted in extensive information about HBV, its classification as a hepatotropic DNA virus (Hepadnavirus) and the development of a safe and effective vaccine for the prevention of HBV infection.

In 1970, HDV known as hepatitis delta virus was identified as nuclear antigen in the liver cells of patients infected with HBV. The antigen was not a component of HBV and it was distinct from HBV. This virus measured 35 to 37nm and contained an inner core composed of HDV antigen with RNA genome and its outer cortex was made of HBsAg. The RNA sequences were different from any known RNA sequences. Thus, HDV was found to be a defective virus requiring helper function of the HBV for its expression. The possibility of relation of HDV to plant satellite viruses and small infectious RNAs has been postulated.

The presence of third etiological agent for serum hepatitis, the hepatitis C virus was recognized with the introduction of specific methods that identified hepatitis A, B and D viruses. In the year 1989, hepatitis C virus was cloned and was found to be an RNA virus that belonged to Flavivirus group. Soon serological tests for the detection of antibodies against hepatitis C virus were introduced and with the introduction of PCR technology, the quantitation of viral load became a routine investigation for all hepatitis viruses. The existence of other etiological agents for viral hepatitis is currently under active investigation.

Etiological Identification and Transmissibility

During early period of 20th century, McDonald predicted a viral etiology for epidemic jaundice. However, all attempts to isolate the virus in cell culture systems, in experimental animals or in embryonated eggs were not successful. Nevertheless, the infectious etiology was strongly suggested based on epidemiology and nature of epidemic form of the infection. In 1931, a laboratory worker got infected while handling the serum sample from an infected patient. Transmission of infective hepatitis through blood transfusion was recorded in 1938. Japanese scientists succeeded in experimental transmission in 1940. MacCallum and his team of workers from England, Havens and his colleagues from New Haven, Neefe and his coworkers from Philadelphia demonstrated the properties of HAV and HBV. The clinical features and the pathological changes produced by these two viruses were closely identical but their epidemiological behavior and mode of transmission were quite different. Detailed immunological studies of HAV and HBV resulted in the discovery and identification of D, C and E viruses as separate entities. The differentiating features of these various hepatitis viruses are shown in the Table 22.1. The earlier nomenclature such as infectious hepatitis, serum hepatitis, short incubation and long incubation period hepatitis or MS-1 and MS-2 hepatitis were replaced by HAV and HBV by the first expert committee on viral Hepatitis by World health Organization in 1952.

Apart from the size of the virus particle and its nucleic acid composition, the most fundamental immunological basis for differentiation of these various etiological agents of viral hepatitis is the lack of antigenic similarities to provide cross protection on re-challenge. Homologous immunity to HCV infection is either weak or absent. Hepatitis A and E spread mainly by feco-oral transmission, while percutaneous transmission is characteristic of HBV, HCV and HDV. Chronic infection and long-term carrier status is not seen with HAV and HEV infection, whereas the other viruses can produce chronic infection and long-term carrier status is variable. Case fatality rate with HAV and HEV infection is very low except that pregnant women infected with HEV may have a mortality rate as high as 20 percent. The morbidity rate with HBV, HCV and HDV infection is more than that of HAV and HEV infections. Hepatitis D super infection with HBV carriers or HDV coinfection with HBV may be an important factor contributing to the variable case fatality rate. Fulminant co-primary HBV and HDV and fulminant HDV super infection of HBV carriers with case fatality rate as high as 17 percent have been described.

Table 22.1: Differentiation of the etiological forms of viral hepatitis

Feature	*HAV*	*HBV*	*HCV*	*HDV*	*HEV*
Size of the virus	27 nm	42 nm	30–60 nm	35–37 nm	32 nm
Nucleic acid	RNA	DNA	RNA	RNA	RNA
Incubation period	15–49 days	28–160 days	15–160 days	21–140 days	15–45 days
Mean period of incubation	30 days	70–80 days	50 days	35 days	42 days
Heterologous immunity	No	No	No	No	No
Homologous immunity	Yes	Yes	Yes	Yes	Yes
Viral excretion in feces	Yes	No	No	No	No
Fecooral transmission	Yes	No	No	No	Yes
Percutaneous transmission	No	Yes	Yes	Yes	No
Carrier state	No	Yes	Yes	Yes	No
Risk of chronic hepatitis	No	Yes	Yes	Yes	No
Risk of cirrhosis	No	Yes	Yes	Yes	No
Risk of primary hepatocellular carcinoma	No	Yes	Yes	No	No

Prevention of Hepatitis A

Hepatitis A virus infection to some extent can be prevented by good personal hygiene, proper treatment and disposal of human waste and by provision of safe drinking water. The specific measures of prevention include administration of pooled human immunoglobulin and vaccination.

Pooled human immunoglobulin in doses of 0.2 mL/kg body weight is useful for post-exposure prophylaxis which is usually given to household members and sexual contacts of an infected individual. Administration of pooled immunoglobulin of human origin may not prevent infection but remarkably reduces or eliminates the clinical symptoms by reducing the levels of viremia. The pooled human immunoglobulin should be given within two weeks of exposure. It is also effective as pre-exposure prophylaxis for individuals traveling to endemic areas. Pre-exposure prophylaxis with pooled human immunoglobulin can prevent infection depending upon dose, time of administration and the magnitude of viral inoculum.

Inactivated whole virus vaccines are available worldwide. The inactivated vaccine contains purified HAV particles both complete virions and empty capsids produced in cell cultures and inactivated with formalin. The inactivated vaccine is adsorbed to an adjuvant like aluminum hydroxide and administered intramuscularly. They are safe and highly immunogenic. Single dose of vaccine produces antibody levels exceeding that produced by single injection of pooled human immunoglobulin. Booster dose given after one month following primary immunization enhances the titers of virus neutralizing antibody. Inactivated virus vaccines do not produce any secretory antibody but prevent intrahepatic viral multiplication that significantly reduces the fecal excretion of virus rendering the individual unable to transmit the infection if exposed to the virus. The major disadvantage of inactivated vaccines is that they are expensive and not suitable for mass vaccination programs.

Several attenuated vaccines have been evaluated in clinical trials but in general the immune responses to these attenuated vaccines are very slow and produce low antibody response. This is probably due to the fact that these virus strains are highly restricted in their ability to replicate in human host. Virus candidates with large deletion mutations within the 5′NTR of a virulent but minimally cell-culture adapted variant have been tried with not much success. Chimeric HAV strains containing selected sequences of human and simian HAVs are also tried. There has been little success in the development of recombinant vaccines against hepatitis A virus because the protective epitopes present on this virus are conformationally defined by interactions between the individual capsid proteins in the assembled virus particle. Nevertheless, it has been demonstrated that it is possible to produce immunogenic, assembled virus-like capsids by recombinant vaccinia virus following expression of the P1 protein precursor and $3C^{pro}$. Preliminary studies with synthetic peptide mimotopes indicate that certain peptide motifs appear to mimic the conformational immunodominant antigenic site of HAV. This observation may lead to the development of synthetic peptide vaccine in future (Table 22.2 to 22.10).

Table 22.2: *In vitro* techniques for detecting HAV and anti-HAV

Technique	HAV	Anti-HAV	Remarks
Immunoelectron microscopy	+	+	
Complement fixation	+/–	+	Less useful for detecting HAV in unpurified clinical specimens
Immune adherence hemagglutination	+/–	+	Less useful for detecting HAV in unpurified clinical
Radioimmunoassay	+	+	
Immunofluorescence/immunoperoxidase	+	–	Detection of HAV in liver cells
ELISA	+	+	

Table 22.3: Histological diagnosis of viral hepatitis

Histological feature	Hepatitis A	Hepatitis B	Hepatitis C and sero-negative non-A, non-B hepatitis
Portal (mononuclear) inflammation	Marked	Modest	Minimal
Limiting plate	Disrupted	Preserved	Preserved
Periportal inflammation	Simulate chronic active hepatitis	Minimal	Minimal
Bile ductular lesions	Rare	Occasional	Common
Zone 3 cholestasis	Common	Occasional	Occasional
Parenchymal necrosis	Moderate	Marked	Mild
Pleocytosis	Moderate	Moderate	Mild
Sinusoidal lining cell activity	Minimal	Moderate	Marked
Sinusoidal inflammation	Mild	Mild	Marked
Fat	Rare	Mild	Common
Ground-glass hepatocytes	Absent	Rare	Absent

Table 22.4: Hepatitis B nomenclature

Preferred term	Comment
Hepatitis B	A specific etiological entity, defined serologically rather than epidemiologically
Hepatitis B virus (HBV)	Agent responsible for hepatitis B, a 42 nm spherical DNA virus classified as hepadnavirus (hepatotropic DNA virus type I)
Hepatitis B surface antigen (HBsAg)	Antigenic determinant on surface of HBV that is smaller, 22 nm spherical particles and tubular forms, representing excessively produced coat material. Major envelope polypeptide encoded by the S gene of HBV DNA
Pre-S1 and pre-S2 antigens	Large and middle proteins of HBV envelope encoded by pre-S region of HBV DNA; present with HBsAg on surface of HBV and on 22 nm spheres and tubules.
Antibody to HBsAg (anti-HBs)	Antibody to surface determinants on HBV and small spherical and tubular particles; individual antibodies to subdeterminants are designated as anti-a, anti-d, anti-y and so on
Antibody to pre-S antigens (anti-pre-S)	Antibody to large and middle sized polypeptides found on HBV coat and small spheres and tubules
Hepatitis B core antigen (HBcAg)	Antigenic determinant associated with core of HBV, detectable in the nucleus of infected hepatocytes or after removal of the coat of HBV; HBcAg is not associated with small HBsAg spheres and tubules, and it is encoded by C gene of HBV DNA

Contd...

Contd...

Preferred term	Comment
Antibody to HBcAg (anti-HBc)	Antibody to core antigen of HBV
Hepatitis B e antigen (HBeAg)	Soluble non-particulate antigen, immunologically distinct from HBsAg, HBcAg and subdeterminants of HBsAg. Three specificities have been identified; associated with core of HBV but not small HBsAg particles; HBeAg appears to be formed by cleavage of a precursor of HBcAg – related polypeptide
Antibody to HBeAg (anti-HBe)	Antibody to hepatitis B e antigen with three specificities designated as anti-HBe/1, anti-HBe/2 and anti-HBe/3
Hepatitis Bx antigen (HBxAg)	Gene product of X gene of HBV with transcriptional and transactivating function
Antibody to HBxAg (anti-HBxAg)	Antibody to HBxAg

Table 22.5: HBsAg subdeterminants and antibodies

Preferred term	Comment
HBsAg/adr or ayr or adw1-4 or ayw1-4	Recognized sub determinants of HBsAg include a group specificity labeled *a* and sets of sub determinants designated *d, y, w1, w2, w3, w4* and *r*, these and other less well-defined antigenic sub determinants of HBsAg are found on HBV and small spheres and tubular forms
Antibodies to sub determinants	Antibody to surface sub determinants on HBV and small spherical and tubular particles; individual antibodies are designated as anti-a, anti-d, anti-y and so on

Table 22.6: Classification of human blood products according to risk of transmitting viral hepatitis

Average risk products	High risk products	Safe products
Whole blood	Factor IX complex	Albumin
Packed, washed or frozen red blood cells	Anti-hemophilic factor (factor VIII concentrates)	Immune globulin
Fresh frozen plasma	Multiple donor platelet concentrates	Hyperimmune globulin (Hepatitis B, Rho D)
Single-donor platelet concentrates		
Single unit cryoprecipitate		

Table 22.7: Serological parameters for HBV infection

Parameter	Serological marker
Prevalence	Anti-HBc
Infection	HBsAg
Time of infection	IgM anti-HBc (Quantitative)
infectivity	HBV DNA
Natural immunity	Anti-HBc and Anti-HBs
Immunity after vaccination	Anti-HBs (Quantitative)

Table 22.8: Categories in HBsAg carriers

Parameter	Immune tolerance	Chronic disease	Healthy HBsAg carrier
HBsAg (μg/mL)	30–150	< 30	< 30
HBeAg(PEI units/mL)	2000–10,000	< 2000	Negative, anti-HBe+
HBV DNA (GE/mL	10^9–10^{10}	3000–30,000	10^6–10^9
pg/mL	< 3000	< 10^6	< 3
Anti-HBc	+ to ++	+++	+ to ++
IgM anti-HBc (PEI units/mL)	< 50	10–500	< 10
ALT (IU/mL)	< 60	> 60 variable	< 25
HBcAg + cells in liver	90–100%	Variable, low	Negative
HBsAg+ cells in liver	90–100%	Variable, low	Variable, frequent ground glass cells, LHBs+
Dynamics	Stable	Unstable	Stable
Interferon response	Transient or none	Often sustained	No treatment required

Table 22.9: Hepatitis vaccine recommendations

Category	HBIG	Vaccine
HBV Before Exposure		
Health care workers	–	+
Institutions for mentally retarded:	–	+
a. Staff	–	+
b. Clients	–	+
Hemodialysis patients	–	+
Homosexually active males	–	+
Intravenous drug abusers	–	+
Recipients of certain blood products	–	+
Household and sexual contacts of HBV carriers	–	+
Contacts of populations with high HBV endemicity	–	+
HBV After Exposure (Source HBsAg Positive)		
Perinatal	+	+
Sexual	+	+
Percutaneous	+	+
Previously unvaccinated	–	+
Previously vaccinated	–	–
Responders	+	+
Nonresponders		
Booster		
Normal hosts < 7 years since complete immunization	NA	–
Hemodialysis patients (Anti-HBs <10 mIU/mL)	NA	+

Table 22.10: Recommendations for use of immunoglobulins

Virus exposure	*Time of evaluation*	*Nature of exposure*	*ISGa*	*HBIGb*
HAV	Before exposure	Travel to endemic area	+	NA
	After exposure	Household or day care center	+	NA
		School or work place	–	NA
		Primate handler	+/–	NA
		Medical and paramedical personnel	–	NA
		Common source epidemic	+	NA
HBV	Before exposure	Personnel or family members	–	+
	After exposure	Parenteral transfusion of HBsAg-positive blood	–	
		Accidental needle stick injury or contact with blood on open wound or mucous membrane	–	+
		Non-parenteral Intimate contact	+	+
HCV		Parenteral transfusion	+	NA
		Accidental	+	NA
HDV	—	—	–	NA
HEV	—	—	–	NA

HUMAN IMMUNODEFICIENCY VIRUS (HIV-I AND II)

During early 1983, scientists at Pasteur Institute, Paris, isolated a novel retrovirus from a young homosexual man with lymphadenopathy, and named it as lymphadenopathy associated virus (LAV). This virus was distinct from known human retroviruses (Fig. 22.2). Soon Robert Gallo and his team isolated a biologically and molecularly similar virus from patients suffering from a clinical syndrome called 'Acquired Immunodeficiency Syndrome' (AIDS) and named the virus as 'Human T lymphotropic Virus III (HTLV-III). Further studies confirmed that the LAV isolated at Pasteur Institute, Paris and HTLV-III isolated from USA were same and differed from HYLV-I and II in that they replicated quickly in T-lymphocyte cell cultures with distinct cytopathic effects and they were unable to transform the cells and showed unique antigenic and molecular properties. In 1986, a subcommittee of the International Committee on Taxonomy of Viruses (ICTV) recommended that this new subfamily of viruses be named as human immunodeficiency viruses (HIV). The committee also suggested that the various strains of the virus be designated by a code with geographically informative letters and sequential numbers be placed in brackets or as subscript like HIV-1_{SF33} for San Francisco isolate 33.

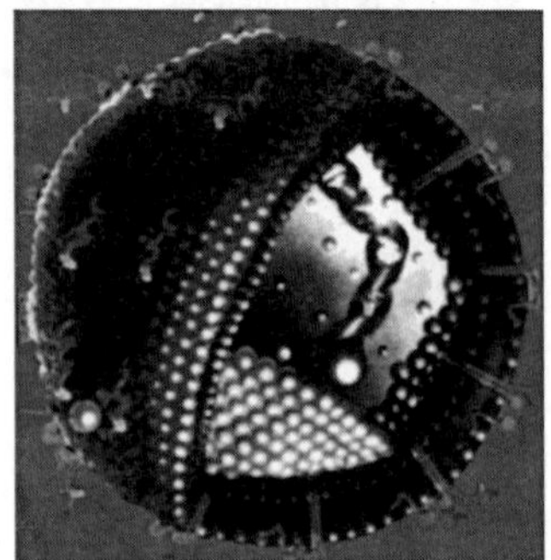

Fig. 22.2: Schematic diagram of human immunodeficiency virus (*For color version, see Plate 6*)

The currently available evidence on the origin of HIV-1 is compatible with a subhuman primate origin for HIV-1. HIV-2 is genetically and biologically different from HIV-1 but it is closer to Simian Immunodeficiency Viruses (SIVs). HIV-2 was identified in West Africa in 1986. Viruses similar to HIV-2 have been isolated from Macaques and Mangabeys monkeys in Africa. A virus that could be a progenitor of HIV-1 has also been isolated from chimpanzees in Central Africa.

Classification

HIV belongs to the family Lentivirinae under the class Retroviruses. The two types HIV-1 and HIV-2 differ in geographical distribution, biological and molecular characteristics and the extent of transmissibility, though both types produce AIDS. The viruses store the genetic information in the form of RNA which must be converted to DNA by a specific enzyme, the reverse transcriptase. HIV-1 is classified into three groups: HIV-1 major main group, outlier group (HIV-1 O) and new group (HIV-1 N). The strains isolated from different parts of the world differ genetically. HIV-1 major group is further classified into several subtypes or clades designated A through H, J and K. These subtypes possess envelope sequences that vary by 20 percent or more. The subtypes differ in geographical distribution, biological characteristics and major mode of transmission. HIV-1 subtype O is distant to all other HIV-1 subtypes but less compared to HIV-2 and so it is classified under HIV-1 and has limited distribution in West Africa (Cameroon). HIV-2 also comprises six subtypes designated as A-F and have been reported from other countries. Genetic studies indicate separate introduction of these groups from animal host into the human population.

Clinical Manifestations

Clinical manifestations in HIV infected patients encompass all organs systems and include a number of infections and malignancies that are rarely observed in immunocompetent persons. The clinical manifestations of HIV infection vary with age, sex, race, geographic location, treatment status and behavioral history. Accordingly the clinical manifestations of HIV infection generally fall into four groups.

1. **Acute HIV Syndrome:** An acute, mononucleosis–like syndrome 3 to 6 weeks after initial infection occurs in about 50 to 65 percent of the patients. The clinical features are nonspecific and may mimic a flu-like illness with fever, sweating, malaise, myalgias, anorexia and diarrhea or pharyngitis. Many patients may show CNS symptoms like headache, meningismus, encephalitis, myelopathy and peripheral neuropathy, or an acute ascending polyneuropathy. These symptoms coincide with plasma viremia and a decrease in $CD4^+$ cell count. The symptoms may subside without any treatment and the $CD4^+$ counts increase in number although they may not reach the original value. Some patients may show lymphadenopathy and truncal rash.
2. **Asymptomatic or Latent Stage:** The average time from the initial infection to developing of the clinical disease is quite variable depending on the geographic area, viral subtype and nutritional status of the patient and on an average this can be 8 to 10 years in developed countries and much less in developing countries. During this period

the viral replication continues, and the rate of progression is directly dependent on HIV RNA levels. Some nonprogressors may have very low HIV RNA levels and a marginal fall in $CD4^+$ counts. In others there are no symptoms despite a progressive fall in $CD4^+$ counts and an opportunistic infection may be the first manifestation. When the $CD4^+$ cell counts fall below or equal to 200 cells/mm^3 the patient is at high risk for clinically apparent disease and is said to be in the stage of AIDS.

3. **Persistent Generalized Lymphadenopathy (PGL):** PGL is defined as the presence of enlarged lymph nodes at two or more extra inguinal sites for which no cause is found, for a minimum of 3 to 6 months. About 50 to 70 of HIV infected patients develop PGL and it may be seen at any time during the course of infection. Mostly posterior and anterior cervical, submandibular, occipital and axillary lymph nodes are enlarged and they are mobile, non-tender and rubbery in consistency. The size may range from 0.5 to 2 centimeters. Abdominal CT-scan reveal enlarged mesenteric and retroperitoneal lymph nodes. Histopathology may show follicular hyperplasia without any specific infection. The natural history of patients with PGL does not differ from those without PGL and patients can be treated without any invasive evaluation.
4. **Symptomatic Disease:** Symptomatic or advanced disease, which involves the major body system such as:

Respiratory system diseases	Dermatological system diseases
Neurological system diseases	Ophthalmological diseases
Gastrointestinal system diseases	Hemopoietic system diseases
Cardiovascular system diseases	Endocrine system diseases
Genitourinary system diseases	Musculoskeletal system diseases

The immunodeficiency of AIDS relates to a primary HIV-1 induced T-cell deficiency, to a secondary dysfunction of B-cells with polyclonal hypergammaglobulinemia and defective specific antibody responses, and to a defective NK cell function.

A number of opportunistic infections routinely occur in patients with advanced HIV-1 infection or full blown AIDS cases. The most common organisms and their common clinical syndromes are *Pneumocystis carinii* (pneumonia), cytomegalovirus (disseminated, pneumonia, retinitis, encephalitis), *Mycobacterium tuberculosis,* atypical mycobacteria (disseminated), *Toxoplasma gondii* (encephalitis), *Candida albicans* (disseminated, esophagitis), herpes simplex (progressive infections), *Cryptococcus neoformans* (disseminated, meningitis) and cryptosporidium (enteritis).

Malignancies develop in AIDS patients and are the hallmark of the syndrome. The most common is Kaposi's sarcoma, an otherwise rare tumor of vascular endothelium that occurs in about 40% of homosexual men with AIDS. Other malignancies associated with AIDS include non-Hodgkin's B-cell lymphomas and carcinomas of rectum and tongue.

An important component of AIDS syndrome recognized in recent times is the occurrence of neurologic syndromes in approximately 40% of patients. These syndromes include encephalitis, progressive dementia, spinal cord degeneration, acute aseptic meningitis, chronic meningitis and peripheral neuropathy. AIDS patients with neurological symptoms show HIV in cells in CSF and in microglial cells and multinucleated gaint cells in brain. This finding is of particular interest since HIV is more morphologically and genetically related to the Visna virus that is responsible for chronic degenerative neurological disease in sheep.

In addition to patients with typical AIDS, there are patients in all risk groups who exhibit an AIDS-related complex (ARC), consisting of generalized lymphadenopathy, constitutional symptoms like fever, loss of appetite, fatigue, diarrhea or low platelet counts. These clinical manifestations can all be a part of the typical AIDS syndrome or may represent a prodrome for development of AIDS.

With an increase in number of women infected with HIV, children with HIV infection are on raise. About 80% of children with HIV infection acquire the infection perinatally either just before or after delivery. Some children present with HIV-induced wasting syndrome, including opportunistic infections and neurological diseases as early as 4 to 8 months after birth. Other children develop HIV-associated clinical manifestations later in the childhood, with lymphoid infiltration in the lung (lymphoid pneumonia) and recurrent bacterial infections.

Laboratory Diagnosis

Blood samples, routinely collected by venipuncture, are generally sufficient for virus detection and serological analyses. To isolate the virus from peripheral blood mononuclear cells (PBMC), heparinized or EDTA-treated blood samples must be collected. HIV can also be isolated from other body fluids like plasma, serum, CSF, saliva, milk, tears, urine and genital secretions and tissue biopsy specimens. Strict precautions should be taken while handling any potentially HIV-infected clinical specimens. Plasma, serum or other body fluids to be tested serologically should be stored at –20°C or –70°C if they are not processed immediately. For best results, virus isolations should be performed immediately after the collection of the specimen. Nevertheless, PBMC or other infected cells may be stored in liquid nitrogen in culture medium with 10% dimethyl sulfoxide.

HIV/AIDS is a complex and unique infectious disease and the infection is life-long and as on to date no permanent cure or successful vaccine is available and relentless transmission particularly through sexual route is going on. A number of moral, ethical, legal and psychological issues are related to HIV testing and anyone attempting to assess HIV status of an individual must be conversant with these issues and strategies of testing, protocols of testing and rationale of using particular tests, technical and other pitfalls as well as quality assurance in practice. The currently available tests for diagnosing HIV in various settings are given in the Table 22.11.

Table 22.11: Tests available for HIV diagnosis

1.	**Antibody blood tests:** HIV ELISA, Rapid HIV tests, Immunofluorescent assays, Western blot (WB), Immunoblot (IB), Recombinant Immunoblot assay (RIBA)
2.	**Antibody tests on other fluids:** Oral HIV antibody ELISA, Urine HIV antibody ELISA
3.	**Other blood tests:** p24 antigen assay, virus isolation from peripheral blood mononuclear cells (PBMC), PBMC HIV DNA detection, plasma/serum viral load (HIV-1 RNA, RT-PCR), b-DNA, NASBA

Antibody Tests (Enzyme Immunoassays)

Screening or confirmatory serological tests to detect antibodies to various HIV proteins are the mainstay of diagnosis of HIV infection since routine culture is not practicable in all clinical laboratories. Blood, plasma and serum are used to detect antibodies by most widely used ELISA assays. Several commercially available ready to use reagents are used in these assays. The assays differ in format, the nature of antigens (whole viral lysates, recombinant antigens or synthetic peptides) used for capturing the antibodies and the conjugates used for detection of antibodies. The matrix used is usually solid like 'wells' 'strips' microplates or beads made of polystyrene or nitrocellulose paper. The conjugates are antibodies of IgG/IgM/IgA type or sometimes antigens are coupled to enzymes. Enzyme immunoassays using HIV antigen conjugates are more sensitive as the antigen conjugates can bind to any type of antibody (IgG, IgM, and IgA). The performance of an assay is defined by its sensitivity (percentage of true positive samples that react positive with the test) and its specificity (Percentage of true negative samples that do not react with the test). The sensitivity should be as close to 100% as possible and the specificity can vary depending upon the type of test and prevalence of infection. Enzyme immunoassay is the most commonly performed test to detect HIV antibodies. There are various kinds of ELISAs based on the principle of the test: (a) indirect ELISA, (b) competitive ELISA, (c) antigen sandwich ELISA, and (d) antigen/antibody capture ELISA. Enzyme immunoassays are also classified on the basis of the antigen used. They are:

1st Generation: Cultured viral lysates is used as the antigen

2nd Generation: Glycopeptides (recombinant antigens) are used as the antigens

3rd Generation: Synthetic peptides are used as the antigens

4th Generation: A mixture of synthetic peptides and recombinant glycopeptides are used as the antigens. p24 antigen and HIV antibodies can be detected simultaneously.

Rapid Tests

Several types of rapid tests based on the technologies like particle agglutination, immunofiltration or immunochromatography are being used which can be performed within 10 to 30 minutes. The sensitivity and specificity of these rapid tests are very close to standard ELISA tests. However, in the field conditions their performance characteristics are low. The sensitivity of these rapid tests is comparatively low on seroconversion panels. These rapid tests are relatively expensive. Nevertheless, these tests can be used in developing countries where lack of technical expertise is a problem.

Western Blot/Immunoblot/RIBA/Immunofluorescence Antibody Assay Tests

Western blot (WB) is used as supplementary test to confirm the result of a reactive sample. These tests are relatively expensive, rather difficult to interpret and can also give a minimum level of false-positive reactions. Several times the persistent indeterminate WB/IB test results are rather confusing. The results of Recombinant Immunoblot assay

(RIBA) are relatively more reliable with reduced indeterminate results. Indeterminate WB results are observed in both HIV infected and non-HIV infected individuals. Early seroconverters and patients with terminal AIDS may give indeterminate results due to low levels of HIV-specific antibodies. It may take several weeks to several months to develop antibodies to all antigens of HIV after an acute infection. Some of the causes for false-positive WB results in non-HIV infected individuals include, infection with other human retroviruses, antibodies to mitochondrial, nuclear and T-cell antigens, high concentrations of serum bilirubin, hypergammaglobulinemia due to polyclonal gammopathy and normal ribonucleoproteins. Serum samples giving indeterminate results need to be retested 8 to 12 weeks later. Consistent indeterminate results are to be confirmed by other diagnostic tests.

Recently the criteria of interpretation given in the kit literature by the manufacturer are usually followed to arrive at the test result. An alternative supplemental/confirmatory test which can be used is Immunofluorescence antibody assay (IFA) particularly to resolve indeterminate or discordant results. Results of IFA and WB are usually concordant. However, IFA assay is seldom used because the technique is more demanding and expensive (Table 22.12).

Interpretation of Serological Tests

Serum samples which give negative results in enzyme immunoassays are reported as 'non-reactive' provided the individual is not indulged in any risk behavior during the last six months prior to testing. Those sera which are repeatedly reactive with different test systems (e.g. two different types of ELISA kits) are reported as 'reactive' for HIV antibodies. The serum samples which are reactive in the first system and nonreactive in second system are unlikely to be positive, especially in low prevalence areas and they are reported as nonreactive. Some serum samples may give discordant result in ELISA and indeterminate or negative WB test. This could either be a false-positive reaction or may be an evidence of recently acquired HIV-1 infection. Such individuals are retested after a couple of weeks taking into consideration of risk behavior, presence of other infectious disease or any other pathology that can be attributed to HIV-1 infection. Some of the serum samples even though repeatedly reactive give atypical band pattern in WB testing. Such results are interpreted taking into account of clinical history and behavior of the individual. Results which remain indeterminate for one year should be considered as negative. False-positive results may be due cross-reacting antibodies due to rheumatoid arthritis, SLE, syphilis and malaria and other diseases. Inconsistent serological results may be due to technical error

Table 22.12: Criteria used by various organizations to interpret a positive Western blot

Organization	*Criteria*
American Red Cross	Three or more bands from each gene: *gag, pol, env*
Consortium for Retrovirus Serological Standardization	Two or more bands: p24, or p31/34 and gp41 or gp120/160
World Health organization	Two *env* bands with or without *gag* or *pol*
Center for Disease Control	Any two: p24, gp41, gp120/160

or due to poor quality of reagents which should be minimized by proper quality assurance programs and documented preventive measures. False-negative results may be due to the early seroconversion window, or emergence of divergent strains of the virus with altered antigens which are not present in the assay system.

Other Blood Tests

Detection and quantification of **p24 antigen** in specimens like serum, plasma, CSF and cell culture supernates can be done using commercially available kits manufactured on the ELISA principle. The p24 antigen assays are useful for diagnosing primary HIV infection prior to seroconversion, diagnosing infection in neonates, resolving indeterminate serological results, monitoring the response to antiretroviral therapy and detecting window period infections in transfusion services. The p24 antigenemia during primary infection is transient. The p24 antigen may be detected as early as two weeks after infection and it may remain positive upto 3 to 5 months. Persistence of p24 antigen in CSF indicates severe involvement of CNS by HIV-1 infection. The detection of p24 antigen is of limited value in asymptomatic patients. This is due to low antigenemia or may be due to formation of immune complexes with corresponding antibody. The diagnostic and prognostic utility of measuring the immune complex dissociated p24 antigen in plasma using immune complex dissociation assays is controversial. Recently ultra sensitive low HIV-1 p24 antigen detection assays have been developed but they need thorough evaluation in conjunction with other assays. During the course of infection p24 antigen can be detected in 30 to 70 percent of the infected patients. The presence and detection of p24 antigen indicates high level viremia and increased risk of clinical progression. The p24 antigen detection during early neonatal period in a child born to HIV positive mother is helpful in ascertaining the infectious state of the newborn. Though, p24 antigen assay can be used to identify window period infections among voluntary blood donors, because of unpredictable transient antigenemia, low sensitivity of the presently available immunoassays, low frequency of detection of window period HIV infections from the seronegative blood donors, marginal gain of just one week in reducing the window period and HIV positivity and cost involved is not economical, p24 antigen assay for screening the blood in transfusion services has not been approved.

Nucleic Acid Detection Tests

Proviral HIV-1 DNA associated with peripheral blood mononuclear cells and or HIV-1 RNA is detected during window period of HIV-1 infection. Polymerase chain reaction (PCR) is used to amplify the conserved sequences of HIV-1 gag or pol gene and the amplified product is detected by hybridization with enzyme or radiolabeled specific oligonucleotide probes. PCR is highly sensitive and specific in experienced laboratories provided adequate precautions are taken to avoid contamination and maintain high standards of quality assurance. The sensitivity of HIV-1 DNA PCR in clinical practice is 96 to 99 percent. Sensitivity may be lower in individuals with high $CD4^+$ counts, low infected PBMCs in blood and in those on antiretroviral treatment.

Detection of HIV-1 DNA by PCR is useful for early diagnosis of HIV infection in neonates, to resolve indeterminate serological result in high risk group and to minimize the window period transfusions. To maximize the efficiency and minimize the cost, one multiplex nucleic acid detection or mini pool testing can be used. Individual testing can further be done for the members of the pool found to be reactive.

Quantitative HIV-1 RNA assay is useful to monitor the progression of the disease and the response to antiretroviral therapy. It is also used for the primary diagnosis of HIV-1 infection where there is high viremia and serological tests are negative. The sensitivity and specificity of HIV-1 RNA PCR test are 100 and 97.4%, respectively. Because of the possibility of false-positive reactions the use of these assays in the diagnosis of primary HIV-1 infection is controversial. Various modifications of quantitative HIV-1 RNA in plasma include, RT-PCR, Nucleic acid sequence based amplification (NASBA), Nucleic acid amplification and bDNA signal amplification, DNA hybridization and colorimetric detection, and a multiplex transcription mediated amplification are available for routine testing. The lower limit of quantification of HIV-1 RNA by all these modifications is well correlated and ranges from 50 to 80 copies/mL. High viral load predicts rapid progression to AIDS and death. A low level of HIV-1 RNA predicts slow progression to AIDS.

HIV Culture

A definitive test for an active infection is the recovery of HIV from cells of the infected individual. The virus can be cultured *in vitro* by culturing infected PBMC after stimulating them with a mitogen like phytohemagglutinin. More effective viral isolation was observed by omitting mitogen stimulation of the cells in the initial sample. Instead, PBMC from a seronegative donor that have been previously stimulated are directly added to the PBMC from the person under study. The success of this approach is due to the avoidance of a mitogen induced T-suppressor cell activity that may reduce the viral replication. This cocultivation approach permits the isolation of HIV in more than 90% of seropositive patients with different clinical conditions and allows for detection of one productively infected $CD4^+$ cell in a population of more than 10^6 PBMC.

While testing an individual for HIV infection issues related to HIV testing such as technical considerations, ethical and legal considerations, maintenance of confidentiality, providing pre- and post-test counseling should be taken into consideration.

HIV Testing with Saliva and Urine

Oral secretions contain IgG isotype antibodies against HIV at a concentration greater than corresponding serum levels. Commercially available oral HIV tests are comparable with rapid test kits. Oral secretions are collected with the help of a cotton swab placed in the mouth for two minutes and transported in a container with an antibacterial preservative. The sample is tested by an enzyme immunoassay and supplemental tests (ELISA/RAPID/SIMPLE or WB). The sensitivity of oral HIV tests is 99.99% and specificity is 99.99%. However, performance of these tests during seroconversion is not clear. Similarly urine also can be subjected to detect antibodies against HIV using ELISA or any IgG capture particle adherence tests and the results are comparable to that of serum tests. Urine therefore may provide an alternate specimen in patients who are not willing to give serum sample. However, the testing needs further evaluation with respect to its performance and ethical issues.

Treatment

The details of antiretroviral drugs have been described in the previous chapter on 'Antiviral agents.' The drugs are mainly classified into:
1. Nucleoside reverse transcriptase inhibitors (NRTIs)
2. Non-nucleoside reverse transcriptase inhibitors (NNRTIs)
3. Protease inhibitors (PI)

Other newer drugs under evaluation are:
1. Integrase inhibitors, e.g. AR177
2. Fusion inhibitors, e.g. T-20
3. Replication and packaging inhibitors, e.g. benzamide compounds

Based on these drugs available, combination therapy for HIV can be a convergent approach in which the combination of drugs acts only on one enzyme, the reverse transcriptase. The combination may be 3NRTIs or 2NRTIs + 1NNRTI. The other approach, the divergent type uses drugs that act on both enzymes. Out of 17 antiretroviral drugs currently approved for use in HIV infection management, numerous combinations of three drugs can be designed. The combination used depends upon many factors and it is individualized according to the patient needs. The antiretroviral therapy is useful in:
1. Clinical management of HIV-1 infected patients
2. Prevention of vertical transmission
3. Postexposure prophylaxis for health care workers

Due to widespread use of combination therapy using two NRTIs + one PI, popularly referred as highly active antiretroviral therapy (HAART), a dramatic decline in deaths and hospitalization due to AIDS has been reported from developed countries. Today in the developed countries HIV infection is no longer considered as a fatal illness; rather it is viewed as a chronic manageable disease. The goals of antiretroviral therapy are (a) reduction in morbidity and mortality due to HIV, (b) improvement in quality of life, (c) restoration and preservation of immunological functions, and (d) maximal and durable suppression of viral replication.

In order to understand how to initiate and monitor HAART, one should know that
1. HIV replication is relentless and leads to immune damage
2. Viral load and $CD4^+$ cell counts are important markers
3. The goal of therapy is maximal suppression of viral replication to conserve immune function
4. Drugs are to be used according to optimum schedules and dosages
5. Any change from norm increases future constrains
6. Women receive therapy irrespective of pregnancy status
7. Counsel to sustain sex practices

The durability of viral load suppression is greatest with three drug regimen as compared to monotherapy with zidovudine as practiced during initial stages in 1987 or dual therapy as practiced in 1994. Administration of lower doses of antiretroviral drugs has failed to ensure durable suppression of viral replication. Hence, patient compliance is very important to achieve optimum schedules and doses to ensure long-term success. If a patient fails to respond to one regimen, it is essential to switch over to a second-line regimen early to obtain better response. Indiscriminate use of the drugs will lead to minimal options for the future. While starting the HAART, it is important to inform the patient that:

1. Therapy is not curative
2. It is to be taken life-long
3. It is expensive
4. Long-term adverse events are not uncommon
5. Drug interactions must be kept in mind
6. Several pills per day will need to be taken
7. Adherence to treatment protocols is critical in order to avoid drug resistance

Options for treatment of HIV infection (Table 22.13):

1. 2NRTIs +1PI
2. 2NRTIs + 1NNRTI
3. PIs + 1 or 2 NRTIs
4. 1PI and NNRTI + 1 or 2NRTIs
5. 3NRTIs

Current PI-based regimens lack a balance between potency, tolerability and convenience. They are also associated with severe side effects like lipodystrophy, insulin resistance, hypercholesterolemia, hypertriglyceridemia and osteoporosis. These regimens are also demanding in terms of pill count, cost and fasting requirements. The antiretroviral treatment is currently customized to individual's requirement based on various factors such as base-line viral load, $CD4^+$ cell counts, side-effects profile, previous exposure to drugs, and concomitant use of drugs like Rifampicin. While initiating the therapy, all drugs should be started simultaneously and if the initial tolerance to the drugs is poor

Table 22.13: Comparison of various first-line regimen

Regimen	*Advantages*	*Disadvantages*
2NRTIs +1PI (Strongly recommended)	Most experience Solid clinical data available High genetic barrier to resistance	Complexity and high pill burden Long-term toxicities May compromise future PI based regimens
2NRTIs + 1 NNRTI (Strongly recommended)	Defers PI for future use Equally effective compared to PI Based regimens Low pill burden	Limited long-term data Barrier to resistance is low Long-term toxicities are not very clear
3NRTIs (Recommended and alternative)	Defers two classes Low pill burden	May not be effective in patients with high base-line viral load Limited long-term data May compromise future NRTIs use

all drugs should be discontinued simultaneously, except NNRTI based regimens. Since CNS is an important reservoir of HIV because of local replication, it is essential to choose a regimen, which includes some drugs that penetrate blood-brain barrier and ensure activity within the CNS. There is a considerable debate on when to start treatment for HIV infected patients. Currently available evidence suggests that a tailored treatment strategy to ensure optimal viral suppression is achieved in all patients, starting therapy is probably the most important requirement in determining the success of first-line regimens, rather than when the therapy is started. With the initiation of HAART, it has been noticed that the incidence of opportunistic infections has considerably decreased and if the $CD4^+$ cell count remains steady at $250/mm^3$ for three months or more, the chemoprophylaxis for opportunistic infections can be discontinued. Further with HAART the quality of life is improved with reduction in morbidity and frequent hospitalization. Due to hypersensitivity immune reactions patients on HAART, sometimes may suddenly develop tubercular lymphadenopathy and tuberculosis which is referred to as 'immune reconstitution disease'.

Prevention

Although HIV/AIDS disease has become a manageable disease, HIV infection cannot be eradicated even with HAART because the HIV-specific CD4+ cells do not increase at all. However, memory $CD4^+$ cells and naïve $CD4^+$ cells increase in number following the treatment with HAART. Moreover, HIV infects a variety of cells and body compartments which serve as reservoirs of infection. Efforts to stimulate an HIV-specific immune response in patients on HAART have showed mixed results. Despite all the ingenuity of man and money power, a "cure" or a "vaccine" still eludes mankind and about 11,000 new cases are being infected every minute all over the world. Hence still emphasis on prevention remains even in the developed countries that have enough resources for various antiretroviral therapy regimens.

The HIV/AIDS epidemic has far reaching implications, both for the individual and the community and for the nation as a whole. The social, psychological and economic consequences of HIV infection are immense and they affect the economics of developing countries. To prevent the progression of HIV infection in an individual and in the community, emphasis and focus has to be on the following major issues:

1. Promotion of safer sex behavior through information, education and communication
2. Condom promotion and provision
3. Early diagnosis of sexually transmitted diseases and effective treatment
4. Safe blood transfusion, managing IV abuse and occupational exposure
5. Increased emphasis on care and support of people of people living with HIV and AIDS (PLWHAs)
6. Empowerment of women
7. Prevention of mother to child transmission

Postexposure Prophylaxis

Another mode of transmission though largely undocumented is transmission of HIV infection by needlestick or sharp injury in a hospital or health care setting. Health care personnel (HCP) are normally at very low risk of acquiring HIV infection during the management of an HIV infected patient. But the absence of effective vaccine and curative treatment following an accidental exposure makes the health care personnel apprehensive. Hence, it is necessary to have a comprehensive program to deal with any accidental exposure to blood and body fluids of an HIV infected patient. Professionals that are at risk of frequent exposures to blood are (a) surgeons, (b) emergency care providers, (c) dentists, (d) nurses, (e) labor and delivery room personnel (f) laboratory technicians. Body fluids that are potentially infectious include, blood, semen, vaginal secretions, CSF, amniotic fluid, and other body fluids. Exposure to tears, sweat, urine, feces and saliva of an infected person is not normally considered as an 'exposure' unless these secretions are mixed with visible blood. The risk is normally very low but not zero. The average risk of HIV infection after an occupational exposure is given in the Table 22.14.

Various epidemiological and laboratory studies indicated that the risk of infection varies with several factors such as (a) type of the needle, (b) device visibly contaminated with patient's blood, (c) depth of injury, (d) the amount of blood involved in the exposure, (e) viral load in the infected blood at the time of exposure, (f) whether post-exposure prophylaxis was initiated within the recommended time. The risk can be reduced by observing universal precautions, use of protective barriers like gloves, masks, and eye wear, and aprons. The sharp devices and needles are handled carefully and they are disposed in a puncture-proof container with a disinfectant.

Although it is recommended that immediately following exposure, needlestick injuries and cuts should be washed with soap and water and the pricked finger should not be put in to the mouth reflexly. The splashes to the nose, mouth, eyes and skin should be flushed with plenty of water or saline. No scientific evidence is available to the fact that the use of antiseptics for wound care or squeezing the wound will reduce the risk of transmission of HIV. However, use of antiseptics is not contraindicated. All exposures must be reported immediately to the appropriate authorities and the condition must be considered as emergency. Post-exposure prophylaxis if required should be started immediately within few hours and initiating the treatment after 72 hours of exposure is not recommended. The decision to start PEP is made on the basis of extent and severity of exposure (See exposure code) and the HIV status code (See HIV status code) to arrive at a decision regarding initiation of PEP (Table 22.15 and 22.16).

Table 22.14: Average risk of HIV infection after an occupational exposure

Small amount of blood on intact skin	*No risk*
Risk with damaged skin/prolonged exposure	1:1000
Exposure on eyes, nose or mouth	1:1000
Needle-stick or sharp injuries	1:300

Table 22.15: Determination of the PEP recommendation

EC	*HIV SC*	*PEP recommendations*
1	1	PEP may not be required
1	2	Consider basic regimen
2	1	Follow basic regimen
2	2	Follow expanded regimen
3	1 or 2	Follow expanded regimen
	Unknown	In case the source is unknown, if the setting suggests a possible risk for HIV exposure and the EC is 2 or 3 consider basic PEP regimen

EC = Exposure code, HIV SC = HIV status code

Table 22.16: Specific drugs for post-exposure prophylaxis

Basic Regimen	Zidovudine 300 mg twice a day for 4 weeks Lamivudine 150 mg twice a day for 4 weeks
Expanded Regimen	Basic regimen + Lamivudine + Indinavir 800 mg /thrice a day or any other protease inhibitor is added for high risk categories

Though at present there is no vaccine for HIV infection, one such effective vaccine is highly needed because the HIV epidemic has emerged as an epidemic of global proportions. Currently available drugs for treating HIV infection cannot eradicate the infection and the infected persons remain infective for rest of their life and they are the main source of transmission of infection to others. HIV is capable of infecting only humans and the infection results in production of large quantities of antibodies. Among the infected group there is a sub group of nonprogressors who do not develop AIDS even after 10 years. This group shows: (a) high concentration of antibodies, (b) high anti-HIV $CD8^+$ cytotoxic T-lymphocyte activity, (c) low plasma viral load and (d) high levels of antibody dependent complement mediated cytotoxicity directed against HIV infected cells, and (e) high levels of secretory IgA in blood and saliva. Probable correlates of protective immunity for HIV vaccine are (a) neutralizing antibodies, (b) cytotoxic T-cell (CTL) response, (c) a combination of neutralizing antibodies and CTL response, (d) robust T-helper cell response, and (e) mucosal immunity.

One of the major obstacles for development of an effective vaccine against HIV is the high mutation rate of HIV strains resulting in considerable genetic diversity. The most substantial variation is located in the NH_2 terminal of gp120 with variation in the amino acid composition varying from 30 to 50 percent. Scientific challenges in developing a vaccine for HIV are (a) genetic variability, (b) rapid and resistant replication of HIV, (c) spread of HIV by way of cell-associated virus, (d) immunological correlates of HIV protection are ill-defined, (e) long latent period, (f) latency in some cells, (g) lack of an appropriate animal model for HIV infection, (h) possibility of live–attenuated vaccine viruses might recombine with wild strains and revert to the virulent form, and (i) persistent immunity may require persistent expression of the vaccine.

Several studies were conducted using envelope proteins to induce neutralizing antibodies and this was followed by administration of a candidate vaccine through a live-vector such as Canary pox virus to induce strong CTL response backed up by booster doses of recombinant envelop proteins to elicit antibody response. But this technique induced CTL response only in 25% of the vaccinated individuals. A third approach was focused exclusively on eliciting CTL response using HIV-DNA vaccines. It is to be seen which of these approaches will produce a successful or effective vaccine in due course of time.

ARBOVIRUSES

The term *Arbovirus,* derived from an acronym (**AR**rthropod **BO**rne viruses) and it was coined at a time when all the known viruses transmitted to humans by arthropod insect vectors like mosquitoes, ticks, flies were grouped taxonomically under this heading. However, recent studies of virus morphology and genetics have demonstrated that otherwise unrelated viruses are transmitted by arthropod vectors, so that viruses from several different families and genera are now included. Similarly some viruses that are grouped under Arboviruses because of their morphology and molecular characteristics are now known to infect humans without any intermediate arthropod vectors. World Health Organization (WHO) defined the Arboviruses as "viruses maintained in nature principally or to an important extent, through biological transmission between susceptible vertebrate hosts by hematophagus arthropods or through transovarian and possibly venereal transmission in arthropods." Because of dramatic changes in human living habits and practices, during the last two or three decades resulted in many highly pathogenic viruses that emerged not because of mutation from avirulence to virulence. The Arboviruses are widespread and malleable genetic ecologic nature have a great potential for emerging from previously undisturbed and ecological or genetic niches to produce significant human disease.

Structure and Properties of Arboviruses

Arboviruses include three families namely The Togaviridae, Bunyaviridae and Flaviviridae. Togaviridae include four genera, of which only the arthropod-borne is genus *Alphavirus.* Members of the both *Alphavirus* and *Flavivirus* genera have single stranded positive sense RNA genome that approximately measures 4×10^6 in molecular weight, which therefore acts as an mRNA for translation of proteins and the template for the transcription of negative sense RNA. The resultant product is then used to make more positive sense RNA in the replicative cycle of the virion. The Alpha viruses are spherical measuring about 60 to 70 nm in diameter and have three structural proteins—the capsid and the virion surface is composed of glycosylated E1 and E2 proteins. The Flaviviruses are smaller, measure about 40 to 50 nm in diameter and they too have three structural proteins, a capsid, a glycosylated protein and a small membrane associated non-glycosylated protein. Both viruses encode several non-structural proteins that appear to be playing an important role in the viral replication.

Among more than 500 recognized Arboviruses, about 100 are known to infect humans and another 50 or so affect domestic and wild animals. Each group of viruses causes specific illness which can be broadly classified as follows:

Alphaviruses

a. Eastern equine encephalitis
b. Western equine encephalitis
c. Venezuelan equine encephalitis

Flaviviruses

a. Dengue fever
b. Japanese encephalitis
c. Kyasanur forest disease
d. Murray valley encephalitis
e. St. Louis encephalitis
f. Tick-borne encephalitis
g. West Nile encephalitis
h. Yellow fever
i. Hepatitis C virus infection

Bunyaviruses

a. La Crosse encephalitis
b. Reovirus infections
c. Colorado tick fever

Among the three groups of viruses, the Flaviviruses are the most common cause of diseases in humans. A few diseases of high importance are discussed in this chapter. For other viruses the readers are requested to refer to textbooks or reviews.

Flaviviruses belong to the family Flaviviridae that are primarily spread through arhthropods (mainly mosquitoes and ticks). The family gets its name from yellow fever virus, the type virus of the family Flaviviridae (*Flavus* means yellow in Latin). The family Flaviviridae includes the genera, (a) Flavivirus, (b) HepaC virus, (c) HepaG virus, and (d) Pestivirus. Flaviviruses are monopartite, single-stranded, enveloped spherical viruses of 40 to 50 nm diameters. The RNA genome is of positive polarity and measures 9.6 to 12.3 kb in length. The 5′terminus of Flaviviruses carry methylated nucleotide cap which is absent in other viruses of the family Flaviviridae.

JAPANESE ENCEPHALITIS

Japanese encephalitis is the most important form of viral encephalitis in Asia. The causative agent, Japanese encephalitis virus is a member of Flaviviridae. This virus is transmitted to human beings by mosquitoes feeding on reservoir animals like pigs resulting in frequent epidemics of JE. The virus is active over a wide geographical area covering India, China and all of the South East Asia. Approximately 3 billion people reside in the JE virus endemic areas and at least 50,000 cases of JE are reported every year. Of these about 10,000 deaths occur every year and a high proportion of survivors develop serious neurological and psychiatric sequelae. In recent years outbreaks of JE have occurred in several previously non-endemic areas and the virus has been isolated from newer geographical areas like Pakistan and Australia. The high fatality rate and the frequent residual neuro-psychiatric complication in survivors make JE a considerable public health problem in many Asian countries and it has become an emerging pathogen in Australia. In India JE infection is common in Uttar Pradesh and several part of South India.

Nearly 40% of cases occur in children below 5 years it would be necessary to vaccinate 2- to 4-year-old children in all areas of transmission in any future vaccination program. The seroepidemiological survey of primary school children has revealed annual seroconversion rates of 47 to 75 percent indicating subclinical infection with Flaviviruses, predominantly JE virus. Repeated exposure to subclinical infections due to Flaviviruses has been shown to provoke anamnestic reactions and therefore the need for a booster dose in such circumstances has to be defined. Studies conduction at National Institute of Virology (NIV), Pune have demonstrated that JEV can cause persistent infection in porcine kidney cells. This has been attributed to the development of temperature sensitive mutants. Indian researchers have demonstrated persistence and latency of JEV in the muse model. The virus can persist in thymus and brown fat of pregnant mice upto 16 weeks. Inducing immunosuppression can reactivate the virus. Reports of recurrence of symptoms in children who had acute JE infection 8 to 9 months earlier have been documented and the virus was found in the peripheral T lymphocytes JE virus that is remaining latent in peripheral T lymphocytes could be recovered only upon cocultivation of T cells with mouse embryonic fibroblasts. Studies conducted at NIMHANS, Bangalore confirmed the presence of JE virus in a latent state in 12 patients out of 323 laboratory confirmed cases by demonstrating JEV specific IgM antibodies in the CSF beyond 6 to 8 weeks of illness, presence of JE antigen in CSF beyond 30 days of infection. Virus isolation from CSF beyond 3rd week of illness has not been reported in literature. Persistence of JEV has been noted to occur despite a vigorous immune response as evidence by the presence of significantly high titers of virus specific antibodies in the serum and CSF of some of the patients. The incidence of persistence is about five percent. The generation of suppressor T lymphocytes on the other hand, has been attributed as the primary mechanism in mice infected with JEV. The role of blocking factors such as antigen excess or immune complexes in the persistence of JEV has not been demonstrated. Apart from the host factors, the alterations in the viral properties such as generation of temperature sensitive mutants have been attributed to the persistence of JEV. JE virus is capable of persisting in the nervous system even in the presence of vigorous humoral response, tempting us to postulate that a defective cell-mediated immunity may be the important cause. However, it must be added that the quality of antibodies produced, their affinity for JE viral antigens and their ability to neutralize the virus *in vivo* and their ability to modulate the antigenic expression *in vivo* need to be scrupulously investigated in humans before the drawn conclusions are confirmed. The secondary immune response although offers some protection, it is not sufficient to clear the virus from the body and the result in persistence.

At present there is no specific treatment for JEV infection. Infection can be prevented by formalin inactivated of JEV cultured in infant mouse brain. Persistence of immunity in volunteers after administration of indigenously prepared vaccine was studied by estimating the levels of neutralizing antibodies by plaque reduction assay. This study in volunteers showed a seroconversion rate of 100% after two primary doses and the levels of antibody titers increased after the third booster dose. Seroconversion remained upto three years. However, this vaccine cannot confirm long-lasting immunity and there are practical difficulties in the production of large amounts of vaccine needed for mass immunization in endemic areas. Further mouse brain vaccine if used repeatedly might cause hypersensitive reactions. A live attenuated JEV vaccine using SA 14-14-2 strains is licensed in China and it recorded excellent safety and efficacy. However, WHO did not approve this vaccine for human use. Using molecular cloning techniques, several vaccines have been developed of which plasmid DNA vaccine and chimeric yellow fever/JEV based vaccine are showing promising results.

Dengue Fever

Of all the arthropod-borne viral infection dengue fever that is transmitted by female Aedes spp mosquitoes is spread worldwide. It is one of the most important diseases of tropical and subtropical regions affecting urban and peri-urban areas. The geographical distribution of the disease greatly expanded during the last 30 years and nearly half of the world population is exposed to the risk of dengue infection and it has become an epidemic disease is more than 100 countries. It is estimated that approximately 100 million cases of dengue fever and 25000 cases of dengue hemorrhagic fever occur annually. These figures may be much high because there is no surveillance system for dengue fever in many countries. Tropical areas of Asia, Africa and oceans, Australia and USA are reporting dengue fever cases of which Southeast Asia reported 1,19,707 cases with 452 deaths in 2001. In temperate areas, infection occurs in summer season. Dengue is an important cause of paediatric morbidity and mortality in Southeast Asian countries. All four serotypes have been detected circulating in all countries but the transmission potential different both at the macro and micro levels. The ecological and climatic factors influence the seasonal variation of vector species, while factors related to human ecology determine the extent and intensity of breeding. Based on the climatic factors the countries of the region have been grouped under four categories.

Group A

Tropical monsoon and equatorial climatic zone, comprising of Indonesia, Myanmar and Thailand. In these countries, dengue is a major public health problem and the predominant vector responsible for the transmission is *Aedes aegypti*. Thailand succeeded in bringing down the case fatality rate to below one by 1985 and to < 0.5 by 1990 and since then it is being maintained at that level. In Indonesia and Myanmar, the case fatality rate is between two and four percent.

Group B

Deciduous and wet climatic zone, which includes India, Bangladesh and Sri Lanka. These countries recorded serious outbreaks in 1980 (Sri Lanka), 1990 (India) 2000 (Bangladesh). The case fatality rate during the epidemics remained at 3 to 4 percent in all the three countries. During interepidemic period it fluctuated between one and two percent. The disease incidence, did not exceed high numbers, except the 1996 outbreak (Delhi), the figures crossed 15,000.

Group C

Sub-Himalayan foothill regions that include Bhutan and Nepal, where no cases of dengue were reported because the high altitude appears to be a barrier for the survival of *Aedes aegypti.*

Group D

The temperate climatic zone is nonepidemic for dengue (DPR – Korea).

In India over the last few years, DF, DHS/DSS have spread dramatically in many parts of the country. Seasonal and cyclic epidemic pattern of dengue is the recent phenomenon in North India. The new dengue paradigm, viz. the burst of sudden disease has secured firm foot indifferent areas. Dengue related deaths have been reported in the country. In 1996, 16,517 cases and 545 deaths were reported. During the subsequent years the incidence decreased. In 2001 there was a rise in the incidence (3175 cases and 53 deaths) of dengue infection. A large number of cases regularly occur in urban and suburban and rural areas with increasing proportion of DHF and DSS. Both adults and children were affected with higher occurrence in children below the age of 6 years. In our country thirteen states experienced dengue epidemic so far. The details are as follows Kolkata (West Bengal) 1965, 1983, and 1990. 1965 epidemic was caused by serotypes 1, 2 and 4. 1983 and 1990 outbreaks were due to serotype 3. In Rajasthan dengue serotype 3 was responsible for the outbreak. The unusual picture of this epidemic was that it occurred during summer. In Maharashtra state the outbreak in Parbhani district was due to serotype 2. The outbreaks that occurred in Gujarat and Karnataka were due to serotype 2.

Serological studies revealed the presence of antibodies to all four types of dengue virus. However, higher incidence of positivity was observed with serotype 3 and 4. A close association was seen between IgM response and also mixed immune response (IgM + IgG secondary) and severity of the disease. The association was significant. IgM response could be seen in 16% of cases of DHS/DSS. In addition DHS/DSS was seen in infants suggesting that infants with dengue virus infection may have acquired IgG antibodies passively from mother and subsequent exposure to primary infection at an early age leading to DHS/ DSS. However, the role of viral virulence cannot be ignored in the disease mechanism.

KYASANUR FOREST DISEASE

Kyasanur forest disease is another hemorrhagic fever of viral etiology first observed in 1957 in Karnataka State of India. Initially several dead monkeys were noticed in the Kyasanur forest area which was soon followed by illness among the villagers in the area. A year later similar illness was noticed in the locality. The new Arbovirus transmitted by the bite of tick was closely related to Russian spring summer encephalitis (RSSE) and it was named after the Kyasanur forest. The epizootic and the endemic activity confined to areas of contiguous to its original origin in Sagar for many years. Between 1972 and 1975 a few other foci were noticed in northern Karnataka and antibodies were demonstrated in humans and animals in the Kutch and Saurashtra areas indicating the wide distribution of the virus. In 1982, the situation changed suddenly with the appearance of epizootic and epidemic infection in Belthangadi area of south Karnataka. This followed the clear falling of part of evergreen reserve forest in the area in September 1982. Following the observation of dead monkeys in October, the first human case occurred in late December. During the next five months a total of 1142 cases were recorded of which 104 died of the infection.

WEST NILE ENCEPHALITIS

Emerging of arboviral encephalitis in the Western world is a classical example of changing trends in the viral infections. The recent outbreaks of West Nile encephalitis in New York and Israel have drawn the attention of western world. Till recently West Nile virus was considered as benign virus causing nonspecific self-limiting disease but the present epidemiological studies point out that West Nile virus has changed and causing increased number of encephalitis cases. The virus was first discovered in 1937 in Uganda. It is a member of JE antigenic complex and is represented by single serotype. Antigenic analysis differentiated the strains isolated from Africa, Europe, former USSR, Middle East, India and Far East. Nucleotide sequencing of E gene revealed two lineages. Lineage I comprises of strains from Europe, Middle East, West Africa and Central Africa and distinguishable clades representing strains from India and Australia. Lineage II comprises of strains from various regions of Africa and the virus emerged in New York in 1999 and strains from Middle East (Israel). West Nile virus is present throughout Africa, Middle East, Continental Europe, former USSR, India, and Indonesia and since 1999 in Australia and Mid Atlantic USA. Apart from transmission by Culex mosquito, the virus has been isolated from ticks in Russia but their role in virus transmission is not defined. Laboratory infections to humans by respiratory route are documented. The case fatality rate of West Nile infection of CNS is 5 to 10 percent. Younger patients are more likely to develop encephalitis. Fatality rate is more at both extremes of age. CSF IgM antibody titers appear to be high in fatal cases. CD4 and CD8 T-cell count were lower in Romanian patients with encephalitis suggesting impaired cell-mediated immunity. IgM capture ELISA and RT-PCR is useful in the early diagnosis of infection.

CHANDIPURA VIRUS INFECTION

In the **year 2003** several part of Andhra Pradesh witnessed an outbreak of encephalitis like illness, which affected approximately 383 children below the age of 10 years. The mortality rate was high and most of the deaths occurred within 48 hours. The local teams as well as teams from National Institute of Virology, Pune, and WHO, investigated the outbreak. Although the epidemiological investigations were patchy and inadequate, the scientist from National Institute of Virology, Pune isolated Chandipura virus in a few clinical samples and also demonstrated viral RNA from clinical samples and also from a brain biopsy specimen taken from a deceased child. Sequencing of G, N and P proteins of isolate showed 97% identity with previously isolated virus in 1965. They also demonstrated IgM antibodies against Chandipura virus in some serum sampled obtained after 4 days of illness. IgM antibodies were also present in two family contacts of patient with encephalitis suggesting the virus may remain asymptomatic or may lead to fever without encephalitis. Neurological findings were limited to the territory of middle cerebral artery either unilaterally or bilaterally vasculitis of middle cerebral artery resulting in either occlusion of spasm was proposed as the cause of acute encephalitis due to vascular endothelial damage by viral invasion or inflammation.

Chandipura virus was first isolated from fever cases that occurred in the village Chandipura near Nagpur in 1965. Sero surveillance at that time revealed the presence of antibodies in general population. But subsequent surveillance programs were lacking and there was no report on Chandipura virus infection till 2003, the virus returning with full vigour almost after 40 years. This is in fact a puzzle to epidemiologists and virologists. During the same outbreak some serum samples showed antibodies of dengue virus. It was hypothesized and speculated that the cause of epidemic of brain involvement due to Chandipura virus may be due to presence of a second virus that may be responsible for the pathogenesis. It was postulated that the second virus involved could be one of the member of JE group. However, the cause of the epidemic and the reason for the re-emergence of Chandipura virus was largely remained as an unsolved puzzle.

CHIKUNGUNYA FEVER

In the year **2005** Andhra Pradesh state reported the occurrence of Chikungunya virus infection and the state was one of the worst affected, one with a figure of 80,000 suspected cases. Chikungunya virus is not a new virus that entered India. It was isolated in Kolkata way back in 1963 and several reports on this viral infection from different parts of the country were recorded. The last outbreak occurred in 1971 and since then no active or passive surveillance was done and it was assumed therefore that the virus disappeared from the country. But recent reports have confirmed the re-emergence of this viral infection. Several districts of Karnataka, Maharashtra states also reported the occurrence of Chikungunya virus disease during February-March, 2006. During the same period Orissa state also reported 490 cases of fever associated with myalgia and headache. The sero surveillance studies conducted by NIV, Pune in Andhra Pradesh demonstrated antibodies to the virus in 139 serum samples out of 362 sera collected from various districts as well as from Secunderabad of Andhra Pradesh. Apart from India several small countries like French reunion Islands, Mauritius, and Seychelles have also reported on Chikungunya virus disease in the recent times. The clinical symptoms resemble that of dengue virus infection but hemorrhagic manifestations of shock are rare with Chikungunya. Most often it is a self-limiting disease and rarely can cause meningoencephalitis. The factors responsible of the re-emergence of Chikungunya are worth investigating. Serosurvey conducted at Kolkata a decade ago showed only 4.3 percent sero positivity to Chikungunya virus and maximum sera belonged to the age group of above 50 years indicating the lack of herd immunity to Chikungunya virus. Genetic analysis of earlier isolated of Chikungunya virus showed two distinct lineages one containing all isolated from Western Africa and the other one comprising all southern and eastern Africa strains and strains from Asia. Similar studies from the present outbreak are useful to know if any mutations have occurred in the virus. For this infrastructure facilities are needed in more laboratories (At present only NIV, Pune is conducting studies) and networked to get rapid diagnosis as such outbreaks.

The clinical manifestations caused by Arboviruses are diverse and span the entire spectrum of clinical infectious disease. Most infections produce a mild or subclinical illness with fever, headache, orbital pain, myalgia, back ache, flushing of the skin or rash, conjunctivitis and anorexia. Some viruses may cause nausea, vomiting and leukopenia is often a feature indicating a transient immunosup ression. Most infections subside without any localizing symptoms or complications and in most cases neutralizing antibodies can be demonstrated along with life-long immunity. However, the immunity is type-specific and reinfections with closely related viruses are common. The reinfections are usually mild or asymptomatic with notable exception of dengue. Studies on cellular immunity are virtually very few, which may be important both in virus clearance and protection against reinfection. Nearly all agents of Arbovirus group are capable of producing severe disease, although the mechanisms involved are not very clear.

Viral encephalitis may be caused by members of Alphaviruses, Flaviviruses and Bunya viruses. The clinical manifestations include fever, headache, vomiting, tremors, confusion, and somnolence and generalized seizures. Focal neurological manifestations and paralysis are uncommon. Some of the viruses like St. Louis encephalitis, Venezuelan encephalitis and Japanese encephalitis carry high mortality rates or enormous number of affected individuals (e.g. Japanese encephalitis).

Arboviruses can cause acute fulminant hepatitis. In addition to yellow fever, Crimean-Congo hemorrhagic fever (CCHF) and West Nile viruses may be associated with severe fatal hepatitis, although the numbers of studies are very few and the laboratory and histological data are limited.

Five arboviruses, namely dengue, Hantaan virus hemorrhagic renal syndrome (HFRS), CCHF, yellow fever and Kyasanur forest disease are mainly responsible for viral hemorrhagic fevers with shock. Although shock may develop at any stage during infection due to arboviruses, the distinct syndrome of clinical shock associated with volume depletion, extravasation of protein into the tissues; pericardial and pleural and sometimes pericardial spaces and proteinuria is usually seen as complication of the infection due to the five viruses mentioned. Nevertheless, other viruses also can cause similar syndromes occasionally. Although the shock in these infections may be associated with hemorrhagic diathesis, it is attributable mainly to the loss selective fluid and macromolecules through a dysfunctional capillary endothelium, but not to the loss of blood into the extravascular spaces. In most instances, the loss of fluid and the macromolecules appears to be due to reversible biochemical dysfunction of the endothelium rather than the destruction of cells by the invading virus or vasculitis. Patients are typically diaphoretic, restless, with cold extremities. The blood pressure decreases and respirations become shallow and rapid. Patients may develop frank adult respiratory distress with interstitial pneumonitis mainly due to vascular leakage. In addition they may also develop pericardial and pleural effusions, ascites and facial edema. Intravenous fluid therapy may be life-saving but fluid balance is a delicate problem and patients may die due to overhydration, especially those with dengue and HFRS.

Some arboviral infections especially dengue, HFRS, yellow fever and CCHF may begin with disordered hemostasis. The patients may show petechiae, especially in dengue and HFRS. Frank hemorrhage with epistaxis or mucosal bleeding may develop only in a very few patients. Intractable bleeding and intracranial hemorrhage remains as the main cause of death due to dengue or HFRS. Other signs include bleeding from the puncture sites and bruising. Bleeding in yellow fever may be severe and in CCHF extensive ecchymoses may be seen which indicate poor prognosis.

The pathogenesis of dengue is distinct and it may be immune-mediated. Presence of antibodies to dengue serotypes 1, 3 or 4 early in life or maternal antibodies in low titer may in fact enhance the infection by serotype 2 of dengue virus. On the basis of currently available evidence, it appears that the immune complexes of dengue type 2 attach to the Fc receptors of macrophages and other cells of immune system, thereby increasing the number of virus particles that infect the cells of reticuloendothelial system. Thus dengue type 2 infections which are normally mild as a primary infection, may be made more virulent by immune enhanced entry into the target cells and subsequently increase in virus multiplication. A rapid increase in the levels of cytokines and chemical mediators apparently play a key role in inducing the plasma leakage, shock and hemorrhagic manifestations. It is likely that the entire process is initiated by infection with so called virulent dengue virus, often with the help of enhancing antibodies in secondary infection and then triggered by rapidly elevated cytokines and chemical mediators produced by intense immune activation. Further, concurrent infections by two dengue serotypes may also increase the severity of the disease. Similarly simultaneous isolation of dengue virus as well as chikungunya virus from the same patient has been reported. Still our understanding of the dengue hemorrhagic fever (DHF) pathogenesis is far from complete.

Severe systemic manifestations of the arboviral infections may be associated with acute renal failure especially yellow fever and acute renal failure is unique component of HFRS. Renal angle tenderness and copious proteinuria is common. Hypotension may occur within four days after the onset of infection followed by a rapid phase of oliguria or anuria. A polyuric phase heralds a prolonged phase of convalescence.

There is no specific treatment for arboviral infections. However, the broad spectrum drug Ribavirin may be effective against HFRS and CCHF but not against yellow fever. It may be effective against encephalitis viruses but the effective therapy depends on the penetration of the drug to the brain. Specific immune serum therapy has been advocated for severe diseases like CCHF but its benefits are uncertain and the risk of using unscreened immune serum has to be considered carefully. Infections are usually self-limiting and those requiring hospitalization need good medical supportive care. Management of fluid and electrolyte balance is a problem in patients with hypovolemic shock and success depends on careful rehydration without risking fluid overload. Heparin therapy is potentially dangerous if there is no evidence for a primary role for disseminated intravascular coagulation. Low platelet counts do not predict clinically significant bleeding in dengue. Platelet or blood transfusion should not be administered based on platelet counts alone. Dengue hemorrhagic syndrome (DHS)/dengue shock syndrome (DSS) cases frequently have compensated consumptive coagulopathy that seldom needs treatment.

The 17-D strain of yellow fever virus has been an effective and safe vaccine since 1940s. It has been widely used and is responsible for a great degree of the control of yellow fever. Single injection is highly effective for life-long. Effective vaccine is available for Japanese encephalitis and for some tick-borne encephalitides. Japanese encephalitis vaccine is a purified inactivated mouse brain vaccine that is given in three doses for reliable protection. An effective attenuated live vaccine is available for immunizing animals but it is not yet tested in humans. CCHF vaccines have been used in Bulgaria and China but its safety and efficacy has not been well documented. To be effective, arbovirus vaccines should be administered early in life preferably with the childhood vaccine programs. Because of the zoonotic reservoirs, eradication of Arbovirus infections is impracticable and continuous surveillance, control of insect vectors, environmental sanitation, and health education will be needed to achieve control.

HERPES SIMPLEX VIRUS

Herpes simplex virus belongs to the group herpes viruses. These are large DNA viruses, contain double stranded DNA. These are enveloped viruses. They are ether sensitive. They are sensitive to heat, chemicals and high temperature. Herpes simplex infection is prevalent throughout the world. The virus spreads by direct contact with the highly infectious lesions. Infants may be infected during the delivery by exposure to the virus in the birth canal.

The herpes simplex virus enters the human body through mucous membranes or through skin abrasions. The virus undergoes multiplication in the epithelial cells. Due to multiplication of virus in the epithelial cells, the cells undergo lysis and form a vesicle. The vesicle contains clear fluid and this fluid contains millions of virus particles. After multiplication in the epithelial cells, the virus migrates to dorsal nerve root ganglion and establishes lifelong latency and under favorable condition the virus returns to the skin and causes recurrent infection.

Primary infection with herpes simplex virus occurs in preschool children. The incubation period is 2 to 12 days. The virus causes pain in the mouth, excessive salivation, redness of the pharynx and edema. This is followed by appearance of vesicles, which rapidly become shallow ulcers. In young adults it may cause tonsillitis (Fig. 22.3). Healing occurs in 1 to 2 weeks.

Herpes viruses can sometimes cause infection of the genital organs. The infection may be asymptomatic or it may be severe. Vesicles and ulcers are formed along with vaginal or urethral discharge. Recurrent infections are common. The herpes simplex

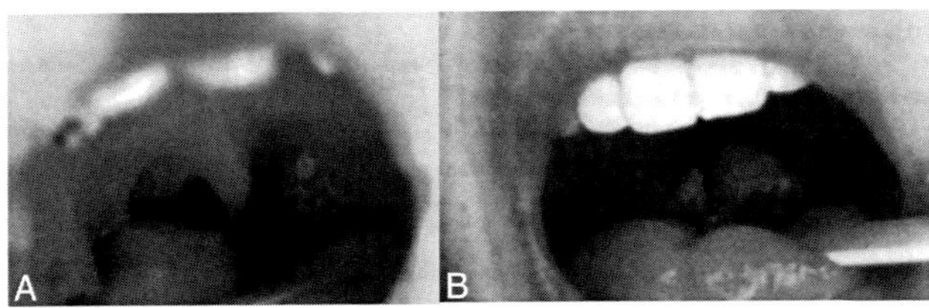

Fig. 22.3: Streptococcal pharyngitis and infectious mononucleosis
(*For color version, see Plate 6*)

virus can cause infections of skin resulting in 'herpetic whitlow' resembling paronychia. There will be severe pain at the affected region, and regional lymph nodes are enlarged. Patients with eczema develop serious form of infection known as eczema herpeticum. Infection of the brain results in encephalitis. Infection of the eye results in corneal ulcers or follicular keratoconjunctivitis. Congenital infection may result in convulsions, hepatosplenomegaly, bleeding, infection of the eye (chorioretinitis), pneumonia and skin vesicles. In immunosuppressed patients or patients undergoing transplantation of kidney, liver or heart, the infection may be fatal Herpes simplex virus infection is also common in patients having AIDS.

The laboratory diagnosis comprises of isolation of virus from the clinical specimens. The vesicular fluid inoculated into tissue culture results in the growth of virus within 24 to 48 hours. Other methods include demonstration of antibodies against herpes simplex virus antigens using techniques like ELISA and neutralization tests. Prevention of the infection can be achieved by good handwashing practices. No vaccine is available till today.

CYTOMEGALOVIRUS

Cytomegalovirus infection is very common with a wide spectrum of illness ranging from asymptomatic to life-threatening disease. The infection virus belongs to herpes viruses.

The infection is endemic and there is no seasonal variation. The virus is transmitted by person-to-person contact. The virus is present in saliva, urine, semen, breast milk, blood, transplanted donor organs, cervical and vaginal secretions. Infection spreads by mother-to-child transmission and by sexual contact. During pregnancy the latent virus can get reactivated and may transmitted to the fetus *in utero*. Infection can also be transmitted by breast milk. Transmission of infection due to contact with saliva can occur among the schoolchildren. Primary or recurrent infection due to cytomegalovirus can occur due to blood transfusion or organ transplantation.

The infected person may develop hepatosplenomegaly, jaundice, chorioretinitis, respiratory distress, neurological abnormalities such as microcephaly and focal calcifications in the brain. Congenitally infected infants are asymptomatic at birth but later they may develop loss of hearing and mental retardation. In normal persons, the virus may not cause any clinical symptoms or sometimes may produce mild 'flu' like illness with headache, body pains, fever and mild hepatitis. The virus can cause myocarditis, meningoencephalitis, pneumonia, leucopenia, hemolytic anemia and thrombocytopenia.

In patients with immunosuppression, the virus can cause severe infection resulting in leucopenia, retinitis, pneumonia, or graft rejection. Superadded bacterial fungal or parasitic infection might occur because cytomegalovirus infection itself can induce immunosuppression.

The virus is spherical in shape with cubical symmetry. It contains double stranded DNA. The virus is sensitive to chemical disinfectants and heat. The virus classically produces large intranuclear inclusions resembling like owl eye because of the cell enlargement. The virus isolation in primary cell lines, electron microscopy, histological examination for the presence of intranuclear inclusions and serology establish the diagnosis. Antibodies against cytomegalovirus antigens can be detected by ELISA technique or by complement fixation. Detection of IgM type of antibodies in the newborn indicates active infection. Two live attenuated vaccines have been shown to offer partial protection against cytomegalovirus infection. Immunoglobulins having high concentration of anti-CMV antibodies reduce the severity of disease especially in bone marrow transplanted patients.

CHICKENPOX (VARICELLA)

Chickenpox is an acute highly infectious disease caused by varicella zoster or human herpes virus 3 belonging to DNA group of viruses. The source of infections is secretions from nose, throat and skin lesions of an infected case. Unlike smallpox, the crests or scabs formed on the vesicles are not infective. The incubation period is 14 to 16 days, and infection occurs in children below the age 10 years. After the recovery from the infection, the virus may be present in sensory ganglia for years and get reactivated to produce zoster, i.e. painful vesicles along the distribution of sensory nerves. Chickenpox usually occurs during the last six months of the year, and it is transmitted by droplet infection (respiratory route) or by person to person contact.

The infected person may show mild illness with few eruptions or severe fever with widespread rash. The patient may have back pain, chills, weakness for a day or two before the rash appears. The rash is typically seen on the trunk, and then on face and arms (centripetal distribution). Vesicles may be seen in pharynx and mouth. Palms and soles are not affected (affected in small portion). Rapidly the rash passes through the stages of macules, papules (elevated part of the skin), vesicles. The vesicles may be infected resulting in pustules. The vesicles on the skin appear like dew drops. The vesicles heal by scab or crust formation. Pleomorphism is the characteristic feature of chickenpox, i.e. at a given time one can see rashes, macules, papules, vesicles, pustules, crusts, simultaneously (Fig. 22.4).

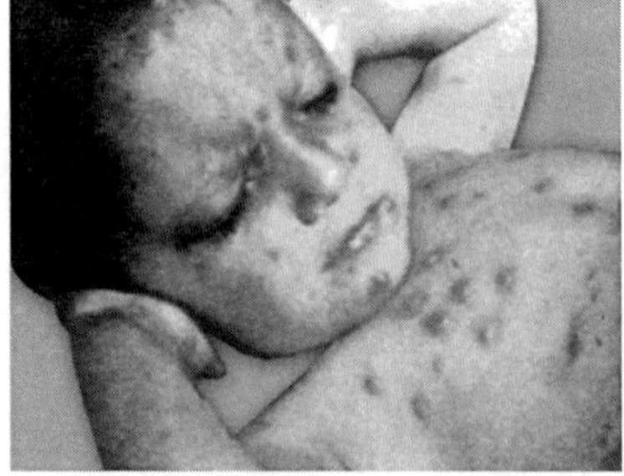

Fig. 22.4: A baby with chickenpox. Note the erythematous papules and pustules mostly on chest and abdomen. Less number on the face (*For color version, see Plate 6*)

Chickenpox is usually mild and self-limiting disease but in persons who undergo kidney transplantation, steroid therapy, cancer therapy, immunosuppression, it may be very severe with involvement of brain and liver. Chickenpox occurring in pregnant women may cause abortion or congenital defects in infant. The virus can produce cancer. The diagnosis and confirmation of chickenpox is very important to differentiate it from smallpox, a disease which got eradicated in 1977.

MEASLES (RUBEOLA)

Measles is acute viral infection caused by measles virus belonging to paramyxovirus. It is a RNA type of virus. Measles is endemic all over the world and tends to occur as epidemic especially in children. In developing countries death due to measles among preschool children are very high. It is estimated that 2 to 15 percent of infected children die of complications due to measles. Subclinical infections can occur. The source of infection is a case of measles. The infection occurs due to entry of virus through respiratory tract and the secretions from nose, throat and respiratory tract contains large number of viruses which are shed into the environment by sneezing and coughing. Usually children of three months to three years age are affected. One attack of measles results in lifelong protection and secondary attacks in already suffered person are rare. Newborn children are protected from measles through mother's antibodies which are present in breast milk. The incubation period is 10 days. The disease is characterized by fever, flowing nose, cough and sneezing. Increased production of tears, redness of eyes, photophobia, diarrhea and vomitings can occur. In the mouth characteristic rashes known as 'Koplik's spots' appear in a day or two before the onset of rashes (Fig. 22.5). During the eruptive phase, typical rash or maculopapular rash appears behind the ears and spreads rapidly throughout the body. Measles is usually self-limiting disease but neurological complications like febrile convulsions, encephalitis, progressive mental deterioration due to subacute sclerosing panencephalitis (SSPE). Occasionally measles and chickenpox may occur together.

RUBELLA (GERMAN MEASLES)

Rubella an acute viral infection caused by rubella virus belonging to RNA group of viruses. Transmission is by respiratory route through droplet infection from a case. Rubella occurs worldwide. Fetal infection occurs secondary to viremia in the mother and this results in congenital defect which is popularly known as 'congenital rubella syndrome'. The

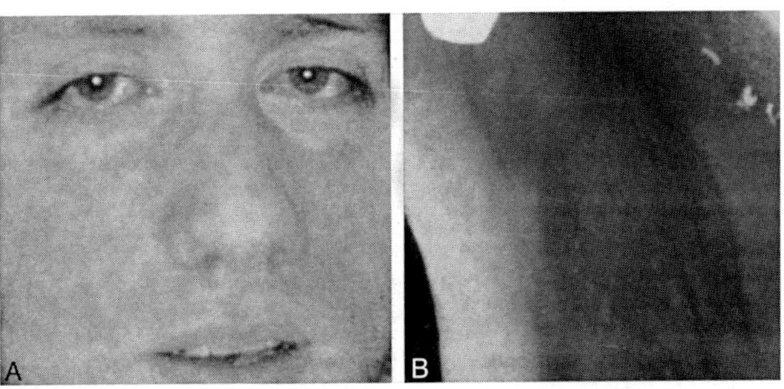

Fig. 22.5: Rash, conjunctivitis and Koplik's spots due to measles infection (*For color version, see Plate 6*)

incidence and the type of defects are related to the age of the fetus at the time of infection. Approximately 16 percent of the infected infants have major defects at birth if the rubella infection occurs in the carrying woman during the 1st trimester.

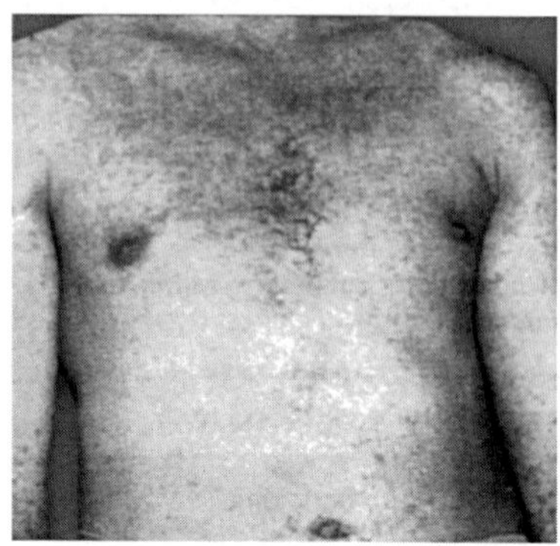

Fig. 22.6: A patient showing skin rash due to rubella infection *(For color version, see Plate 6)*

The infections is characterized by mild fever, and rash in 50% cases which is not blotchy (Fig. 22.6). Most of the patients are systematically well and recover without much complications. The complications include polyarthralgia (pains in multiple joints) in young women, encephalitis (infection spreading to the brain) and neurological problems. The rash is mainly seen on trunk and disappears in three days. Sore throat, enlarged tonsils and lymph node can be seen in some cases.

Congenital rubella is characterized by cataracts, infection of the retina of the eye, glaucoma, microphthalmia (incompletely developed eyes) arterial defects, defects in heart, deafness, enlargement of liver and spleen, hepatitis, mental retardation and bone defects.

The clinical diagnosis of rubella is wrong in 50% cases. Only estimation of antibodies (protective proteins known as globulin) is acceptable evidence of immunity.

MUMPS

Mumps is an acute infection frequently seen in children in the age group of 5 to 15 years but it can occur in any age group. The infection (i.e. undiagnosed cases by clinical examination) is very common. The infection is caused by RNA virus Myxovirus parotiditis, and it belongs to myxovirus family. The source of infection is both clinical and subclinical cases. The virus is seen in saliva and can be isolated from it. The incubation period is 2 to 3 weeks. Second attack of mumps can be seen in 86 percent of cases. It is largely an endemic disease and more number of cases occur in winter season. Epidemics are often associated with overcrowding. The infection is transmitted by droplet infection or person-to-person contact.

The infection is characterized by pain and swelling of parotid glands (salivary glands). There may be earache and pain and stiffness of the mouth. Complications include painful swelling of the testes, pancreas, ovaries and prostate. The infection may sometimes affect the brain as meningoencephalitis, or it may involve heart. Infection of the pancreas may lead to diabetes. There is no specific treatment for mumps. A highly effective vaccine is available but whether it gives lifelong immunity against infection is not known.

INFLUENZA

Influenza is a highly contagious viral infection caused by influenza virus A, B, C types. The infection is spread by droplet infection or by person-to-person contact. The incubation period is 1 to 4 days and epidemics occur every year mostly during winter months. Most infections occur in children and young adults. Influenza infection in older age group may be severe and requires hospitalization.

The typical influenza syndrome is characterized by sudden onset of fever, cough, increased nasal secretions and tears, redness of eyes, body pains, headache, weakness. Complications include secondary bacterial infection, pneumonia, asthmatic attacks, etc. The illness subsides in 3 to 6 days. In children fever, vomiting, diarrhea, nasal secretions can occur. The illness in children may mimick meningitis. In old age group acute infection may cause respiratory failure.

Epidemics of influenza occurs with both influenza A and B viruses. Type C influenza virus causes milder sporadic cases. Pandemics occur due to antigenic variation resulting in new strains to which the population have immunity or resistance to overcome the infection. Deaths due to complications are common during pandemic. Patients with underlying heart and lung disease will have more serious complications due to influenza virus infection. Influenza virus have been isolated from a wide variety of animals such as birds, dogs, horses, cats which act as the reservoir of infection. In India epidemics have occurred in summer. Influenza vaccines are not useful in the prevention of epidemics but they are indicated in elderly people with chronic underlying diseases to prevent complications.

POLIOMYELITIS

Polio viruses belong to picorna group of viruses. They are small RNA viruses. There are 3 types of polio viruses. These viruses cause an acute viral infection which is about 1 percent of cases causes central nervous system infection resulting in varying degrees of paralysis and possibly death. In India poliomyelitis continues to be a serious problem and an estimated 2,00,000 cases occur every year. The disease has been almost eradicated from developed countries due to widespread use of vaccine. Lameness surveys (Surveys based on lameness due to poliomyelitis in children) in North India indicate that the annual incidence rate is 2 to 5/1000 rural preschool children and 1 to 3/1000 urban preschool children. Similar surveys in South India suggest the prevalence rates as 3.5/1000. Poliomyelitis can occur sporadically, endemically or epidemically. Currently the originally sporadic disease has evolved itself into epidemic form and what was predominantly a disease of infants has shown a tendency to affect higher age groups.

The infection is caused by taking contaminated food or water with poliovirus from a case. The virus enters through alimentary tract. Males are more frequently affected than females and the age group is usually below 5 years. Fatigues, trauma, injections during epidemics may increase the risk of infection with poliovirus. Majority of cases occur between June to September. The incubation period is 7 to 14 days. Infections can also be transmitted through droplet infection.

The infection is characterized by subclinical infection or abortive polio or minor illness or nonparalytic polio characterized by stiffness of neck and back followed by rapid recovery and lastly paralytic polio in which the virus enters central nervous system and particularly destroys motor neuron cells resulting in flaccid paralysis, which is asymmetrical. Complications include extension of the disease to medulla resulting in respiratory paralysis (also known as bulbar polio). There is no specific treatment for polio. Good nursing care, early physiotherapy and supportive appliances like calipers may be able to rehabilitate the affected persons. Live attenuated oral vaccine prevents polio infection.

RABIES

Rabies is one of the major public health problems. This viral disease is transmitted mainly by the bite of a mad dog. Since the disease once gets established has no cure and ultimately leads to fatal death. Physicians, microbiologists, public health workers are more concerned seriously about its prevention and control.

Rabies is an acute, usually fatal virus infection of all warm-blooded animals characterized by inflammation of the central nervous system and manifested by abnormal behavior. The virus belongs to the family Rhabdoviridae and it is bullet shaped virus of 60–40 to 60–85 mm in size with a single stranded RNA as the genome. The virus is ether sensitive and relatively stable at 4°C for weeks and in the presence of glycerol it is stable at room temperature for weeks. The virus has 4 major proteins, namely glycoprotein, polypeptide, and 2 membrane proteins. The composition of virus comprises of 74% protein, 22% lipid, three percent carbohydrate and 1 percent RNA. Glycoprotein is responsible for virus neutralization; antibody and nucleoprotein antigens are for complement fixation, precipitation and fluorescent staining.

Mongoose is the major reservoir in Greneda. Except frugivorous, insectivorous, and vampire bats, in all warm-blooded animals species virus may be found in varying concentrations in central nervous system, saliva, urine, lymph, milk, blood and droppings. The incidence of rabies infection varies with respect to geographical area. In USA from 1972 to 76,82,000 cases were diagnosed in the laboratory and 1 million people received postexposure treatment. Finland, Ireland, UK, Malta, Sweden are free from rabies. Various types of rabies like sylvatic rabies, canine rabies, canine with sylvatic rabies, etc. are known to exist.

Lowest susceptible animal is opposum. Incubation period varies from 3 to 8 weeks depending upon the site of the bite. Bites on the face are more dangerous with less incubation period. Virus remains at the site for 2 weeks. There are 4 serotypes among the rabies virus. The virus multiplies in muscle or connective tissue and is propagated through the endoneurium of the Schwann cells or associated tissue spaces of the sensory nerves of the central nervous system. After multiplication it may then spread through peripheral nerves to the salivary glands and other tissues. It is not found in the blood of infected persons. When freshly isolated in the laboratory the strains are referred to as street virus, which have a long incubation period and regularly produce intracytoplasmic inclusion bodies. Inoculated animals may exhibit a long periods of excitement. In rabbits yield a "fixed" virus, which does not multiply in the extraneural tissues. The "fixed" virus multiplies rapidly with shorter incubation period and inclusion bodies are found only with difficulty.

Clinical Course

In India dogs are mainly responsible for maintaining the disease and transmitting it to human beings. Jackals, foxes, wolves, etc. maintain the disease in sylvatic areas. The possibility of rabies should always be kept in mind when wild animals, which normally avoid human beings, lose their fear of man and appear tame and attack him. Once the symptom of rabies develops in the animal it rarely survives more than a week. The saliva may be infective 3 or 4 days before the onset of clinical symptoms and during the course of illness till death. Although reports of death from rabies (hydrophobia) due to apparently healthy dog appear from time to time, unequivocal evidence has not been documented so far. Hence it is necessary to keep the dog under observation for at least 10 days, and the risk of rabies involved from the bite of an apparently healthy dog after 10 days observation period is remote indeed. Infected dogs may be excitative or paralytic.

In humans the clinical course is divided into 4 phases, a short prodromal phase, a sensory phase, a period of excitement and a paralytic or depressive phase. Usually there is an abnormal sensation at the site of bite. General sympathetic overactivity is observed. The throat muscles go into spasm on swallowing saliva or water.

Because of the patients apparent fear of water the disease has been known as hydrophobia since ancient days. Finally the patient develops convulsive seizures, coma and death within 3 to 5 days after the onset of the disease. A form of Landry's ascending paralysis was the predominant clinical picture in cases of rabies transmitted by vampire bats in Trinidad and Latin America. Penetration of the virus through digestive tract is possible. Virus travels centripetally through cell. Penetration occurs within 15 minutes.

Laboratory Diagnosis

The laboratory diagnosis comprises of:

a. Direct microscopy
b. Culture
c. Serology.

Direct Microscopy

The diagnosis of rabies has long been based on the finding of cytoplasmic inclusions known as "Negri bodies" in the nerve cells of an infected patient or animals or in the brains of inoculated laboratory animals. Impression smears of the brain tissue are often used in the microscope examination for Negri bodies. Negri bodies contain rabies virus antigens and they are variable in size and shape. They are acidophillic and intracytoplasmic.

Currently tissues infected with rabies virus are identified by direct fluorescent antibody technique with antirabies hamster serum. This is the method of choice as regards speed and accuracy of identification. Fluorescent antibody technique can be applied for corneal impressions taken from the patient for rapid diagnosis. If the examination of the animal brain by fluorescent antibody technique is negative for inclusion bodies, the bitten person need not be treated unless the bite scratch is from a bat.

Culture

Virus can be isolated from the infected tissue or saliva by intracerebral inoculation of mice or intramuscular inoculation of hamsters. The inoculated laboratory animals develop flaccid paralysis and their brains will be positive for Negri bodies. The virus can also be propagated in chick embryos, baby hamster kidney cells and human diploid cell cultures. Serially passaged flury strain in chick embryos can be used as attenuated vaccine.

Serology

Humoral response to rabies infection can be detected by detecting the specific IgG, IgM type of antibodies by virus neutralization test in laboratory mice or in cell culture system. Other techniques like complement-fixation text, detection of antibodies by immunofluorescence, ELISA or RIA. Plaque reduction technique in agarose gel suspended BHK-21-S cell line if used results will be available in 5 to 6 days instead of 12 to 14 days of mouse neutralization test. Passive hemagglutination test (PHA), complement-fixation test (CFI), hemagglutination inhibition (HAI) tests are less sensitive.

Immunofluorescence, radioimmunoassay (RIA), ELISA are more sensitive and specific. Immunolysis of rabies infected cells in the presence of complement and specific antibody can be measured by counting staining cells with trypan blue, colony inhibition of the infected cells or measurement of Cr^{51} from infected cells are some of the other techniques available for the estimation of virus specific antibodies.

Management

Since there is no specific cure for an established case of rabies, the management of rabies infection is carried out in two steps:

a. Treatment of wounds
b. Immunization.

Treatment of Wounds

In majority of cases the infection occurs through salivary contamination of the wounds caused by the bite of the animal. Hence, it is necessary to remove as much saliva as possible from the wound by proper wound toilet without causing additional trauma. After this the residual virus should be inactivated by cauterization by using either heat (in the form of applying heated needle for scortching the wound) or chemical cauterization or by applying hyperimmune antirabies serum. Immediate and appropriate wound toilet minimizes the risk of rabies greately and it is therefore, repeatedly emphasized that physicians and health workers must pay attention to it.

Wounds should be flushed thoroughly with soap and water. Then the wounded part should be cauterized with carbolic acid and neutralize it with surgical spirit for 1 minute. Other compounds like one percent benzalkonium chloride or tincture of iodine may be used. Quarternary ammonium compounds should not be used in the presence of soap. Wounds on the face should not be cauterized with strong chemicals. For such wounds hyperimmune serum or tincture iodine should be applied. Wounds should not be sutured immediately or within 24 hours of the bite. Suturing can be done after 48 to 72 hours. Wound sepsis should be prevented with appropriate antibiotic therapy. If the patient is already immunized against tetanus, a booster dose of tetanus toxoid is sufficient and there is no need for antitetanus serum (ATS) otherwise both tetanus toxoid and ATS should be administered.

Immunization

Active immunization: This is achieved by administration of inactivated virus, which may be:

a. Nervous tissue vaccine.
b. Duck embryo vaccine.
c. Purified chick embryo cell vaccine.
d. Vero cell rabies vaccine.
e. Human diploid cell culture vaccine (HDCC).
f. Hamster kidney cell vaccine.
g. Fetal bovine cell culture vaccine.
h. Dog kidney cell culture.

The above vaccines are useful in humans.

Choice of vaccine: Since there are no known side effects of HDCC vaccine it is most preferable for routine use. But this is costly and many may not be able to afford it in countries like ours. When there is a history of definite exposure the choice can rest between nervous tissue vaccine and duck embryo vaccine since the inactivated chick embryo vaccine is not an efficient immunizing agent for primary vaccination. Of the two types of vaccines, nervous tissue vaccine is the best in conferring active and efficient immunity against rabies. The antibody response with nervous tissue vaccine is preferred for the post-exposure prophylaxis. It should be remembered that the type of exposure encountered in India is definitely much more severe than that seen in Europe or America. The use of duck embryo vaccine, on the other hand, may be considered in cases where the risk involved is minimum or negligible. Inactivated chick embryo vaccine though not useful as primary immunizing agent, but it can be used for those who have to discontinue the nervous tissue vaccine due to adverse reactions. Nevertheless, nervous tissue vaccine has stood the test of time.

When to give treatment: Antirabies vaccines occasionally cause severe complications, and hence the treating physician should make sure that the exposed person really needs the post-exposure prophylaxis and at the same time since delay is dangerous, treatment should be started immediately before laboratory tests become available to know the status of the biting dog. Clinical judgment plays pivotal role. Treatment should be given:

a. If the biting animal is known to be rabid.
b. If the animal has bitten the persons indiscriminately.
c. Laboratory tests on the brain of the suspected animal are positive though the clinical signs were not typical.
d. The biting animal cannot be traced or identified.
e. If the biting animal is ill or runs away during the 10 days observation period.
f. All unprovoked bites by wild animals.
g. When a fresh wound gets soiled by the saliva of any one of the above-mentioned animal.

Not to Give Treatment

a. A bite through the clothes without tearing or piercing it and when the skin is *unbroken* though a bruise may be present.
b. Handling of animals bitten by rabid animal or contact with fomites (utensils, bedding, etc.) of rabid animals.
c. Drinking of boiled or unboiled milk from rabid animal. Class I type of treatment may be given to persons who give the history of drinking unboiled milk and if they are excessively apprehensive.
d. If the biting animal remains normal and healthy for a minimum period of 10 days after the bite in class I and class II cases only.
e. Many a time physician is in dilemma whether antirabies treatment is to be given to a person bitten by an apparently healthy dog that remained healthy for more than 10 days. Since the risk of rabies from such bites are very remote and neuroparalytic complication which is a serious personal, familial and social handicap is more frequent (1 in 7000 to 10000 in treated cases), instruction to treat every individual bitten by dog irrespective of its rabid status will not be safe. The physician should carefully assess the situation after taking full history, before starting the antirabies treatment.

Classification of Exposures and Treatment Schedule

Antirabies treatment when required should be started immediately. Since rabies has prolonged incubation period, active immunization induced is expected to prevent the development of the disease.

The incubation period and the chance of developing rabies are directly related to the amount of virus induced, site of the wound and the number of wounds inflicted by the biting animals.

Antirabies hyperimmune serum should be given to all cases of class III type together with vaccine. In such cases two more booster doses at 10 days and 20 days after the completion of full vaccination schedule is required to overcome the interference.

Class I exposure: Negligible exposure. All cases of licks (excepts those on fresh cuts or scratches). These people be given antirabies vaccine only at the rate of 2 mL, daily for 7 days irrespective of age and weight.

Class II exposure: Moderate exposure with definite risk. All bites except those on hands, neck, face, palm and finger and less than five minor wounds in number. Licks and scratches on fresh cuts drawing blood. For these patients the treatment consists of antirabies vaccine. Adults should receive 5 mL/day for 14 days. This should be followed by one booster of same dose 3 weeks after 14th injection.

Class III exposure: Severe exposure. Definite and grave risk. All bites on the neck or above palm and finger lacerated wounds anywhere in the body. Multiple bites, wolf, jackal and other wild animal bite. These cases should receive combined antirabies serum and vaccine treatment (Full course of vaccine as per class II category) upto 7 days of bite otherwise antirabies vaccine only.

Control of Rabies

In endemic countries like India both urban and sylvian forms of rabies are prevalent. The urban cycle is maintained by the stray dogs and the sylvian cycle by the carnivorous wild animals. Urban cycle is responsible 99% of the cases. Hence, control of rabies depends upon eradication of stray dog population. The pet animals can be vaccinated to prevent the infection in them.

Three types of vaccines are available for preimmunization on pet animals:

a. Veterinary avianized live virus antirabies vaccine prepared by Central Research Institute, Kasauli and it contains 33% of the infected chick embryo suspension. It should be stored at 4°C and can be used for pet dogs and cats but not for other animals.
b. Veterinary BPL antirabies vaccine which is a 20 percent suspension of sheep brain infected with modified virus and it is inactivated by β-propiolactone (BPL). It is available in 5 mL single dose. It should be given as single injection every year.
c. Veterinary BPL antirabies vaccine (multiple dose) also prepared from sheep brain and the vaccine contains five percent suspension of sheep brain infected with rabies virus and inactivated by BPL. It is used in multiple doses. For detailed vaccination schedules for various domestic animals veterinary expert should be consulted rabies infection. Bats can be controlled by using anticoagulants.

There are reports where rabies cases have recovered from infection though at present there are no specific antiviral agent to treat the established disease. Proper precautions while handling the animals, vaccination of the domestic animals, prompt post-exposure treatment and accurate maintenance of patient records, control or eradication of stray dogs will control the disease to the maximum extent. Neuroparalytic complications due to nervous tissue vaccine or serum sickness due to administration of hyperimmune serum can be avoided by careful selection of the cases after taking the full history.

Chapter 23

Parasitic Infections

INTRODUCTION

Scientifically speaking the term 'parasite' can be applied to all types of infectious agents such as bacteria, viruses and fungi. However, by convention, the name is restricted to infections caused by protozoa and helminths and excludes the other infectious agents. The grouping of protozoa and helminths is scientifically not correct because they have little in common except that they are all eukaryotic. Nevertheless, parasitology is a well-established specialization and it continues to embrace both protozoa and helminths and the same tradition is being followed for convenience in all textbooks.

Diseases due to protozoa and helminths are well known to our ancestors. Some evidence regarding the existence of parasitic diseases is available even before the written history began. Characteristic lesions of parasitic worms were found in the early sculptures and the eggs of parasites were found in Egyptian mummies and other human remaining. Apart from Greek physicians including the descriptions of Hippocrates in 5th century BC, physicians of the other civilizations such as China (3000–300 BC), India (2500–200 BC) and Rome (700 BC–400 AD) made significant contributions to human parasitology. Even, Arab authors Rhazes (850–923 AD) Avicenna (980–1077 AD) wrote important medical works pertaining to the diseases caused by various parasites. Tropical diseases emerged as a distinct branch of medicine by 1898, when Sir Patrick Manson published his first classical book on tropical diseases and he is considered as 'Father of tropical medicine.' He described many diseases like malaria, sleeping sickness, amebic dysentery, kala azar that are due to parasites invading the humans. Subsequently between 1870 and 1920 several workers, succeeded in establishing the etiologies of the classic group of vector-borne parasitic diseases.

Parasitic diseases have been always fascinating to travelers, clinicians and scientists. Some of the parasitic diseases are unique to tropical countries, while others are not only important to tropical countries but also even to temperate regions. Finally, some parasitic diseases are worldwide in distribution. Improved hygiene and living conditions played an important role in the control of many of these diseases in the developed countries. Thus, many parasites that were once widespread are now found only in warmer and developing countries of the world and considered as exotic diseases when imported in to the cooler northern and southern latitude where they were once prevalent.

Discoveries in parasitology with respect to protozoa and helminths have followed the parallel pathways and converged at the turn of the 19th century when Patrick Manson published his textbook on 'Tropical diseases.'

Because of their small size, protozoa could not be appreciated until the discovery of microscope by Antoni van Leeuwenhoek toward the end of 17th century. All the members of scientific community agree that the first person to see parasitic protozoa was Anthony van Leeuwenhoek, who observed *Giardia* spp in his own fecal specimen. Curiously, it was only after 140 years later the other parasitic protozoa were described.

Helminthic worms are large and easily recognizable and are the common parasites of the domestic pet animals as well as wild animals. Thus, they were well studied by zoologists who were interested in comparative zoology and treated these parasites in the same way as other group of animals. Nevertheless, the clinicians and veterinary experts soon noticed the implications of these infections in domesticated animals and in humans. The history of parasitology embraces some of the most exiting discoveries ever made in medicine and these findings paved the way to the discovery of other diseases such as vector-borne filariasis, malaria and the mosquito-borne yellow fever, the whole field of arboviruses, trypanasomiasis, borreliosis and plague.

Remarkably most of the great discoveries in parasitology were made within a short period of 30 years spanning 1885 to 1915, the period during which major advances were also made concerning other infectious agents. In short, the history of parasitic diseases has a number of phases: the recognition of the disease, the identification of the organism involved, establishing the common connection between the organism and the disease, consolidation of all these observations and application of the knowledge to control schemes.

ENTAMOEBA HISTOLYTICA

The motile form of *E. histolytica,* the trophozoite is highly dynamic and pleomorphic cell and its motility is influenced by several factors like changes in temperature, redox potential, pH and osmolarity. The trophozoite form is actively motile with protruding lobopodia and trailing uroid. The resting stage of the trophozoites is spherical. The size of the trophozoites varies from 10 to 60 µm. The cell surface has numerous circular micropinocytic vesicles which are absent from the large protruding stoma of macropinocytic channels and lobopodia. The uroid if present appears as tail with irregular folds of membrane and filiform processes called filopodia (Fig. 23.1).

The plasma membrane, which is 10 nm thick, is covered with uniform surface coat mainly composed of glycoprotein. The lectin concanavalin A binds to the surface of the trophozoites indicating the presence of high content of sugar residues. Interaction of the plasma proteins with specific ligands results in capping of sugar molecules that may be one of the mechanisms of evasion of host humoral immune responses. The capping mechanism involves actin and myosin regulated by calmodulin and myosin light chain kinase. The cytoplasm of

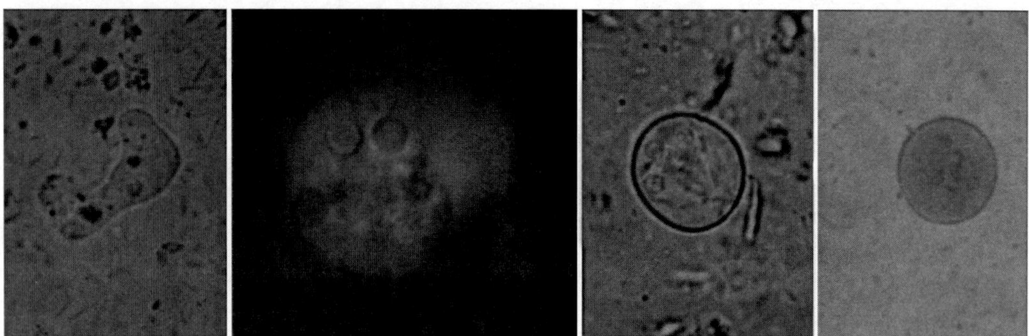

Fig. 23.1: Trophozoite and cyst form of *Entamoeba histolytica*. Note the presence of RBC within the cytoplasm of *E. histolytica* trophozoite form *(For color version, see Plate 7)*

E. histolytica is devoid of mitochondria, Golgi apparatus, endoplasmic reticulum, centrioles and microtubules. Instead, it contains a number of vacuoles that are variable in size. The vacuoles include phagocytic vacuoles, macro- and micropinocytic vacuoles, lysosomes, residual bodies, autophagic vacuoles and food vacuoles. Food vacuoles contain starch and bacteria. Amoebae recovered from dysentery stools contain ingested red blood cells that are considered as the best evidence for invasiveness. The lysosomes of *E. histolytica* differ in that the enzymes are bound to lysosomal membranes. Ribosomes are mostly arranged in helical arrays that are 300 nm length and 40 nm width. In resting trophozoites and cysts, the helices aggregate into large crystalline inclusions that can be several micrometers in length forming classical chromatoid body with an hexagonal packing pattern. The biological significance and the nature of the cylindrical particles present in the cytoplasm is not known.

The nucleus of *E. histolytica* is 4 to 7 µm in diameter, and the nuclear membrane appears to be a double membrane interrupted by several nuclear pores and lined by thin uniform layer of granules that gives the nucleus, the appearance of ring in optical sections. The karyosome is small spherical mass located centrally in the nucleus. The significance of intranuclear bodies that are seen is not known.

The cysts are round or oval hyaline bodies surrounded by refractile cell wall. The plasma membrane frequently shows invaginations. The polyribosomes and vacuoles filled with dense fibrogranular material are found close to cytoplasmic space. As the cyst matures, the food vacuoles disappear. Chromatoid bars, which are aggregated ribosomes, can be seen *within* the cytoplasm as rod-shaped structures with blunt or round ends. The cyst contains 1 to 4 nuclei depending upon its maturity.

Under unfavorable conditions, the trophozoites undergo encystation and produce four nucleated mature cysts.

These spherical, hyaline structures with refractile wall are excreted along with the feces.

The cysts can survive in the environment for several days. They are relatively resistant to chemicals like mercuric chloride, chlorine and temperature.

The cysts are ingested along with the contaminated water, food and raw vegetables. The cysts pass the stomach unchanged.

In the terminal ileum, each cyst releases 8-uninuleated amoebulae that mature and are capable of invading the intestinal epithelium. Thus, the cycle continues (Fig. 23.2).

The cystic forms of the parasite are ingested through contaminated water and food, and the transmission of infection is by feco-oral route. The cysts traverse the stomach unchanged since they are resistant to the action of hydrochloric acid of the stomach. The cysts once they reach the terminal part of the ileum undergo excystation, and each of four nucleated cyst releases eight amoebulae. The amebulae mature and become trophozoites. The trophozoites get attached to the epithelial cells of the intestinal mucosa with the help of the adhesion molecules present on its surface. The lytic factor causes dissolution of the cells and the matrix. As a result, the trophozoites gain entrance into the submucosal layer and initiate inflammatory reaction due to invasion. The trophozoites actively digest the mucosa and submucosa producing flask-shaped ulcers. Invasion of the colonic and cecal

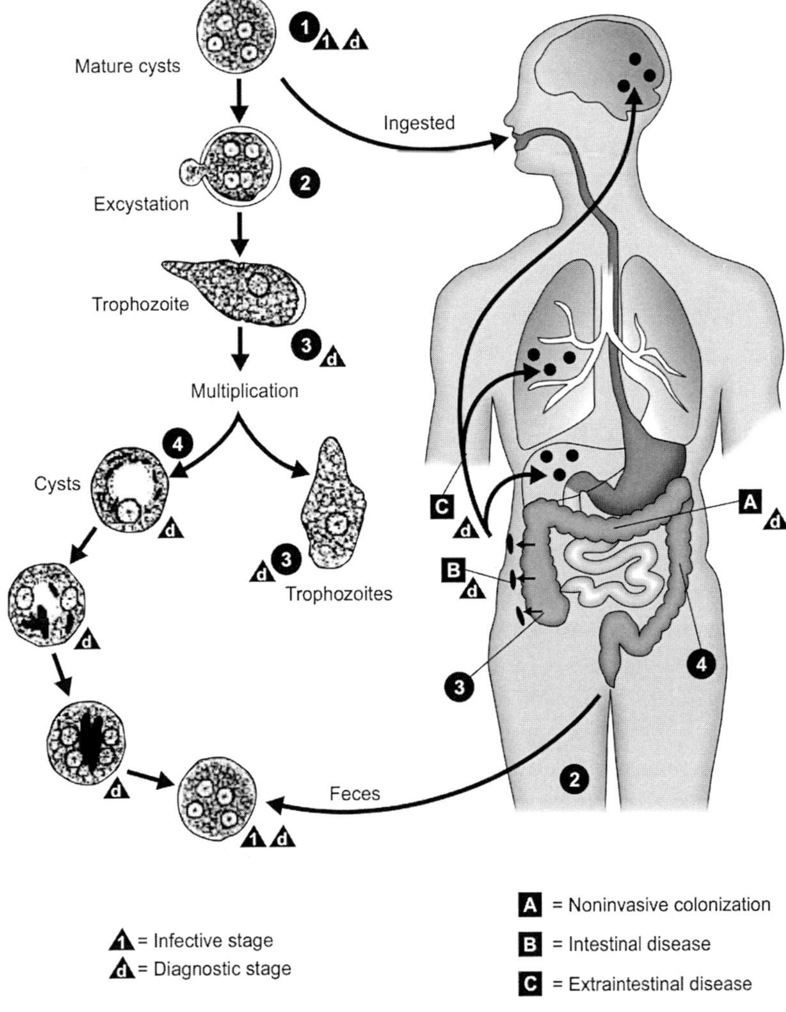

Fig. 23.2: Life cycle of *Entamoeba histolytica*

mucosa begins in inter glandular epithelium. The trophozoites produce rapid lysis of the surrounding inflammatory cells and the tissue that results in necrosis.

Because of rapid lysis of the inflammatory cells, acute inflammation is seldom seen in invasive amebiasis. The ulcers are pinhead in size but under the mucosa, flask-shaped ulcers are seen. The ulcers are extended into submucosa and produce abundant microhemorrhages. The trophozoites often show erythrophagocytosis. The mucosa between the ulcers is normal. The ulcers are initially superficial, hyperemic with a necrotic base. The ulcers may further invade muscle layer and serosa. Complications of intestinal amoebiasis include perforation, direct extension to the skin and hematogeneous dissemination. The presence and the extent of liver involvement are no way related to the severity of intestinal amebiasis and these two conditions need not coexist. The initial pathology of amebic liver abscess has not been studied in humans. In experimental animals, inoculation of trophozoites into the portal vein results in multiple foci of infection in the liver with neutrophil infiltration around the parasites followed by focal necrosis and granulomatous infiltration. As the infection progresses, the granulomas become necrotic and coalesce and the necrotic tissue occupies the major portion of the liver. Hepatocytes that are close to the lesion are degenerated and necrosed. Direct contact of trophozoites with hepatocytes is rare. Finally, infection progresses to a large area of liquefied necrotic material surrounded by a thin capsule.

Infection due to *E. histolytica* is ubiquitous with an incidence of 10% among the world population. The infection is very common among the communities with poor socio-economic background, lack of safe drinking water, inadequate sanitation and poor hygiene. According to World Health Organization (WHO), about 500 million people (except those in China) are infected and upto 100,000 deaths can be attributed to the complications of invasive amoebiasis. The exact incidence of amebiasis is difficult to estimate because there is a tendency of over diagnosis in endemic areas and in low endemic areas, there is a tendency to overlook the diagnosis. The main reservoir of *E. histolytica* is human population. Human susceptibility to infection is widespread but most of the individuals harboring the parasite remain asymptomatic. Most of the asymptomatic carriers harbor *E. dispar* but some individuals may carry *E. histolytica* without any clinical symptoms. Follow-up studies showed that 90% of the carriers remained asymptomatic and underwent spontaneous cure. Only 10% of the infected population may develop amebic colitis depending upon the host and the parasite relation-ship. Luminal amebiasis has shown an increased incidence among the homosexuals. Most reported cases are asymptomatic or present with diffuse symptoms except in homosexuals in Japan. *E. dispar* is most commonly identified. The available data on invasive amebiasis based on microscopy and sigmoidoscopy are very divergent. The figures vary from 2.2 to 16.2 percent among the patients with diarrhea or dysentery. The case fatality rate also ranges from 0.5 to 40.2 percent depending upon the development of complications. Liver abscess is a reliable marker of rates of liver infection and two percent of adult amebiasis patients develop amebic liver abscess. Amebic liver abscess is at least 10 times more common in adults than in children and it is three time more common in men than in women of the same age group between 20 and 60 years. The reason for the age and sex predilection of the infection is not known Table 23.1.

Table 23.1: Clinical features of amebiasis

Classification	*Characteristics*
Asymptomatic intestinal infection	Colonization without tissue invasion
Symptomatic intestinal infection	Tissue invasion
Amebic dysentery	Fulminant ulcerative intestinal disease
Nondysentery colitis	Ulcerative intestinal disease
Ameboma	Proliferative granulomas of the intestine
Complicated intestinal amoebiasis	Perforation, hemorrhage and fistula
Post-amebic colitis	Unknown mechanism
Nonspecific hepatomegaly	No demonstrable invasion accompanies intestinal infection
Acute nonspecific infection	Amebae in the liver without abscess
Amebic abscess	Focal structural lesion
Amebic abscess complicated	Direct extension to pleura, lungs, pericardium and peritoneum
Amebiasis cutis	Direct extension to the skin
Visceral amebiasis	Metastatic infection of the lung, brain and spleen

Morbidity and mortality due to invasive amebiasis have greatly reduced with the use of amebicidal drugs. The most useful luminal amebicidal drugs are diiodohydroxyquin, 650 mg three times a day for three weeks or diloxanide furoate 500 mg three times per day for 10 days. The amebicidal drugs effective in tissues are emetine and dihydroemetine but currently they are not in use because of their cardio toxic effects. Chloroquine, which acts in the liver, is a useful tissue amebocide. Metronidazole, tinidazole and ornidazole are useful both as luminal and tissue amebicidal drugs. There is no drug resistance in amebiasis. Surgery is indicated in cases of appendicitis and toxic mega colon. Amebic lesions heal without any scarring once adequate treatment is initiated.

Food handlers should be frequently checked. Personal hygiene should be improved with adequate washing of the hands before serving the food or beverages. Houseflies and cockroaches should be controlled. Only those asymptomatic individuals carrying *E. histolytica* should be treated with appropriate antiamebic drugs. *E. dispar* carriers are closely monitored for the possibility of developing *E. histolytica* infection. Continuous training is required for the technical persons to improve their accuracy in identifying the cysts in the fecal specimens. The physicians are periodically appraised of the advances in the diagnostic and therapeutic modalities of amebiasis.

GIARDIA LAMBLIA

The genus *Giardia* has two names. The term *Giardia* is used in Western countries and *Lamblia* in USSR and Eastern Europe. Approximately 40 species have been identified based on morphology. Among them *Giardia duodenalis* is the common species that infects humans frequently. However, there is no rigid host specificity. *Giardia* holds a special place in the affection of all protozoologists because it was the first animal parasitic protozoan ever to be seen. *Giardia* was first discovered by Antoni van Leeuwenhoek in1681 in his own fecal specimen but this observation did not gain any attention until 1859, when Vilem Lambl described the parasite. The parasite received little attention until the World War II.

Giardia species are worldwide in distribution apparently more prevalent in children and more common in areas with warm climate. It is most commonly diagnosed flagellate in the intestinal tract and it is the most commonly diagnosed intestinal pathogen in some parts of the world. Although, several parameters such as morphology, host specificity and other structural variations have been used to differentiate the species of *Giardia*, there is still no common understanding over the nomenclature and classification of this group of organisms. Filice, based on structural variations, proposed three groups; amphibian *Giardia* (*Giardia agilis*), *Giardia muris* from rodents and birds, *Giardia intestinalis* from humans, birds and reptiles. Parasitologists use the terms, intestinalis and lamblia. Meyer preferred the term intestinalis. *Giardia lamblia* is commonly used and this tends to eliminate any confusion. Some are of the opinion that *Giardia duodenalis* is taxonomically correct name for the species and refers to many species containing the duodenalis double medial bodies.

The parasite exists in two forms namely the trophozoite and cyst. The trophozoite is usually seen as teardrop shaped from the front with posterior end being pointed. The trophozoite when seen from the side resembles the curved portion of a spoon. The concave portion is the area of the sucking disk. The trophozoite has 4 pairs of flagella and it is binucleated. It has two axonemes and two slightly curved bodies called median bodies. The trophozoite measures 10–20 µm in length and 5 to 15 µm in breadth. It stains well with trichrome and iron-hematoxylin. The cyst is either round or oval and it contains 4 nuclei, axonemes and median bodies. The cyst normally measures 11 to 14 µm × 7 to 10 µm in size. Some cysts appear to be shrunk and one may see two halos, one around the cyst and the other inside the cyst wall. The halo effect is particularly prominent in permanently stained smears (Fig. 23.3).

The trophozoites are intestinal dwelling stages and attach to the intestinal epithelium of the host villi by means of the ventral disc. The attachment process probably involves multiple mechanism involving microtubule mediation, hydrodynamic action and contractile protein activity. The trophozoites are mainly seen in the crypts of duodenum. Cyst formation

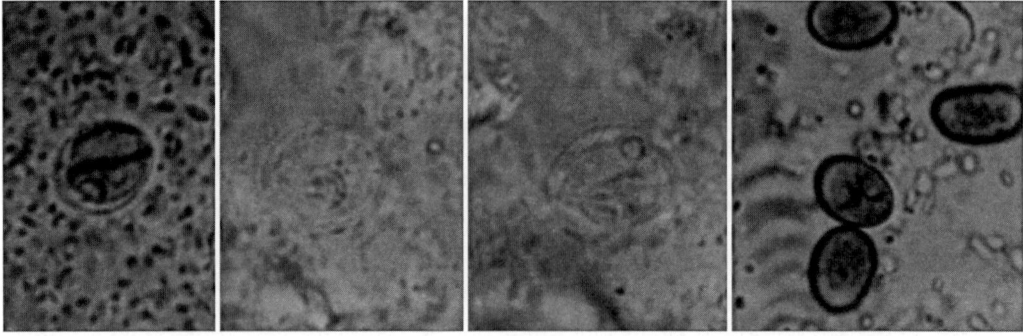

Fig. 23.3: Trophozoites and cysts of *Giardia lamblia* (*For color version, see Plate 7*)

takes place as the organism moves down through the colon. Conjugated bile salts are known to promote encystation. Cholesterol starvation may also stimulate encystation. The trophozoites retract flagella in to axonemes and the cytoplasm is condensed. The cyst wall is secreted. The cyst matures and the internal structures are doubled so that when excystation takes place, two trophozoites are produced. The encystation occurs in the duodenum or in the appropriate culture medium *in vitro*. The cysts are ingested through the contaminated food and water and they reach duodenum where they are transformed in to trophozoites. The trophozoites, as they move down through the colon they become encysted and are excreted in to the feces (Fig. 23.4).

An inflammatory reaction in the lamina propria is the frequent finding in acute *Giardia infection*. Sensitized lymphocytes may be responsible for mucosal damage. The organism may be found in large numbers in the crypts of duodenal mucosa but they may not cause any pathological changes. The organisms feed on mucosal secretions and do not penetrate the mucosa.

High incidence of giardiasis has been shown to occur in individuals with immune deficiencies such as common variable hypogammaglobulinemia. Giardiasis is the most common cause of diarrhea in these patients and it is associated with mild to severe villous atrophy. Successful treatment of giardiasis results in symptomatic cure and improvement in mucosal abnormalities except nodular lymphoid hyperplasia. Acute and chronic inflammatory cells have been found in the lamina propria together with increased mitoses. In the lamina propria, the plasma cells producing IgM and IgG are increased whereas local production of IgA is decreased. Patients with decreased immunoglobulin levels show more severe damage to the villi. Direct damage to enterocytes triggers both humoral and cell-mediated immune response in the lamina propria as well as in the lumen. Deficiencies of disaccharidases, peptide hydrolases and enteropeptidases activity has been documented. Vigorous immune response results in the elimination of the organism. This may contribute to the intestinal alterations with acute explosive and frequently self-limiting infection on one hand, to asymptomatic cyst passers on the other hand. Humoral immunity plays important role in the elimination of the organism. Re-infection is very common and chronic infection is more marked in patients with defective humoral immune response. Acute inflammatory response within the epithelial cells of intestine, destruction and thickening of villi, high turnover of intestinal epithelium suggests hypersensitivity to antigens of *Giardia* species.

All diagnosed cases of giardiasis should be treated. However, the therapy is controversial depends on the geographical region. In most of the cases of giardiasis, the infection can be eliminated with quinacrine but its side effects like nausea, vomiting, headache, dizziness, vertigo, hyperhidrosis, fever, pruritus, corneal edema and myalgias may result in discontinuation of the treatment. Metronidazole is very effective but it has potential carcinogenic effect. Tinidazole has been proven more effective than metronidazole as it can be given as single dose therapy. Furazolidone is often used for treating the children, and paramomycin has been suggested for pregnant women.

In the absence of clear-cut parasitological diagnosis, the treatment of suspected cases of giardiasis is a common question with no clear-cut answer. The most commonly

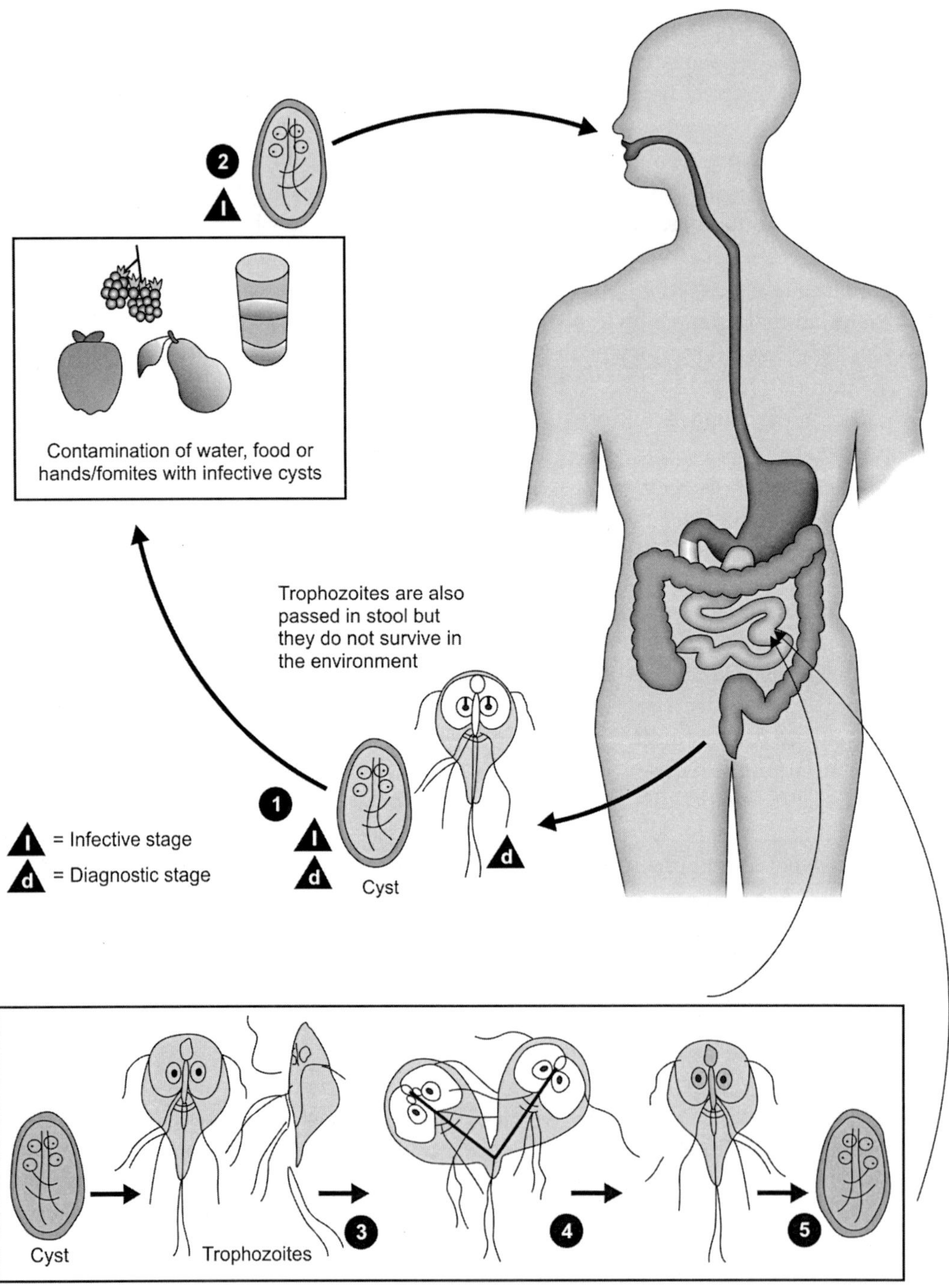

Fig. 23.4: Life cycle of *Giardia lamblia*

used drugs for treating giardiasis are also effective against other organisms including *Entemoeba histolytica*. With respect to the treatment of asymptomatic patients, generally it is recommended that all proven cases of giardiasis should be treated because the infection is known to cause sub-clinical malabsorption, symptoms are often periodic and may appear later and carriers are potential source of infection to others. In high endemic areas, the benefit for cost ratio has to be kept in mind.

Personal hygiene, improved sanitary measures use of iodine compounds to disinfect drinking water, use of appropriate effective filtration systems, proper handling of cooked food, use of boiled water for drinking purpose, control of insects are some of the measures that would lead to decrease in the overall numbers of the infection.

TRICHOMONAS VAGINALIS

The genus *Trichomonas* described by Donnē in 1837, comprises of trophozoites with four free flagella, one along the outer margin of the undulating membrane, a costa at the base, an undulating membrane and an axostyle. Of the 3 to 5 Trichomonad species found in the humans, only *Trichomonas vaginalis* has the capacity to produce disease in humans. Human trichmoniasis is essentially a cosmopolitan, sexually transmitted disease and persists despite the availability of effective therapeutic agents and little evidence of development of significant drug resistance. The clinical symptoms range from a mild or in apparent to one resulting due to chronic and substantial level of inflammation in the female reproductive system. Significant urethritis in men has been described. Rare cases of perinatal infections of female children born to infected mothers have been documented.

Honiberg and King first documented the classical description of the morphology of this urogenital flagellated pathogen in 1964. The parasite is typically pyriform in shape but ameboid-shaped trophozoites are seen in parasites adhering to the mammalian cells. The parasite may vary in size and shape with an average length and width being 10 µm and 7 µm, respectively. In axenic cultures, the shape tends to be uniform. The non-dividing parasite possesses 4 anterior flagella. The parasite also has an undulating membrane and a costa, which originate in the kinetosomal complex at the anterior position of the parasite (Fig. 23.5). It has a single ovoid nucleus at the anterior end and in the cytoplasm, the chromatin granules are typically arranged in two rows along the costa and in three rows along the axostyle. These granules are known as hydrogenosomes. The life cycle of the organism is simple and it multiplicates by longitudinal binary fission. There is no cystic form in the life cycle of *Trichomonas vaginalis*. Different morphological forms without flagella, observed in cultures are thought to be the developmental forms preceding the appearance of mononuclear flagellate, rather than the different stages of the life cycle.

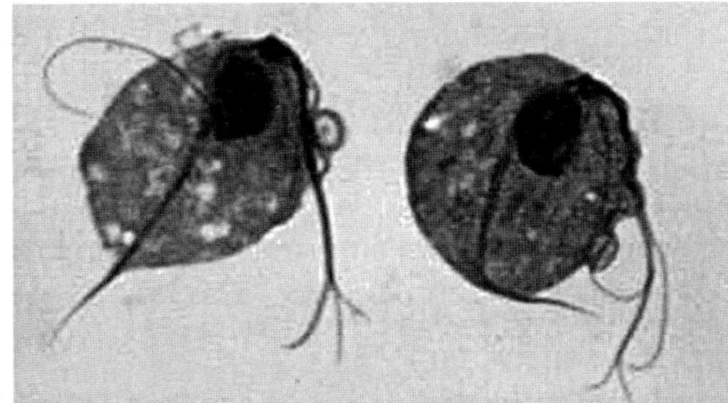

Fig. 23.5: *Trichomonas vaginalis*
(For color version, see Plate 7)

Although Donne described *Trichomonas vaginalis* in 1836, Hohne recognized its role as a cause of vaginitis only after 80 years in 1916. Hogue in 1943 reported the pathogenic effects of the parasite on the cells in cultures and suggested that the parasite directly damages host cells. Trichmoniasis is a frequently reported sexually transmitted disease and a common cause of vaginitis and endocervicitis. Children born to infected mothers may show low birth weight probably due to tissue damage by the cytopathic effect of the parasite on the mammalian cells. The 'strawberry cervix' appearance of the exocervix is due to extravasations of blood resulting in petechiae (not ulceration) and is not generally due to inflammation.

Human trichmoniasis is worldwide in distribution and it is one of the sexually-transmitted diseases that causes significant morbidity, emotional and economic burden on the community. The parasite was considered as harmless for a long time, but at present, its role as primary pathogen of human genitourinary tract is undisputable.

In recent years, the incidence of human trichmoniasis is increasing and has emerged as the most common sexually transmitted disease of parasitic origin and common cause of non-viral sexually transmitted disease. In India, 6.8 to 10 percent of the women attending the gynecology clinics are infected with *Trichomonas vaginalis.* The incidence of the infection is significantly high among the contraceptive users (7.3%), antnatal women (7.5%) and in women with gynecological disorders it is 9.2%. It is lower in postnatal women (3.6%) and in infertile women it is 2.8 percent.

Most of the infected men are asymptomatic and the infection is generally self-limiting. Though the exact incidence in men is not known, some studies suggest a median prevalence of 11% among the men with non-gonococcal urethritis. It has been observed in India that one out of 40 gonococcal urethritis cases has been found to harbor *Trichomonas vaginalis.* The rate of transmission from men to women appears to be higher than the other way round. In men, it appears that the disease is often self-limiting and the parasites are cleared spontaneously. About 2 to 17 percent of female offsprings acquire infection during the perinatal period.

Person infected with *Trichomonas vaginalis* may be asymptomatic yet may still suffer from infection. In females, the vaginitis may be of varying severity. Asymptomatic patients may develop infection at a later stage. Clinical symptoms in females include purulent vaginal discharge, pruritus and dyspareunia. Leukorrhea and dysuria are rarely observed. Vaginal discharge may be malodorous only in 10% of the infected females. The vaginal discharge may be yellow-green and frothy in about eight percent of the patients. About 50% of the infected females may show purulent discharge. Diffuse vulvar erythema and copious discharge are often present. Punctate hemorrhages of the cervix may result a strawberry-like appearance in a very small percentage of the patients. Pruritus, particularly vulvar itching is frequently reported clinical finding.

Metronidazole, tinidazole and ornidazole are the choice of drugs for the treatment of trichmoniasis. However, WHO recommends only metronidazole. Tinidazole and metronidazole have comparable efficiency when used in single dose regimens. The single dose treatment is highly effective when both partners are treated simultaneously but it will not protect them from reinfection from an untreated sexual partner. Systemic treatment is preferred to treat trichmoniasis because of its multifocal nature. Local treatment may fail because of endogenous reinfection by the parasite harbored in urethra and periurethral glands.

Control of trichmoniasis should include:

1. Thorough examination to detect the infectious status of the patient
2. Continued surveillance by public health agencies
3. Appropriate treatment to all infected individuals and their partners
4. Studies should be conducted to understand the role of certain surface antigens and secreted antigen molecules in the protective immunity against the organism
5. New target antigens should be identified and the antigens responsible for effective protection are to be characterized for development of effective vaccine.

LEISHMANIA

Several species of the genus *Leishmania* are the causative agents of the disease leishmaniasis that is transmitted by an insect vector, sand fly. The disease is prevalent in various forms both in the New World and in Old World. Human leishmaniasis can occur as an accidental infection acquired from naturally infected wild animals. Hoare in 1938, Garnham in 1986 and Manson-Bahr in 1996 described the history of Old World leishmaniasis. William Leishman and Charles Donovan are considered as first discoverers of the intracellular parasite known as Leishman-Donovan bodies. By middle of 1910, enough evidence was accumulated to incriminate sand flies belonging to the genus *Phlebotomus* as the vectors of transmission of the parasite causing leishmaniasis. Because of the small size of the vector, it took several years to confirm its role in the transmission of Leishmania parasite and in 1921 experimental proof of transmission from a sand fly to human being was documented by Edourd Sergent and Etienne Sergent (Known as Sergent brothers). The final proof for the transmission of infection by the bite of sand fly was established in 1941.

The New World leishmaniasis has been recognized in the sculptures since 5th century and in the writings of Spanish missionaries since 16th century. Earlier it was thought that the New World form of leishmaniasis and the Old World form of leishmaniasis were the same but in 1911 Gaspar Vianna found that the parasites in South America were different from those in Africa and India and he created a new species, *Leishmania brasiliensis*. Initially there was some controversy about the status of the New World visceral leishmaniasis, nevertheless in 1937, a separate species of *Leishmania chagasi* named in the honor of the great Brazilian pathologist Carlos Chagas and the species was confirmed by molecular and biochemical studies as separate species. Apart from the genus *Phlebotomus,* the species of the genus *Lutzomyia* were also involved in the transmission of the Leishmania parasites. The complex pattern of species of the parasite, the vector, reservoir host and the disease pattern have been elaborated by Ralph Lainson in 1996.

At present there are five species of Leishmania that are responsible for Old World leishmaniasis; *Leishmania major, Leishmania tropica, Leishmania aethiopica, Leishmania donovani* and *Leishmania infantum*. Among these five species, the first three are the causative agents of cutaneous leishmaniasis and the rest two species are the predominant agents of visceral leishmaniasis. In addition to these five species, there are other species, some of which are closely related but not identical to the well-established species.

The genus *Leishmania* one of the several genera within the family Trypanasomatidae (Class: Kinetoplastida; Order: Trypanosomatida). The differences between *Leishmania* and *Trypanasoma* are listed in the Table 23.2.

The parasite, *Leishmania* spp exist in two morphological forms. The amasitogote form is oval, nonmotile and it is largely intracellular. The promastigotes are elongate, spindle shaped, motile and it is mainly extracellular. The amasitogote form, which is oval, measures 3 to 5 µm in size. Giemsa stained smears under light microscope show central round nucleus and a row or rod-shaped kinetoplast. The surface membrane is a conventional unit membrane under which is a corset of microtubules are seen that serve as the cytoskeleton and makes the cell robust (Fig. 23.6). Flagellum emerges from flagellar pocket, which is an infolding of the surface membrane. The flagellum is nonfunctional and the amasitogote form is nonmotile. The kinetoplast is a dense mass of mitochondrial DNA. The kinetoplast DNA is composed of several circular DNA molecules, which can be grouped in two sizes. The cytoplasm contains both rough and smooth endoplasmic reticulum, Golgi complex and lysosomes with unique glycosome. The promastigotes are introduced in to the skin of humans by the bite of a sand fly. The promastigotes are soon transformed to amasitogote forms. The precise mechanism involved in the transformation of promastigotes form to amasitogote form and their uptake by the skin macrophages remains unclear. The transformation takes place mainly in the host cell and the time taken for complete transformation varies from 12 to 24 hours according to *in vitro* studies. The parasite remains as amasitogote form for the rest of the mammalian phase of the life cycle. The parasite grows and multiplies within the cells and is intermittently released to infect new macrophages. This phase is chronic and may last from months-to-years or even lifetime. The further course of infection varies widely between individuals ad there is a strong influence of the host genetics on the susceptibility to infection. The location of the infected cells varies with the type of the disease.

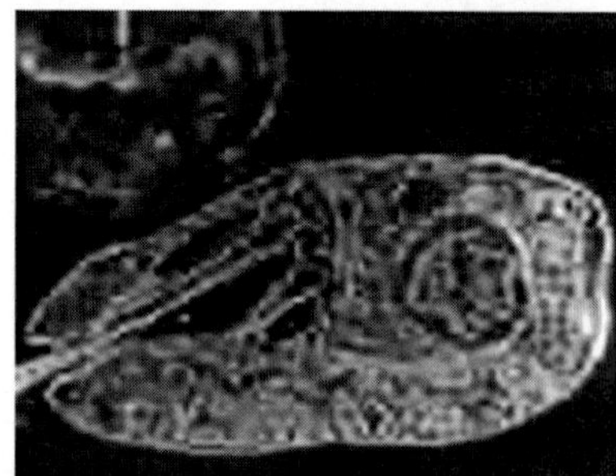

Fig. 23.6: *Leishmania*
(*For color version, see Plate 7*)

Table 23.2: Comparison of leishmania and trypanosoma

Leishmania	*Trypanosoma*
Species infecting the mammals are homogeneous	Trypanosomes are more heterogeneous
Only two morphological forms are seen	Morphologically three forms are seen. The trypomastigotes are extremely variable in size and shape
All species are transmitted by sand flies belonging to the genera Phlebotomus and Lutzomyia	The species are transmitted by a wide variety of vectors like leeches and insects
The range of mammalian species that they infect is comparatively restricted	The range of mammalian hosts are very wide
Invades only mononuclear phagocytic system	Invades all types of cells especially muscle, glial vascular endothelium and mononuclear cells

From the infected mammalian host, the parasite is transmitted to sand fly when a female sand fly bites the infected host for its blood meal. Sand flies are poor feeders. They possess cutting mouthparts that slice in to the skin and they feed from the small pool of the blood that seeps into the wound. Parasites causing the cutaneous lesions enter sand fly along with the blood meal if the fly feeds on a cutaneous lesion. In visceral leishmaniasis the parasites are predominantly found in the liver, spleen or bone marrow and the sand fly gets infected from the infected macrophages or monocytes released from the bone marrow. Infected monocytes may reside in the skin to act as a source of the parasite. It is to be noted that in most of the endemic foci the acquisition of *Leishmania* parasites by individual sand flies is a rare event and a vast number of sand flies are uninfected. Those that are infected are the efficient vectors.

The phase of life cycle of the parasite in sand fly is relatively acute and the flies that acquire the *Leishmania* infection remain infected for life. The transformation of amasitogote forms in to promastigotes forms in the sand fly is relatively rapid and it may be as short as 5 to 7 days under optimal conditions. Development occurs exclusively in the gut. The infected macrophages disintegrate to release amastigotes or free amastigotes may be found in the blood meal. Their transformation to promastigote forms occur within 48 hours and might be completed within 5 to 7 days. The promastigotes grow and multiply in the sand fly gut. The mammalian infective forms, the metacyclic promastigotes are accumulated in the anterior mid gut and the foregut of the sand fly. When the infected female sand fly is ready to take the blood meal the transmission to a mammalian host occurs. The number of promastigotes required to initiate infection in a mammalian host is not known and it varies with the host. It is generally believed that the required number may range from 10 to 100 although a single infective promastigote is sufficed to cause the infection (Fig. 23.7).

Clinical diagnosis mainly depends upon awareness and a recent history of travel to an endemic area. Visceral leishmaniasis does not show any unique signs and symptoms. Diagnosis by therapeutic trial is commonly practiced but it is not satisfactory because the drugs are expensive. Visceral leishmaniasis may be mistaken for malaria that failed to respond to treatment. The patient in the late stage may present with low-grade fever, loss of weight and hepatosplenomegaly. The patient is remarkably alert and feels well considering his condition. The skin sometimes appears 'muddy' or dark. Persistent diarrhea is frequently seen. Lymphadenopathy is an irregular finding. Blood picture may show neutropenia, pancytopenia, anemia and hypergammaglobulinemia. Several diseases like malaria, trypanasomiasis, brucellosis, schistosomiasis, tularemia, tropical splenomegaly, amoebic liver abscess, myeloid leukemia, lymphoma, histoplasmosis and thalassemia are to be considered in the differential diagnosis. Diagnosis of leishmaniasis in HIV infected patients is difficult due to atypical presentation, serological tests are not reliable, and they may be negative.

All forms of cutaneous leishmaniasis are usually present without any systemic disease. Typical lesions of oriental sore are easily recognized with raised edges, necrotic exudative center with granulomatous base, long duration and its painless nature. Less typical lesions may present in various forms that require differentiation from basal cell carcinoma, tuberculosis, fungal infections and lepromatous leprosy. Leishmaniasis recidivans may be

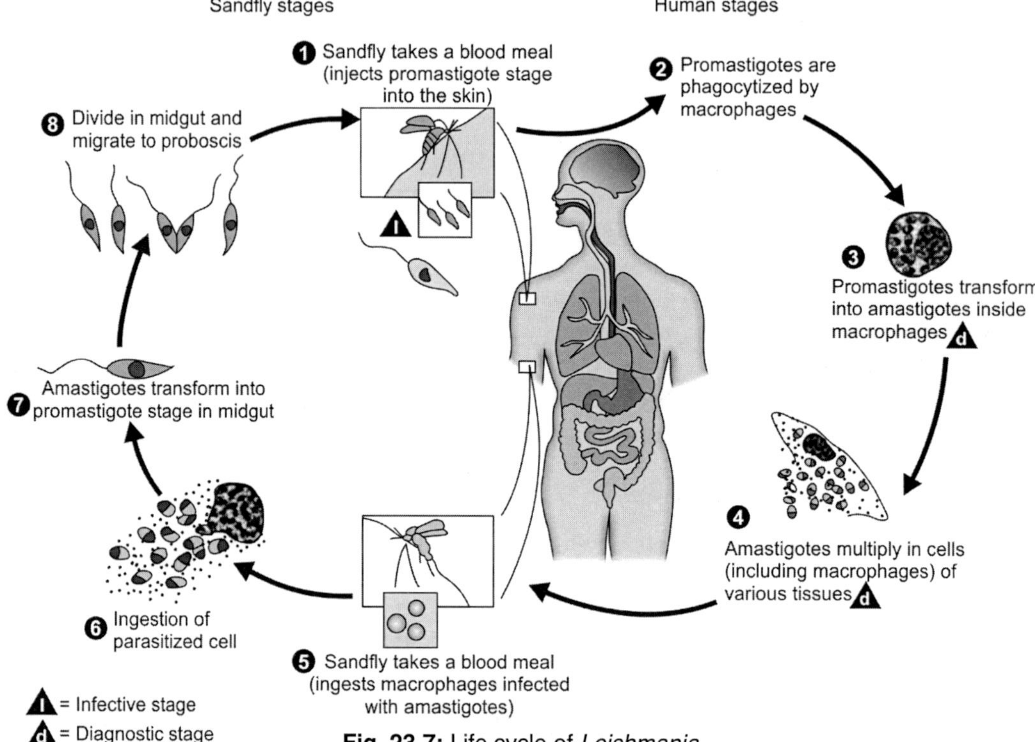

Fig. 23.7: Life cycle of *Leishmania*

indicated by the presence of scar or a positive skin test. Diffuse cutaneous leishmaniasis shows no ulcerations and may be negative for a skin test with *Leishmania* antigen.

The drug of choice at present is meglumine antimonate or sodium stibogluconate, which replaced tartar emetic many years ago. Intraleisonal infiltration is useful for simple lesions but intramuscular injection is preferred in all other types of disease. Even though the treatment is prolonged, the drug is relatively safe and free from toxicity if administered in correct dosage.

The second drug of choice is pentamidine as isethionate or dimethyl sulfonate and it is used in cases that are not responding to the antimony compounds. This drug has serious side effects due to sensitivity at the site of intramuscular injection, too rapid intravenous administration, accumulation of the drug or due to over dosage. The drug may cause intractable diabetes due to disruption of blood-sugar homeostasis.

The antibiotics like monomycin, paromomycin or aminosidine can be used either as intraleisonal injection or as a topical application for cutaneous leishmaniasis. The drug is incorporated in collagen and applied to the lesions lightly. Topical application causes too severe irritation or inflammation. These antibiotics show synergism when used in combination with antimalarial drugs both in visceral and cutaneous types of leishmaniasis.

Amphotericin B is useful in cases where other drugs have failed to cure the infection. The drug is too toxic and administered slowly by intravenous route. The initial doses must be reduced to minimize the side effects. The drug is rarely indicated for Old World leishmaniasis.

Control of leishmaniasis greatly depends upon local information about the prevalence of the disease. Avoiding the areas of risk is the simplest method that could be applied to military and other activities involving entry in to semi-arid areas where zoonotic *L. major* can be a serious risk. As a part of environmental management, destruction of desert rodent colonies in inhabited areas has been attempted with great success. In areas where transmission peridomestic is seen with *L. tropica* or *L. donovani* in Asia, sand fly numbers can be greatly reduced by appropriate insecticides. In fact antimalarial campaigns were credited with near eradication of kala-azar in India. Experiments with insecticide impregnated bed-nets or curtains have given promising results. Where transmission is sylvatic, little can be done other than the provision for active case detection and treatment and use of insecticide impregnated bed-nets or curtains with no guarantee that the latter will be effective. These measures are almost impracticable in poor socio-economic countries.

PLASMODIUM

The four species of the genus *Plasmodium* are responsible for malaria disease, which ranks among most important infectious diseases of the world. Its history extends to antiquity and had been reviewed many times by several authors. Malaria certainly evolved with humans during development from our primate ancestors. Similar parasites are commonly seen in monkeys and Apes. The disease appears to be originated in Africa and spread with human migration throughout the tropical, subtropical and temperate regions of entire world. The classical description of malaria fever can be seen in the records of every civilized society from China in 2700 BC through the writings of Greeks, Romans, Assyrians, Indians and Arabic and European physicians upto 19th century. The earliest detailed descriptions are those of Hippocrates of 5th century BC.

The science of malariology could not progress until the end of 19th century. The discovery of malaria parasite and its mode of transmission were full of triumphs, disappointments and rivalries. In 1880, French surgeon Charles Leveran first described the malarial parasite in the human blood smear and it was casually linked with malaria. The mode of transmission was not at all clear but by intuition Sir Patrick Manson suggested that mosquito could be the possible vector. Manson in 1877 demonstrated the role of mosquito in the transmission of lymphatic filariasis and Bruce in 1894 implicated tsetse flies in the transmission of African trypanasomiasis. Based on these findings Manson thought that a vector might be involved in the transmission of malaria too and further he postulated that it could be mosquito. This was later confirmed by Sir Ronald Ross, an Army Surgeon working in Secunderabad, Andhra Pradesh, India. In 1897, Ross succeeded in demonstrating developing parasites in the mosquito belonging to the genus *Anopheles*, fed on an infected patient after a number of putative attempts with mosquitoes belonging to other genera like *Culex, Aedes* and so on. Soon the rest of the life cycle in the mosquito was described by the Italian scientists Amico Bignami, Battista Grassi and Giovanni Bastianelli.

The genus *Plasmodium* comprises of more than 125 species that can infect reptiles, birds and mammals. The genus *Plasmodium* is further subdivided into 10 subgenera. The human and primate malarial parasites are all included in the subgenus *Plasmodium (plasmodium)* and *Plasmodium (laverania)*. The four species of malarial parasite that are of human importance are *Plasmodium (laverania) falciparum, Plasmodium (plasmodium) malariae, Plasmodium (plasmodium) vivax,* and *Plasmodium (Plasmodium) ovale*. The major criteria used in Garnham's classification is shown in the Table 23.3. However, the analysis of sequence homologies of circumsporozoite gene (CCS) in different species and comparison of small sub unit ribosomal RNA genes revealed that murine plasmodia have segregated from other

Table 23.3: Differential diagnosis of human *Plasmodium* species

Property	*P. falciparum*	*P. malariae*	*P. vivax*	*P. ovale*
Appearance of the infected red blood cell (Size, shape)	Both normal	Normal shape; size normal or smaller	1 1/2 to 2 times larger than normal; shape normal or oval	As per *P. vivax*; but some have irregular, frayed edges
Schuffner's dots (Eosinophilic stippling)	None but presence of occasional comma-like red Maurer's dots	None	Present in all stages except in early ring forms	As for *P. vivax*
Red cells with multiple parasites per cell	Common	Rare	Occasional	As per *P. vivax*
Stages present in peripheral blood	Rings and gametocytes; Schizonts are rarely seen	All stages	All stages	All stages
Ring form (Young trophozoite)	Delicate, small ring, Scanty cytoplasm. Some times at the edges of the cell Accolé form	Ring 1/3 rd diameter of the cell; heavy chromatin dots; vacuole sometimes filled in	Ring 1/3 rd to ½ of the cell; heavy chromatin dots;	As per *P. vivax*
Schizont	Rarely send in the peripheral blood; 16–18 merozoites	6–12 merozoites in rosette; Coarse pigment clump in center	12–24 merozoites rosette filling the entire RBC central pigment	8–12 merozoites in rosette
Gametocyte	Crescent shaped	Round or oval; coarse pigment	Round or oval	Round or oval
Main criteria	Only rings and crescent-shaped gametocytes in the blood; multiple infection. Infection level is high. Normal RBC shape. No Schuffner's dots	All stages are seen in the blood; trophozoites compact and intensely stained; band forms suggestive; coarse pigment: Normal or small RBC. No Schuffner's dots	Large pale RBC. Presence of Schuffner's dots; Round gametocytes; large amoeboid trophozoite with pale pigment	Similar to *P. vivax*. Oval RBC with fimbriated edges; characteristic but not always present

mammalian malarial parasites and *Plasmodium falciparum* is more closely related to avian species than mammalian plasmodia.

The morphological features of various stages of malaria parasite vary dramatically, reflect both on different functions, and to various microenvironments inhabited. Only sporozoite, merozoite and ookinete, which invade hepatocytes, erythrocytes of humans and the midgut epithelium of the mosquito respectively, possess a surface coat and a specialized apical end that is characteristic of Apicomplexa. Surface coat recognizes the host's cell and responsible for adherence. The invasion organelles allow the parasite to enter the target cell. The sexual stages undergo complex differentiation and get equipped for fertilization process, which takes place within the midgut of the mosquito. Meiosis is seen only in ookinete and it is diploid.

Life Cycle in Humans (Cycle of Golgi) (Fig. 23.8)

The infection starts with the bite of an infected female *Anopheles* mosquito and the infective stage, the sporozoite of the parasite enters into the skin of the host together with saliva of the mosquito. The sporozoites rapidly travel and reach the liver where they invade the hepatocytes.

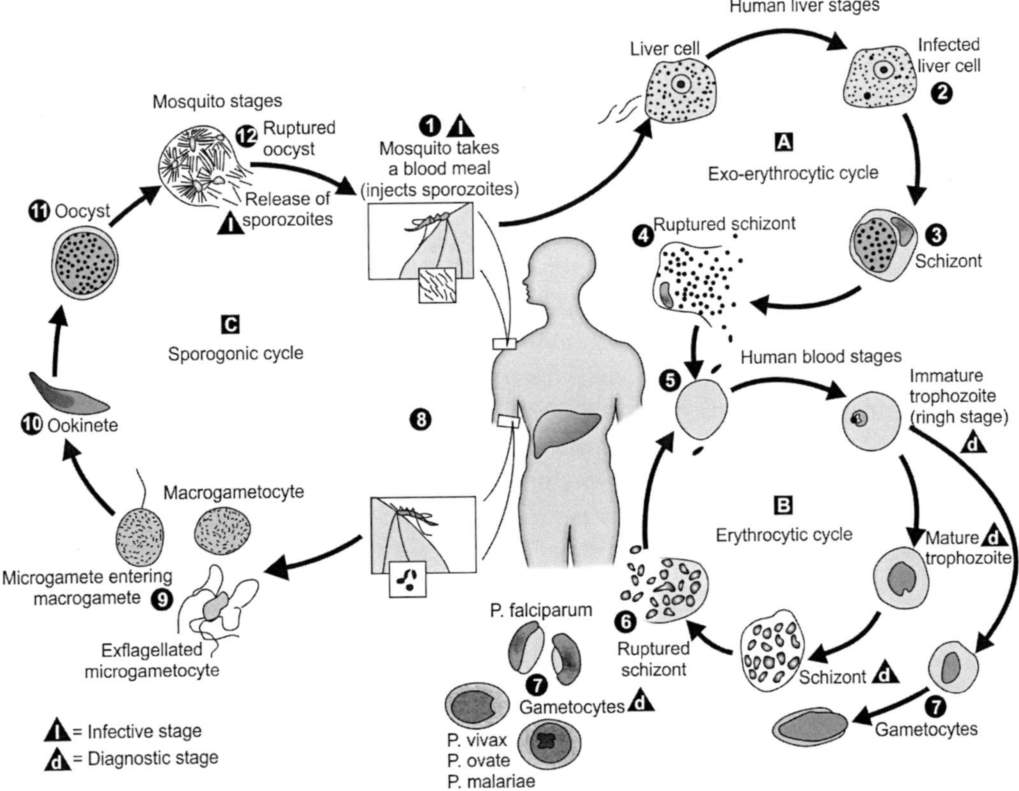

Fig. 23.8: Life cycle of *Plasmodium*

Exoerythrocytic Stage

The sporozoites reach the liver through the blood stream and invade the hepatocytes. Following the invasion of the hepatocytes, the morphology of the parasite changes drastically. It looses the apical complex and the surface coat. The sporozoites become round or oval. Development takes place within the parasitophorous vacuole of the hepatocytes. The nucleus of the parasite undergoes schizogony. The number of nuclear divisions and the duration of schizogony vary with the species. In mammalian plasmodia, the merozoites arising from the exoerythrocytic schizogony invade only the red blood cells.

Erythrocytic Stage

The merozoites from the liver invade the erythrocytes. After invasion, the invasion organelles are lost and the merozoite becomes around trophozoite that is located in the parasitophorous vacuole in the red blood cell cytoplasm. The young trophozoite now known as ring stage grows and undergoes several nuclear divisions. The duration of schizogony varies with the species. As the parasite develops within the host's red cell, it brings out a series of alterations in the red cell of the host that include formation of vacuole in the red cell or clefts and morphological changes on the surface of the red cell membrane (knobs or caveolae). These morphological alterations are visible in stained parasites as Maurer's clefts in *Plasmodium falciparum* or Schiffner's dots in *Plasmodium vivax*. The distribution of hemozoin pigment, a waste product of hemoglobin metabolism is another distinguishing feature.

Life Cycle in the Mosquito (Cycle of Ross) (Fig. 23.8)

Some merozoites instead of attacking the fresh blood cells to continue schizogony develop in to male and female gametocytes. The underlying mechanisms and the factors that induce sexual differentiation are not still clear. Matured gametocytes of *P. vivax, P. malariae,* and *P. ovale* are round whereas the gametocytes of *P. falciparum* are elongated, crescent or sickle shaped. The half-life of these gametocytes in the blood stream is only 2 to 3 days, while waiting in a suspended animation state to be taken up by the mosquito. When a suitable mosquito vector takes these gametocytes along with the blood, the gametocytes become gametes within the mosquito. This transformation is dependent on factors like changes in the temperature, pH and presence of exflagellation factor. There are no major morphological changes during the maturation of female gametocyte into macrogamete but the male gamete undergoes nuclear division three times and each of 8 nuclei formed combines with cytoplasm to form thread-like microgametes (exflagellation). The highly motile microgametes move actively toward macrogametes and fuse with them resulting in sexual life cycle. The zygote, which forms immediately, elongates to become ookinete. The ookinete slowly moves and crosses peritrophic membrane of the midgut and passes through the single epithelial cell layer and establishes itself beneath the basal lamina, forming oocyst.

The oocyst has a smooth thin wall and grows to reach a size of 40 to 50 µm *within* 4 to 21 days. Each infected mosquito may carry a few hundreds of oocysts. The size and the distribution of pigment of an oocyst is characteristic of each species and can be used as taxonomical marker. From each oocyst, sporozoites are released at the end of maturation; the number of which may vary from 10,000 to 20,000. The immature sporozoites emerge from the cyst wall into the hemolymph and migrate to the salivary glands. When the infected mosquito bites another person, the small numbers of sporozoites that each drop of saliva of mosquito carries, enter into the host. With each bite, the mosquito can introduce five to a few hundreds of sporozoites that are sufficient to produce infection in the host. The time taken for the completion of schizogony varies from 7 days to 8 weeks depending on the species of the parasite, the nature of the vector and the environmental conditions.

Malignant tertian malaria or malaria due to *P. falciparum* is a medical emergency in non-immune individuals. The incubation period is generally 9 to 14 days but it can be as short as one week. The symptoms are generally nonspecific like headache, body pains, anorexia, nausea and feeling of chill rather than a cold phase. Fever is very common but not invariable. Fever is continuous or remittent type. Physical examination shows prostration, mild jaundice herpes simplex on lips and tender hepatosplenomegaly. Opthalmoscopic examination as a part of routine examination may sometimes reveal retinal hemorrhages, which are frequently associated with imminent coma in adults. Cerebral malaria is the most common presentation of severe form of malignant tertian malaria. The other complications include (a) anemia, (b) renal failure, (c) hypoglycemia, (d) malarial hemoglobinuria, (e) hyperparasitemia, (f) fluid, electrolyte and acid-base disturbances, (g) pulmonary edema, (h) circulatory collapse, (i) bleeding and clotting disturbances, and (j) hyperpyrexia.

Benign Tertian Malaria (*Plasmodium Vivax* and *Plasmodium Ovale* Malaria)

The average incubation period of vivax malaria is 17 days but with some strains, it may be as long as 250 to 637 days. During the initial phase of infection, the symptoms may be nonspecific and similar to those described for malignant tertian malaria. After 2 to 3 days, the classical febrile paroxysms with a) cold stage b) hot stage and c) stage of sweating can be seen. The cold stage lasts for 15 to 60 minutes with violent rigors, cold dry skin due to intense vasoconstriction. The core temperature is increased. During the hot stage, the patient has high temperature with throbbing headache, palpitation, prostration, confusion and delirium. The patient looks ill, may be anemic or may show mild jaundice along with tender hepatosplenomegaly. The hot stage lasts for 2 to 6 hours followed by the stage of profuse sweating defervescence and deep sleep. In untreated cases, the febrile paroxysms occur every alternate day. The platelet counts may be low and the only complication that may occur in some cases is rupture of the spleen. Untreated or inadequately treated patients may develop relapse after a period of quiescence at intervals that may vary from 8 to 40 weeks. The incubation period of 'quartan malaria' due to *Plasmodium malariae* is 18 to 40 days. The clinical picture is similar to that of vivax malaria except that the febrile paroxysms occur once in 72 hours. Persistent undetectable parasitemia is a common feature of quartan malaria. Because of this symptomatic recrudescence can occur upto 57 years after first

Table 23.4: Differences between severe malaria in adults and children

Signs and symptoms	*Adults*	*Children*
Cough	Uncommon	Common
Convulsions	Common	Very common
Jaundice	Common	Uncommon
Duration of illness	5–7 days	1–2 days
Pre-treatment hypoglycemia	Uncommon	Common
CSF opening pressure	Normal	Raised
Abnormal brain stem reflexes	Rare	More common
Resolution of coma	2–4 days	1–2 days
Neurological sequelae	Uncommon	Occur in about 10% cases
Pulmonary edema	Common	Rare
Renal failure	Common	Rare
Bleeding and clotting disturbances	Upto 10%	Rare

exposure. This is not due to hypnozoites. Epidemiological studies strongly indicate that *Plasmodium malariae* infection is an important cause of nephritic syndrome in children below the age of 15 years. Children of 6 months to 5 year's age group are more prone to develop cerebral malaria. Differences between severe malaria in adults and children are given in the Table 23.4.

Repeated untreated or partially treated malaria is the common cause of anemia in children of the age group of 6 months to 2 years. The anemia is normochromic with prominent dyserythropoietic changes in the bone marrow. In older children, acute hemolytic anemia with hyperparasitemia may occur. Metabolic acidosis is associated with severe malaria. It may occur individually or in combination with cerebral malaria. Metabolic acidosis is associated with poor prognosis.

Nonimmune pregnant women are susceptible to all the usual manifestations of malaria. They also exhibit increased risk of abortion, premature delivery and low birth weight of the infant. Mortality rate among pregnant women with severe malaria is more when compared to non-pregnant women. Pregnant women are more frequently prone for hypoglycemia when infected with malaria. Congenital malaria is more common in infants born to nonimmune mothers. In endemic areas, its incidence is low even though the prevalence of placental infection is high.

In some endemic regions of malaria, adults develop progressive massive splenomegaly. The liver also may be enlarged. Hypersplenism may result in normocytic anemia, thrombocytopenia and leukopenia. The splenomegaly seems to be an abnormal immune response to recurrent malaria infection with elevated IgM and IgG antibodies. Patents respond well to treatment within 3 months after starting the therapy.

Some sporozoites develop immediately after entering the hepatocytes and a few days later, the merozoites released from the exo-erythrocytic schizonts attack the red blood cells that results in primary infection. This may last for a few weeks to months in the absence of specific treatment. Further waves of parasitemia may follow a few weeks, months or years after the primary attack. In the absence of reinfection, the following causes are responsible for the secondary attacks.

a. A secondary exoerythrocytic cycle of schizogony that is seen with *Plasmodium falciparum* infection in birds and reptiles is not seen in species infecting the mammals.
b. The second cause is presence of dormant stages of the parasite or 'hypnozoite'. Some sporozoites remain dormant for weeks or months. The latent period is variable from one hypnozoite to another and the factors that trigger their eventual growth are not known. Only *P. vivax* and *P. ovale* produce hypnozoites.
c. Parasites that do not produce hypnozoites may nevertheless produce secondary waves of parasitemia called recrudescence either due to long-term survival of the erythrocytic stages or due to low and undetectable levels of erythrocytic schizogony in the peripheral blood stream.

Latent erythrocytic stages require standard chemotherapy whereas hypnozoites need specific therapy. A true relapse is always exo-erythrocytic in nature and it is re-appearance of parasitemia due to sporozoite-induced infection. Infection with blood trophozoites is not relapse (Figs 23.9 to Fig 23.11).

One of the interesting features of clinical manifestations is that the parasites grow in synchrony. The clinical symptoms tend to occur at regular intervals of time. This synchronous life cycle of the parasite is partially due to the host factors. The host's circadian rhythm also contributes for synchronicity. The biological clock of the parasite can be considered as an adaptive mechanism designed to facilitate the transmission of the parasite by the mosquitoes that are nocturnal in their habitat.

Chemotherapy is mandatory in the treatment of malaria and at the same time correct management of complications is also very important. For uncomplicated malaria, oral administration of antimalarial drugs is sufficient and parenteral therapy is recommended for those who cannot tolerate the oral therapy. The various complications of *Plasmodium falciparum* and various drug regimens for all four types of malaria are given in the following Tables 23.5 to 23.10.

During the period 1898-1940, malaria control was mainly achieved by prophylactic usage of quinine and mosquito larval control. During IInd World War several antimalarial compounds were developed both for treatment and for prophylaxis. The first active residual insecticide DDT was used to control mosquito population. Following the next 10 years malaria was eliminated from several countries by the combined use of chloroquine treatment and regular spraying of houses with DDT. From 1956 to 1975 WHO recommended malaria eradication program was pursued but abandoned because the concept of eradication was unrealistic objective due to escalated cost of the equipment, fuel and insecticides, political instability, financial and administrative shortcomings, emerging vector resistance, vector exophils, parasite resistance to drugs and uncontrollable population movements. Malaria control programe at present focused on (a) early diagnosis and prompt treatment, (b) to implement selective sustainable measures against parasite as well as the vector, (c) prevention of epidemics by early detection of infected cases for

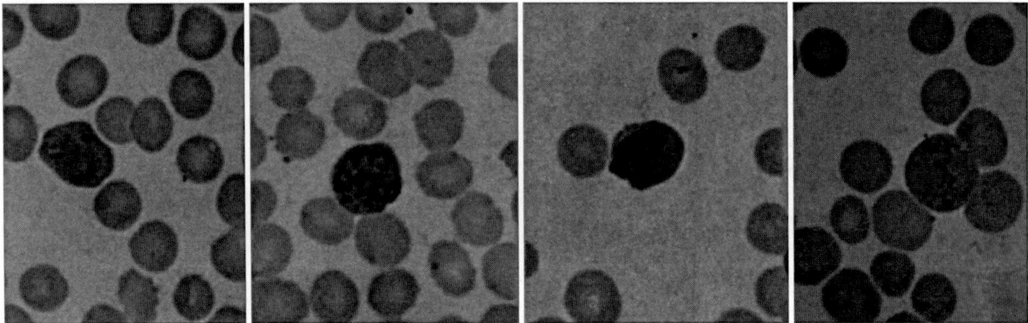

Fig. 23.9: Schizont stage of malarial parasite (*For color version, see Plate 8*)

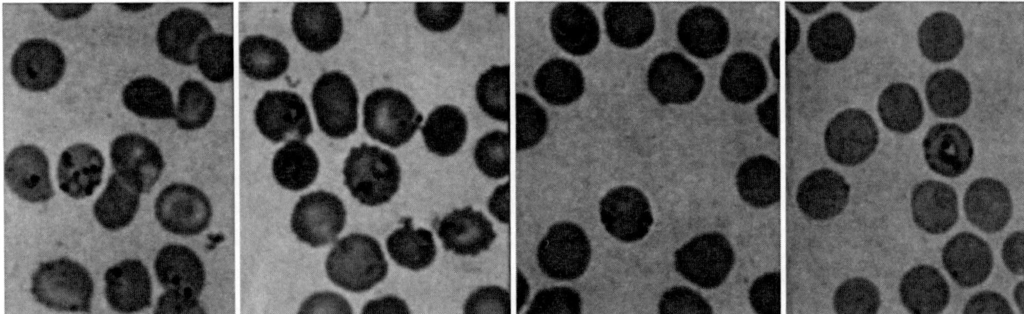

Fig. 23.10: Ring forms and schizont stage of malarial parasite (*For color version, see Plate 8*)

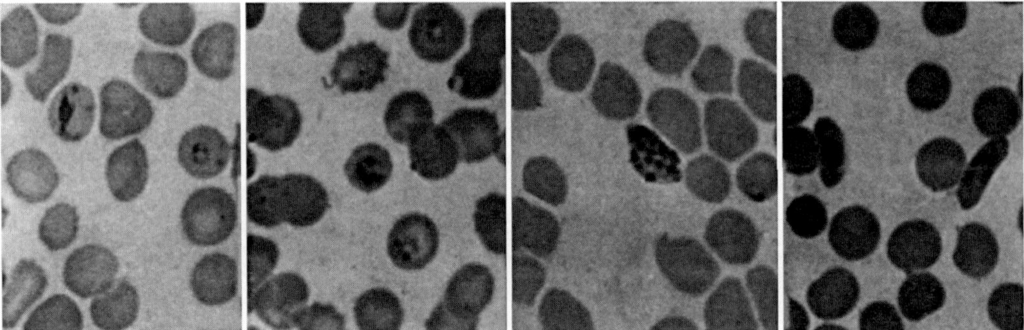

Fig. 23.11: Ring forms and gametocytes of *Plasmodium falciparum* (*For color version, see Plate 8*)

treating them effectively, and (d) to assess the country's malaria regularly with reference to ecological, social, and economic determinants

Awareness programs combined with personal protection using bed-nets, repellents. Chemoprophylaxis at the community level is not recommended due to poor compliance, cot, drug resistance, drug toxicity and lack of adequate supplies. Nevertheless, community based chemoprophylaxis may be useful for children and pregnant women in areas where transmission is seasonal, short and people are cooperative and educated.

Table 23.5: Management of severe complications of *P. falciparum* malaria

Complication	Management
Coma	Maintain airway, exclude other causes of coma, prophylactic anticonvulsants, avoid corticosteroids, heparin or adrenaline
Convulsions	Maintain airway, use anticonvulsants such as diazepam or paraldehyde (0.1 mL through a glass syringe)
Severe anemia	Transfuse packed cells or whole blood
Acute renal failure	Correct dehydration, maintain fluid and electrolyte balance, carry out peritoneal or hemodialysis if indicated
Hypoglycemia	Maintain glucose levels of blood by infusing 50% glucose 50 mL followed by 5% glucose or 10% glucose infusion
Metabolic acidosis	Exclude hypoglycemia or treat hypoglycemia, hypovolemia, gram-negative sepsis, give oxygen, correct arterial pH to 7.2 or above. Blood or crystalloid transfusion may be required
Acute pulmonary edema	Avoid excessive rehydration, patient in prop up position, administer oxygen, diuretics, withdraw 250 mL of blood into donor's bag
Shock or algid malaria	Suspect Gram-negative sepsis, subject appropriate specimens for culture, parenteral antibiotics, correct hemodynamic disturbances
Spontaneous bleeding and coagulopathy	Transfuse blood or clotting factors, vitamin K
Hyperpyrexia	Use tepid sponging, antipyretics
Hyperparasitemia	IV administration of antimalarial drugs, if the parasitemia is >10% carry out exchange transfusion or partial exchange transfusion
Malarial hemoglobinuria	Continue antimalarial drugs, transfuse fresh blood to maintain hematocrit above 20%, give frusemide intravenously
Aspirated pneumonia	Parenteral antimicrobials, physiotherapy and oxygen administration

Table 23.6: Treatment of uncomplicated malignant tertian malaria

Chloroquine sensitive areas	*Chloroquine resistant areas or sensitivity is not known*
Chloroquine	**Mefloquine**
Adults: 600 mg base for first two days. 300 mg base on 3rd day	Adults: 15–25 mg/kg wt in two divided doses 6 hours apart
Children: 10 mg base/kg wt for first two days followed by 5 mg base/kg wt on 3rd day	Children: 25 mg base/kg wt given as two doses 6 hours apart
	Halofantrine
	Adults: 500 mg 6th hourly for 3 days with food
	Children: 8 mg/kg wt 6th hourly for 3 days with food
	Quinine
	Adults: 600 mg 3 times a day for 7 days
	Children: 10 mg/kg wt 3 times a day for 7 days
	Sulphodoxine + Pyremethamine
	Adults: 500 mg + 25 mg 3 tablets single dose
	Children < 5 years: Half tablet, > 5 years < 9 years one tablet < 15 years 2 tablets

Table 23.7: Antimalarial treatment for severe *P. falciparum* malaria

Chloroquine sensitive areas	*Chloroquine resistant areas or sensitivity is not known*
Chloroquine	**Quinine**
Adults: 25 mg/kg wt as continuous IV infusion over 3 hours or	20 mg salt/kg wt diluted in 10 mL/kg wt 5% dextrose saline as IV infusion over 4 hours. Then 10 mg/kg wt in 5% dextrose saline over 4 hours, 8–12 hours until the patient can swallow orally. The 7-day's course is completed with Quinine tablets 10 mg/kg wt 3 times a day or
Chloroquine 2,5 mg/kg wt every 4th hourly IM or subcutaneously or	20 mg salt/kg wt IM in anterior thigh followed by 10 mg salt/ kg wt until the patient can swallow orally. Complete the course as above
Quinine as indicated in the right side column	

Table 23.8: Treatment plan for *P. vivax, P. ovale* and *P. malariae* malaria

Chloroquine: 10 mg/kg wt for 2 days followed by 5 mg/kg wt on 3rd day
For radical cure Primaquine* 0.25 mg 0.33 mg[b] base /kg/wt/day/7days[a]

*Contraindicated in pregnant women.
[a]For G6PD deficient patient 0.75 mg/kg/wt/weekly for 8 weeks
[b]For strains isolated in Ociana and South East Asia

Table 23.9: Treatment of uncomplicated, multi-drug resistant *P. falciparum* malaria

Artesunate or Arthemether* orally 3.2 mg/kg wt on day one followed by 2 mg/kg wt daily for 6 days or Artesunate or
Arthemether orally 3.2 mg/kg wt on day one followed by 2 mg/kg wt orally daily for 4 days. Alternatively mefloquine** 25 mg/kg wt in two divided doses—15 mg/kg wt initially followed by10 mg/kg wt

*Not to be used in first trimester of pregnancy
**Not to be used in severe cases of *P. falciparum* malaria

Table 23.10: Treatment of severe complicated, multi-drug resistant *P. falciparum* malaria

Artesunate 2.4 mg/kg wt given as IV infusion followed by 1.2 mg/kg wt at 12th hourly and then daily for 6 days or
Arthemether* 3.2 mg/kg wt intramuscularly, followed by 1.6 mg/kg.wt intramuscularly, daily for 6 days

*Not indicated in the first trimester of pregnancy

TOXOPLASMA

The history of *Toxoplasma* is relatively recent one, even though the causative agent *Toxoplasma gondii* is the most common human parasite worldwide and the one that infects a wide range of hosts. The history of toxoplasmosis escaped the attention of the major reference books. Charles Nicolle accidentally discovered *Toxoplasma gondii* while he was searching for a reservoir host for *Leishmania* in a North African rodent, *Ctenodactylus gondii* in 1909. During the same time, Alfonso Splendore discovered the same parasite in rabbits at Saint Paulo. Later on, several observers recorded the presence of this parasite in a large variety of animals that belonged to mammals and birds. Wolf and Coven reported first congenital *Toxoplasma* infection in 1937. This initiated interest among the researchers and they soon noticed that *Toxoplasma gondii* is actually a very common parasite of humans but rarely causes disease and it crosses placenta to cause congenital infection. William

Hutchison in 1970 demonstrated that this parasite is a stage in the life cycle of a common intestinal coccidian of cat. Toxoplasmosis subsequently gained new significance as a serious concomitant of HIV infection.

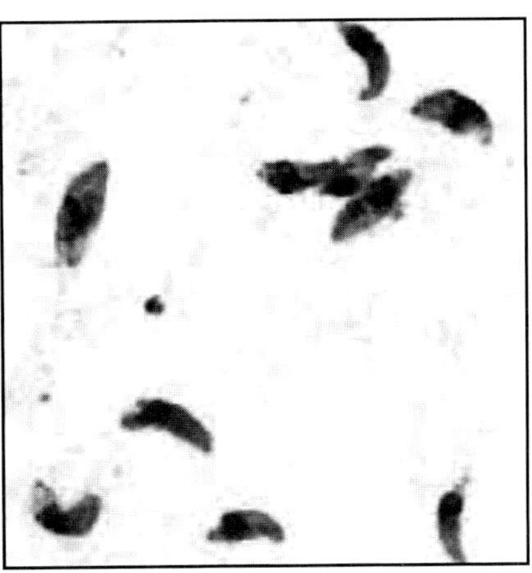

Fig. 23.12: *Toxoplasma*
(*For color version, see Plate 10*)

This coccidian parasite and its related genera are classified in the phylum Apicomplexa (Levine 1970), class Coccidia, Order Eimeridia Leger. Opinions differ regarding the placement of *Toxoplasma gondii* in families and subfamilies.

The name *Toxoplasma* (toxon = bow and plasma = form) indicates the crescent shape of the tachyzoites stage, one of the infectious stage of the parasite. The bradyzoites (tissue cysts) and sporozoites (in oocyst) are the other stages of the parasite. The tachyzoites measures 2 × 6 μm and is often crescent shaped but may appear as globular or oval in tissue sections. The anterior (conoidal) end is pointed and the posterior end is blunt or oval (Fig. 23.12). The tachyzoites has an outer covering called pellicle, a polar ring, a conoid rhoptries, microsomes, mitochondria, subpellicular microtubules, endoplasmic reticulum, Golgi apparatus, ribosomes, rough surfaced endoplasmic reticulum, micro pore and a well-defined nucleus. The nucleus is situated at the posterior end or at the central portion of the cell. The pellicle has three membranes. The inner membrane complex is discontinuous at the polar ring, micropore and at the posterior end. The polar ring encircles the conoid (a cylindrical truncated cone with 6–8 fibrillar elements wound like a compressed spring). There are 22 subpellicular microtubules originating from the anterior end running longitudinally almost entire length of the cell. About 4 to 10 club-shaped organelles called rhoptries terminate within the conoid.

The functions of conoid, rhoptries and microsomes are not clear. The conoid appears to be associated with the penetration of the tachyzoites through the host cell membrane by means of boring type of motility. Gliding, rotating or undulating type of movements are seen with *Toxoplasma gondii.* Rhoptries have secretory function associated with host cell penetration. The microtubules probably provide the cytoskeleton.

The tachyzoites enter the host cell by active penetration of the host cell. After entering the host cell, the tachyzoites become oval and surrounded by a phagocytophilum vesicle, which is derived from both parasite and the host cell membrane. The tachyzoites multiply asexually *within* the host cell by repeated endodyogeny (endo = inside, dio = two, genesis = birth), a specialized form of reproduction in which the two progenies form within the parent parasite. Tachyzoites continue to divide by this method until the host cell is filled with the parasites.

After a few divisions, *Toxoplasma gondii* encyst to become tissue cyst, which grow and remain intracellular. The cyst varies in size from 6 to 60 μm or even 100 μm. The younger cyst, which is small, contains only two bradyzoites whereas the larger and older cysts contain hundreds of bradyzoites. Tissue cyst in brain rarely reaches a size of 60 µm; whereas intramuscular cysts elongated and may reach a size of 100 µm. Tissue cysts in unstained live squash preparation vary in size depending upon the pressure applied to squash, the tissue and the medium in which they are suspended. Tissue cysts are mainly present in neural and muscular tissue. However, they are present in other organs also. Intact tissue cyst is harmless and can persist for life of the host.

Tissue cyst wall is thin, argyrophillic and contains hundreds of crescent-shaped bradyzoites. Bradyzoites differ from tachyzoites slightly. Bradyzoites possess nucleus at the posterior end. They contain amylopectin granules that are stained red with periodic acid-Schiff stain (PAS). Bradyzoites are more slender and less susceptible to destruction by gastric juice. Factors responsible for formation of tissue cysts are not very clear. Tissue cysts are more numerous in animals with chronic infection after acquiring immunity. However, current evidence based on *in vitro* studies in cell cultures indicate immunity and formation of tissue cysts are coincidental (Fig. 23.13).

Cats excrete oocysts after ingesting any form of the infectious stage of *Toxoplasma gondii*. The time of shedding of oocysts after initial infection and the frequency of their shedding varies with the stage ingested. Less than 50% of cats shed oocysts after ingesting the tachyzoites or oocysts whereas all cats shed oocysts after ingesting the tissue cysts.

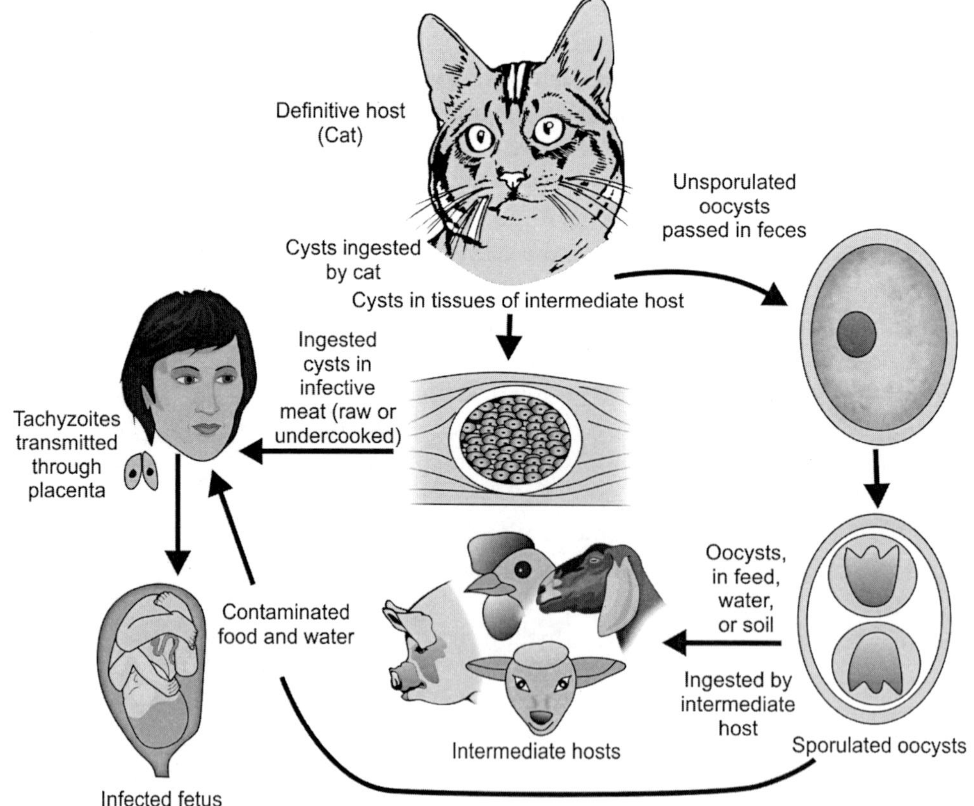

Fig. 23.13: Life cycle of *Toxoplasma*

The tissue cysts are dissolved due to proteolytic action of the enzymes in the stomach and intestines of the cat. The released bradyzoites penetrate the epithelial cells of the intestine and initiate the development of the asexual generation. Five morphologically distinct types of *Toxoplasma gondii* develop in the intestinal epithelial cells before the beginning of the gametogony. The origin of gamonts is not determined yet. Probably they may originate from the merozoites released from meronts of type D or E. The mature male gamonts are oval or elliptical. When microgametogenesis takes place, the nucleus of the male gamont divides to produce 10 to 21 nuclei and moves toward periphery of the parasite to enter into the protuberances formed in the pellicle of the mother parasite. Each microgamete has two flagella with which it swims and penetrates the mature macrogamete. The fusion results in the formation of oocyst wall and subsequently after maturation the oocysts are discharged into the lumen of the intestine due to rupture of the infected intestinal epithelial cells. The oocysts are excreted in the feces of the infected animal.

Unsporulated Oocysts are subspherical or spherical filled with sporonts. The oocyst wall has two colorless layers. Sporulation occurs outside the intestine of the cat within 1 to 5 days depending upon favorable conditions like temperature and aeration. Each sporulated oocyst contains two sporocysts and each sporocyst contains four sporozoites that measure 2×6 to 8 μm in size. Each sporozoite has central or subterminal nucleus, a few PAS positive granules in the cytoplasm. They have most of the organelles found in other Coccidian parasites. While the enteroepithelial cycle is in progress, the bradyzoites penetrate the lamina propria of the feline intestine, multiply as tachyzoites, and may disseminate to extra intestinal tissues where they persist for several months if not for life of the cat.

Toxoplasma infection is widespread throughout the world. Though the exact causes for variations in the incidence in different areas are not known, it appears that environmental conditions, cultural habits of the people and the animal fauna may be contributing to the variation in the incidences in different geographical areas. The infection is more prevalent in hot and humid areas. About one percent of infections occur congenitally. Congenital infections in humans occur only when the mother acquires infection during the pregnancy.

The infection occurs due to ingestion of oocysts or by consumption of raw meat containing tissue cysts. The contamination of the environment with oocysts is widespread because oocysts are excreted by domestic as well as other members of *Felidae*. The oocyst formation is very high in domestic cats and they are the main source of contamination. Oocysts survive for months to years under ordinary environment. Several invertebrates like flies, cockroaches, dung flies and earthworms can spread the oocysts mechanically. Even though, as few as one percent of cats may be shedding the oocysts at any given time, the enormous numbers and their resistance in the environment ensure widespread contamination. Congenital infections can also occur in cats and congenitally infected kitten shed the oocysts. Humans are most probably infected by the ingestion of raw or undercooked meat. Transmission can occur through blood transfusion or after organ transplantation.

Congenital infections occur only when a woman becomes infected during the pregnancy and the severity of the disease depends upon the stage of the pregnancy at the time of the infection. Pregnant women may be asymptomatic but they do have temporary parasitemia.

Focal lesions develop in the placenta and the fetus may get infected. In the fetus, there is generalized infection at first, which later clears from the visceral organs but localizes in the neural tissue. Congenital toxoplasmosis may range from mild to severe type. In cases of mild infection, there is slightly diminished vision whereas if the infection is severe the fetus may develop retinochoroiditis, hydrocephalus, convulsions and intracerebral calcification. Among these clinical manifestations, hydrocephalus is relatively rare but most dramatic lesion of toxoplasmosis. Hydrocephalus due to congenital toxoplasmosis is unique to humans.

Ocular disease is the common manifestation of congenital toxoplasmosis. Involvement of entire eye is very rare and the disease is virtually confined to posterior chamber of the eye. Parasite multiplies within the retina and this produces inflammation in choroid. During acute or subacute stage of the inflammation yellowish–white cotton like patches are seen in the fundus and these lesions are either single or multiple. During the acute stage of infection, the vitreous humor may become cloudy or dense. Once the inflammation subsides, the vitreous fluid becomes clear and the diseased retina and choroid can be visualized with ophthalmoscope. Retinal lesions may be single or multiple with minimal edema and reaction *within* the vitreous humor. The lesions are usually harmless unless they are located in the macular area. Severe infection may be detected at birth but mild infections may be missed until they flare up during adult hood. The socioeconomic impact of toxoplasmosis in human suffering and the cost involved in caring the sick children, especially those with mental retardation and blindness is enormous. The cost benefits of mass screening of all pregnant women are debated in many countries except in France and Austria where the incidence is very high.

Toxoplasma infection acquired afterbirth may be localized or generalized. Infection occurring due to ingestion of oocysts may be more severe than that is due to tissue cysts. Cervical lymphadenitis is the common manifestation of toxoplasmosis occurring afterbirth. The infected lymph nodes are enlarged, tender, discrete but not painful. The infection may resolve spontaneously within weeks to months. Lymphadenopathy may be associated with fever, fatigue, malaise, myalgias, sore throat and headache. The clinical condition is benign but the diagnosis is important in pregnant women. Encephalitis is the most common manifestation in immunosuppressed individuals. The clinical symptoms are nonspecific such as headache, drowsiness, disorientation, convulsions and coma. Diagnosis is aided by serological examination (Table 23.11) but in immunosuppressed patients both inflammatory response and the antibody titers may be suppressed making the diagnosis very difficult. Toxoplasmosis is one of the common causes of death of patients with advanced HIV infection. In HIV, positive patients any organ may be involved with toxoplasma infection but most patients suffer from bilateral headache that is not relieved by analgesics. The predominant lesion in the brain is the necrosis of thalamus.

The choice of chemotherapy is the combination of sulfadiazine and pyremethamine. Both act synergistically and block the metabolic pathway of para-aminobenzoic acid and folic acid synthesis. The combination is well tolerated.

Several compounds such as diaminophenyl sulfone, atovaquone, spiramycin, chlorinated lincomycin analogs, piretrixim, roxithromycin are effective in experimentally

Table 23.11: Serodiagnosis of toxoplasmosis

Interpretation	*Dye test*	*IFA*	*IgM IFA*	*DS IgM ELISA*	*IHA*	*CFT*
Positive titer	1:4	1:10	1:4	1:64	1:16	1:4
Acute infection	>1:1000	<1:1000	1:80	>1:256	1:16–1:256	1:8
Chronic infection	1:4–1:2000	1:8–1:2000	-ve-1:20	>1:64	1:16–1:256	-ve-1:8
Duration of elevation of titers	Years	Years	Weeks–Months	Months	Years	Not studied
Cross reactions	No cross reactions or false-positives	Antinuclear antibody gives false-positive results	Rheumatoid factor and antinuclear antibody may give false-positive results	No cross-reactions	Not useful for congenital infections	No information available

IFA = Immunofluorescence antibody; IgM IFA = Immunoglobulin; IHA = Indirect hemagglutination; CFT= Complement-fixation test.

induced infection in animals or in cell cultures. Spiramycin reaches highest concentrations in placenta. Hence, it can be used in pregnant women without any harm to fetus. But the drug is less effective than sulfadiazine and pyremethamine combination. Clindamycin is effective but it may cause ulcerative colitis. Atovaquone is the most effective cysticidal drug.

Meat handlers should wash their hands well with soap and water before they attend to other works. All instruments that come into contact with uncooked meat should be decontaminated using a detergent and water. Parasites in the meat are killed by exposing them to extreme cold or heat. Tissue cysts are killed at 67°C and –13°C. Tissue cysts are killed by γ-radiation. All meat preparations are well cooked before consuming them. Pregnant women should avoid contact with cats, soil and raw meat. Pet cats should be fed by dry canned or cooked food, and the litter box should be emptied every day. Gloves should be used while working in the garden. The vegetables used for salads are washed well in the running water. *Toxoplasma gondii* can cause severe disease in animals resulting in great loss to live stock industry.

CRYPTOSPORIDIUM

The name *Cryptosporidium* is derived from the observation that unlike other coccidian parasites the oocysts of this parasite do not have sporocyst surrounding the sporozoites (*Cryptosporidium* means hidden sporocyst). The species of the genus *Cryptosporidium* are small coccidian parasites that infect the micro villous region of the epithelial cells of digestive and respiratory organs of vertebrate animals. Clarke in 1855, probably the first person to observe the species of *Cryptosporidium* in the gastric epithelium of mice, which he described as swarming spores. The species *Cryptosporidium muris* was named and described by EE Tyzzer in 1907. Again, Tyzzer in 1929 described the developmental stages of a species of *Cryptosporidium* in the cecal epithelial cells of chickens.

The life cycle of *C. parvum* is similar to that of other true coccidia infecting the mammals. The life cycle has six major developmental stages (Fig. 23.14).

1. **Excystation:** The release of sporozoites those are infective
2. **Merogony:** The asexual multiplication (schizogony) within the infected host cells
3. **Gametogony:** Formation of micro- and macrogametes
4. **Fertilization:** The union of micro- and macrogametes
5. **Oocyst wall formation:** Oocyst wall formation comprises of production of an environmentally resistant stage that transmits infection from one host to another
6. **Sporogony:** The formation of infective sporozoites within the oocyst wall.

The parasitophorous vacuole is confined to microvillous region of the host cell. The oocysts of *C. parvum* undergo sporogony while they are within the host cells and are infective when released in the feces. It has been shown that 20 percent of the oocysts of *C. parvum* within the host enterocytes do not form thick, two-layered environmentally resistant oocyst wall. The four sporozoites of this autoinfective stage are surrounded only by a single membrane. Once these are released from the host cell, the membrane surrounding the sporozoites rupture and the released sporozoites penetrate into the microvillous region of the other enterocytes and re-initiate the life cycle. The thick-walled oocysts that are excreted transmit the infection from one host to another. Autoinfective thin-walled oocysts and type I meronts that can re-cycle are believed to be the life cycle forms responsible for severe infection in hosts exposed to only a small number of thick-walled oocysts and for persistent life-threatening disease in immunocompromised hosts who are not exposed to environmentally resistant stages repeatedly.

Cryptosporidium parvum is transmitted by environmentally resistant oocysts that are completely sporulated and infective at the time they are excreted in the feces. Oocysts are very resistant to commonly used disinfectants. Exposure to 50 percent ammonia or 10 percent formalin for 30 minutes kills the cysts. Similarly, freeze-drying or exposure to temperatures above 60°C or below –20°C inactivates the oocysts. The routine chlorination of drinking water has little or no effect on the viability of the oocysts but the viability of the oocysts is lost following exposure to 80 ppm chlorine at 25°C and pH 7.0 for two hours. Ozone is effective in inactivating the oocysts at a concentration of one percent for 10 minutes.

Calves or domestic animals serve as reservoir hosts. Earlier it was thought that human infections are the result of zoonotic transmission. This may be true for those who live and work in an environment where exposure to fecal contamination from potential reservoir hosts is very likely. However, in urban areas person-to-person transmission is more common. Numerous outbreaks of cryptosporidial infection have been documented in children's day-care centers, hospitals and water-borne infections. This parasite is recognized as one of the causative agents of traveler's diarrhea. Wastewater in the form of sewage and run-off from dairies and grazing lands has been identified as sources of oocysts that contaminate drinking and recreational water. The agricultural sources of oocyst contamination are important because infected calves and lambs can excrete upto 10^9 cysts per day upto 14 days.

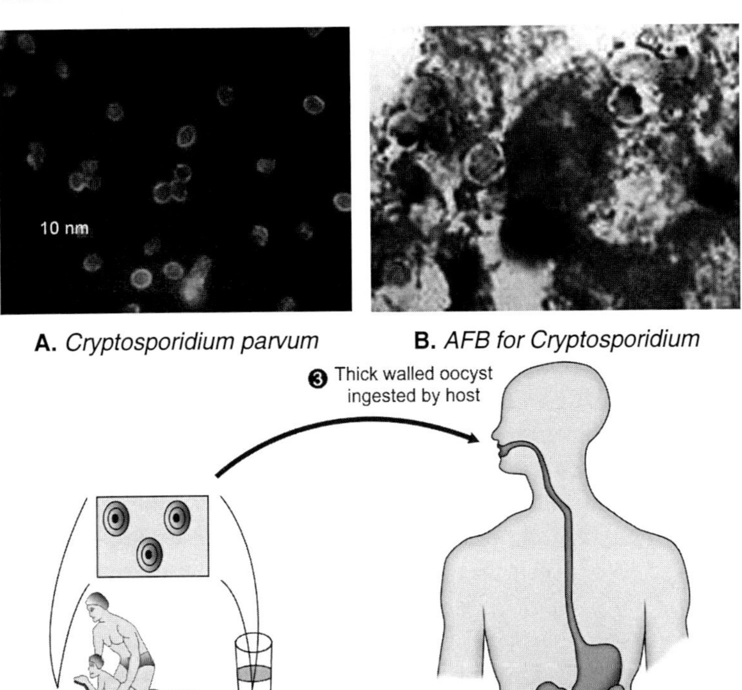

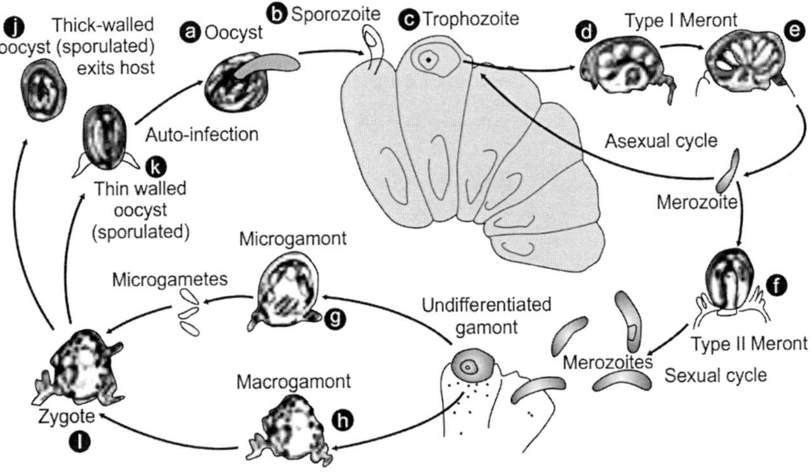

C. 300px-Cryptosporidiosis

Fig. 23.14: Life cycle of *Cryptosporidium* (*For color version, see Plate 9*)

The most common clinical finding of cryptosporidiosis in both immunocompetent and immunocompromised persons is profuse watery diarrhea. It may contain mucus but not leukocytes or red cells. Other nonspecific symptoms include abdominal pain, nausea, vomiting, low-grade fever, myalgias, weakness, malaise and headache. Severity of the clinical manifestations may vary with waxing and waning that corresponds to the shedding of oocysts. Asymptomatic infection can occur in both immunocompetent and immunosuppressed patients. In well-nourished persons, the infection lasts for 3 to 12 days. Cryptosporidiosis is associated with malnutrition.

In immunosuppressed individuals, the infection becomes progressively worse and may lead to death if not treated in time. Initially the parasite colonizes in ileum and jejunum, which later leads to life-threatening condition when large portion of the intestinal mucosa is covered with the parasites. Fluid loss in these patients and in HIV infected patients is very high. In immunodeficient people extra intestinal infections including respiratory tract infection, cholecystitis, hepatitis and pancreatitis may occur.

Intravenous administration (not oral) of spiramycin may be useful in some cases of AIDS with superadded cryprosporidial infection. However, due to adverse reactions and currently available data suggests that spiramycin is of little use in treating human infections due to *Cryptosporidium parvum*. So is the case with azithromycin and the effects of other macrolides are not known. Paromomycin has been used in some patients and the response was dramatic in some of them but many patients continued to pass oocysts, and others showed relapse while still on therapy. Paromomycin being a static agent, treatment with this drug is no better than a placebo.

Since there is no proven consistently effective treatment for cryptosporidiosis, patients should be given good supportive therapy that includes correction of dehydration, maintenance of electrolyte balance, parenteral nutrition. Antidiarrheal compounds may be given to control fluid loss. Subcutaneous administration of octerotide, an analog of somatostatin, may be useful in decreasing the number of daily bowel movements. Currently several compounds are under study both *in vitro* models and in animal models. Reversal of immunosuppression helps in complete resolution of intestinal cryptosporidiosis. The role of specific antibody therapy is not clear. Infants who are breastfed are less vulnerable to infection. Antibody neutralization-sensitive epitopes on the surface of sporozoites of the parasite have been demonstrated and presently several laboratories are investigating the role of immunological intervention in the form of administration of hyperimmune serum and immunotherapeutic efficacy of hyper-immune bovine colostrums.

PNEUMOCYSTIS CARINII

Pneumocystis carinii is the causative agent of pneumocystosis or *Pneumocystis carinii* pneumonia (PCP). The infection is an acute pneumonitis and in 1960s and 1970s, the infection was commonly seen in immunocompromised patients. By 1980, *Pneumocystis carinii* emerged as the most significant opportunistic pathogen in patients with advanced HIV infection. The organism is a unicellular eukaryote that develops extracellularly in the lungs and undergoes encystment during one phase of life cycle. The parasite has many biological characters that resemble those of both fungi and protozoa. As on today, it has not been cultured in the laboratory on artificial media or *in vitro* cultural systems like cell cultures. Presently it is considered as fungus.

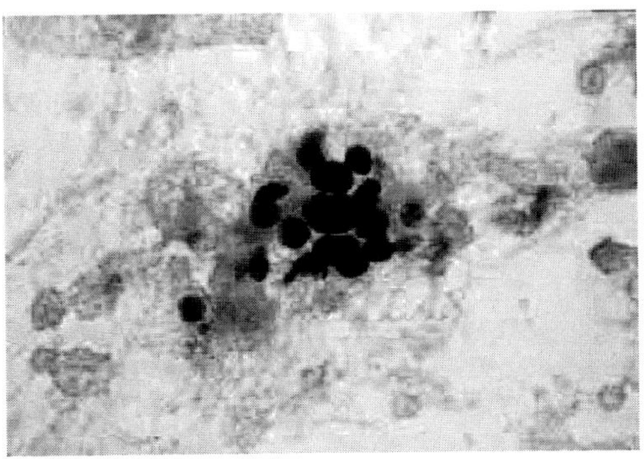

Fig. 23.15: *Pneumocystis carinii*
(*For color version, see Plate 10*)

The currently available knowledge on the life cycle, the mode of transmission, reservoir hosts and the nature of the transmissible form is by and large incomplete. It appears that with some rare exceptions, the primary site of infection is the lungs and it is likely that the entire life cycle of *P. carinii* occurs within the alveoli of the infected lungs. The parasite assumes four basic morphological forms during its life cycle: (a) trophozoite, (b) precyst, (c) cyst and (d) intracystic bodies. The trophozoite form is pleomorphic and it may be oval, spherical or amoeboid. Morphologically, the small trophic forms resemble the intracystic bodies within the matured cysts.

The small trophic form has very few or no tubular extensions on its surface. The pellicle has a thickness of 20 to 30 μm and it has an outer electron dense layer and inner plasma membrane. The cytoplasm has double membrane bound nucleus, single mitochondrion with a few cristae, endoplasmic reticulum, ribosomes and a few osmophilic bodies. The glycogen content is less. The main organelle of this small trophic form is a single mitochondrion with budding area (Fig. 23.15).

The large trophic forms are pleomorphic or ameboid in shape with lobopodic pseudopodia and deep invaginations. The mature forms contain long, thin tubular expansions in large numbers. The trophozoite forms are complicated infolding and intradigitations with type I pneumocytes forming tight cluster of cells on the wall of the alveolar cavity. The large trophozoite has typical unit membrane, covered externally with an electron dense layer. They also show more intermembranous particles. The cytoplasm is less dense and contains single nucleus, a mitochondrion, endoplasmic reticulum, ribosomes, glycogen particles, osmophilic round bodies. The Golgi apparatus is absent.

The precyst is the intermediate stage between trophozoite and the mature cyst. The precyst is oval and measures 4 to 5 μm in size with large nucleus. Initially, the precyst possesses a thin double-layered pellicle that becomes thick as the cyst matures. As the cyst matures, it becomes more spherical and the thickness of pellicle increases. During early stage of development, the precyst contains synaptonemal complex indicative of meiotic prophase. The complex disappears and the nuclear division follows. Each cyst contains eight nuclei. The mature cyst is smooth, round and contains eight intracystic bodies. The cyst wall is very thick and contains three layers namely, an electron dense layer, an electron lucent layer and an inner plasma membrane. The main component of electron dense layer is β-1,3 glucan. The organelles of intracystic body are same as that of trophozoite. After excystation, the empty cysts collapse in to crescent-shaped structures.

During the early phase of infection, the haploid trophozoites without filipodia attach to the type I pneumocytes. These thin-walled stages increase in size upto 100 µm and assume polymorphic shape. The haplophasic trophozoites transformed into diplophasic trophozoites following asexual process. Either the enlarged diploid trophozoites develop by reproducing the asexual forms by binary fission, or undergoes another cycle producing thin-walled cysts that contain pleomorphic daughter cells. The mature trophozoites, which develop after binary fission, possess thin limiting pellicle and they are the pre-cysts and transform into cysts with eight intracystic bodies that remain within the cyst.

The parasite is found in a variety of domestic, wild animals as well as in humans. It is not clear whether, transmission occurs between two different species of animals. Infection is transmitted by inhalation and by close or direct contact between two individuals. Approximately, 19% of the infants below the age of one year show the presence of acquired immunity as seen by the presence of antibody against *P. carinii* in their blood specimens. The incidence increases to 80% at the age of four years. This observation supports the hypothesis that the presence of a reservoir from which the young children become infected.

Although a variety of domestic and wild animals harbor the parasite, it is not clear whether the species of *P. carinii* in all these animals is same or not. *In vitro* studies showed that *P. carinii* can grow in cell cultures incubated at 35–37°C but not at 41°C. This observation indicates that the parasite has specific temperature requirements for its growth and this may well explain why birds do not harbor the parasite whose body temperature is above 40°C.

Epidemiologically human pneumocystosis falls under three categories: (a) classical plasma cell pneumonia in infants, (b) pneumocystosis in immunocompromized hosts, and (c) pneumocystosis in AIDS patients. The classical plasma cell pneumonia is an endemic disease that typically affects malnourished or premature infants. Pneumocystosis in immunocompromised individuals was noticed during 1960s and 1970s and was mainly associated with procedures that control cancer using cytotoxic drugs and procedures and therapies that suppress or compromise the immune mechanisms in transplanted patients. The third type of pneumocystosis was recognized since 1980, and it is prevailed almost in every country that reported AIDS cases. Pneumocystosis in AIDS patients is distinct in that it spreads to organs other than lungs and the recurrence rate is very high even after treatment. It is believed that *P. carinii* is maintained in humans primarily by direct transmission from infected persons to uninfected ones. The source of the parasite in the infected persons is not clear. It may be an exogenous infection or probably a latent infection that is reactivated because of immunosuppression.

Patients respond well to the standard treatment with trimethoprim + sulfamethoxazole if given during the early stage of infection. The dosage is 12 to 20 mg/kg body weight and the treatment is continued for 14 to 21 days. Some of the patients with AIDS may develop severe allergic reactions to this combination. *Pneumocystis carinii* is very sensitive to intravenous administration of pentamidine-isethionate. However, the drug is very toxic and needs close monitoring. To reduce the toxic effects the dosage can be reduced or the drug can be administered as aerosol. A combination of trimethoprim and dapsone has been used in treating mild to moderately severe pneumocystosis in AIDS patients. This combination showed fewer adverse reactions compared to the combination of TMP+SMX. Supportive therapy includes administration of oxygen and corticosteroids.

At present, there is no vaccine available for the prevention of pneumocystosis. The available data suggests that vaccines that induce antibodies against *P. carinii* may be of some use for immunotherapy and immunoprophylaxis. However, such vaccines may of little use for individuals whose immunological system is damaged badly.

Prophylaxis is necessary for AIDS or ARC diseases, transplant patients and patients with lymphoblastic leukemia. In the absence of prophylaxis, 90% of the transplant recipients eventually develop pneumocystosis. Co-trimoxazole or aerosolized pentamidine isethionate are the primary agents for prophylaxis. Aerosolized pentamidine isethionate is used extensively as prophylactic agent (300 mg of the drug to be inhaled every month).

BALANTIDIUM COLI

Claparēde and Lachmann first recognized the genus *Balantidium* in 1858, when they observed this protozoan in the rectum of frog. Since then this organism was described from several other animals and a number of species have been identified. Malmstein in 1857 described a case of acute dysentery in humans and this organism was named as *Paramecium coli* because of its resemblance to *Paramecium.* Leukart in 1861 discovered a similar organism in the large intestines of pig. Stein in 1863, recognized that the human parasite described by Malmstein and the pig parasite described by Leukart were morphologically identical and he named the parasite as *Balantidium coli.*

Balantidium coli is the only ciliate that infects humans. However, human infections with this parasite are rare. On the other hand, this infection is extremely common in pigs and it is generally believed that pig acts as the main reservoir for human infections. The genus *Balantidium* belongs to the phylum Ciliophora. McDonald in 1922 made a proposal to separate the human species from that of pigs by naming the isolates from pigs as *Balantidium suis.* Nevertheless, this separation has not been accepted and the parasite in these two hosts is considered as single species by most authors at present.

The organism exists in two forms; the trophozoite and the cyst. The trophozoite is actively motile, invasive and measures 30 to 300 µm length and 30 to 100 µm in breadth. The shape is generally ovoid but it can vary. The anterior end of the parasite has a funnel-shaped depression through which the food is ingested. The mouth comprises of peristome, cytopharynx and cytostome. The cilia, the organelles of locomotion cover the entire surface of the parasite and are embedded in the pellicle and arranged in the longitudinal rows known as kineties. The peristomal cilia are larger than the somatic cilia. The parasite can ingest a variety of food materials, and the digestion takes place inside the food vacuole. The excretory opening of the parasite is called cytopyge, which is circular and smaller than peristome. The two contractile vacuoles that lie side by side or one above the other maintain the osmotic pressure in the cell by removing the excess water from the cytoplasm and expelling it into the external environment. The trophozoite has a macronucleus and a micronucleus. The macronucleus is situated in the middle of the cell and it is either spherical, curved, elongated or kidney shaped. The micronucleus is enclosed in a nuclear membrane and it can be removed intact from the cell by disrupting the cell membrane. The macronucleus comprises of small nucleoli. The micronucleus is small and lies in close proximity to macronucleus.

The cystic form of the parasite measures 40 × 60 μm in diameter and it is spherical or ovoid in shape. The cyst wall is transparent and thick. The parasite is visible within the cyst and in the immature cyst the movement of the parasite can be seen. As the cyst matures, the cilia are absorbed and the movement of the parasite ceases. The cyst also possesses both micro- and macronucleus (Fig. 23.16).

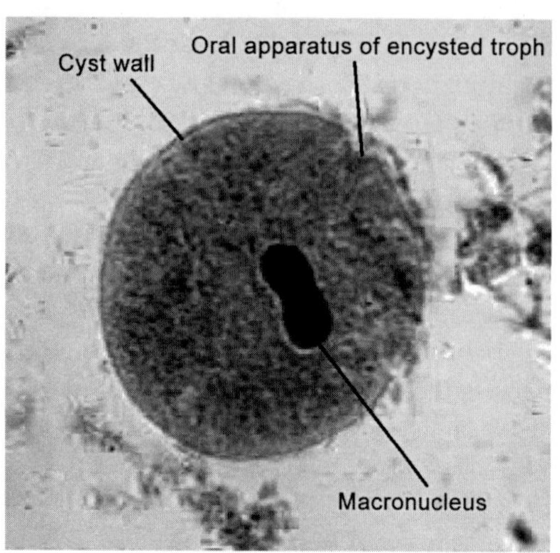

Fig. 23.16: *Balantidium coli*
(*For color version, see Plate 10*)

The infective form of the parasite is the mature cyst which is transmitted by contaminated food and water (fecooral transmission). The cyst is resistant to the action of gastric juices and the excystation probably occurs in the small intestines and the multiplication occurs in the large intestines. The organism multiplies asexually by binary fission. Sexual union (syngamy) is an important aspect in the life cycle of the parasite and this occurs by a process of conjugation. During the conjugation process, the two cells come in to close contact and exchange their nuclear material. The conjugation takes place for a short period and there is no increase in the number of cells due to conjugation. In the infected host, the parasite may be excreted in the feces as trophozoite or as a cyst. The trophozoite degenerates but the cyst survives and it is transmitted to another animal or to humans by contaminated food and water.

Balantidiasis is endemic in tropical and subtropical countries. The incidence varies from 4 to 20 percent, the highest being in Indonesia. McCarey in 1952 reviewed the epidemiology and showed that Iran as an endemic area of unusual interest as there is no pig-farming in Iran because of religious ban on eating pork. The transmission is from human to humans and any other animal if any is not known. The infection is frequently observed in psychiatric wards in USA and in many other countries. The transmission occurs from person-to-person due to poor hygiene.

Tetracyclines, 500 mg 4 times/day for 10 days is recommended as the drug of choice. Clearance of the parasite can occur within 48 hours but treatment should be continued for 10 days. Another useful drug is metronidazole which is given 750 mg three times per day for 5 to 7 days. After successful treatment there is no relapse of the infection and also there is no reported resistance to the drugs that are used for treatment. Treatment is recommended for carriers in institutions to prevent the spread of infection to other members of the institution who may be susceptible to infection.

Prevention

Balantidiasis can be controlled by:

Hygienic rearing of pigs and prevention of human-pig contact.

Improved hygiene in psychiatric institutions to reduce person-to-person transmission.

Treatment of carriers (persons who excrete cysts of *Balantidium coli*).

HELMINTHS OF HUMAN IMPORTANCE

Introduction

Apart from *Protozoa,* there are numerous multicellular animals often referred to as 'Metazoa' that parasitize humans as well as many mammals. These multicellular organisms are generally known as 'Helminths'. Helminth in general means worm and in the present context refers to those animals that belong to groups within the animal kingdom, the *Nematoda* and *Platyhelmenthes*. Nematodes are large single group of cylindrical shaped worms. Two distinct groups of medical importance, Cestodes (Tapeworms) and Trematodes (Flukes or leaf-like flat worms), represent the Platyhelmenthes. The cardinal differences between the groups of these worms are given in Table 23.12.

Phylum Nematoda

Nematodes are the most abundant and widespread animal group, occur in large number in the environment ranging from polar region to hot springs. Many of these are free-living marine, fresh water, soil and parasitic forms (parasitic to both animal and plants). Nematodes are bilaterally symmetrical, unsegmented dioecious worms that are normally filiform. They possess a body cavity with high hydrostatic pressure, a straight digestive tract with an anterior terminal mouth. The anus is situated posterior and it is subterminal. Nematodes are devoid of circulatory system and the excretory system is simple. The body wall is made of outer cuticle and inner longitudinal muscular layer. The phylum is subdivided into two classes; *Adenophoraa* and *Secernentea*. Both the classes have parasitic members. The majority of species that infect animals belong to the class Secernentea. In the *Adenophoraa* group, the first stage larva is infective to the definite host, whereas in *Secernentea* group the third stage larva is infective to the definitive host.

Table 23.12: Anatomis differences between nematodes, cestodes, and trematodes

Nematodes	*Cestodes*	*Trematodes*
Belong to phylum Nemathelmenthes	Belong to the phylum Platyhelmenthes	Belong to the Phylum Platyhelmenthes
Cylindrical	Tape-like, flat and segmented. Each segment acts as a single unit	Flat, leaf-like and unsegmented
Dioecious	Monoecious	Monoecious except *Schistosoma species*,
Well developed buccal capsule is present	Mouth parts contain suckers with or without hooks	Mouth parts contain suckers without hooks
Complete alimentary canal is present	No alimentary canal is present	Incomplete alimentary canal is present

All nematodes have five stages in their life cycle, four larval and one adult, which are separated by a moult of cuticle. The first two moults generally occur within the egg. The life cycle may be direct or indirect. Direct life cycle involves ingestion of fertilized eggs along with food and water or in some cases direct penetration of larva through the skin. The indirect life cycle utilizes an invertebrate host as intermediate host (sometimes vertebrate host). The larvae reside encysted in the tissues of intermediate hosts and the majority of nematodes parasitic to vertebrates reside in the alimentary canal of the host. Some may require migration of larvae through the blood to reach the alimentary canal of the host. Some parasites migrate from the gut into the tissue and back to the gut. This represents vestige of an indirect cycle in its evolutionary process. Whatever may be the mode of transmission, the chance of a particular egg developing into an adult is very slight. This is compensated for many cases by huge output of eggs that may be as high as 20,000 eggs/female/day.

The morphological features by which the nematodes are recognized vary from group to group. The individual species is recognized by the anatomical features of the anterior region of alimentary canal and the features of male tail. At the species level details of the male tail such as arrangement of caudal papillae (sensory structures used during the copulation), the length and the shape of the spicule (sclerotized copulatory aid). The male worms carry more taxonomical information.

ENTEROBIUS VERMICULARIS (PINWORM)

Enterobius vermicularis (E. vermicularis) may have evolved with humans from our primate ancestors. Evidences from early writings, from mummified bodies, and from archeological excavations indicate that pinworm along with other nematodes well established in humans, a few thousand years ago. The Pinworm also known as 'seat worm' is most frequently encountered parasite even in well-developed countries like USA. It is not an exaggeration if we say that nearly everyone at one time or the other has had an infection with pinworm. However, many of the infections are asymptomatic. Although it is rare, many physicians are not aware of the fact that *E. vermicularis* can cause severe ectopic disease in various parts of the body, particularly the urogenital tract of both young girls and women.

Life Cycle (Fig. 23.17)

1. Infection occurs because of ingestion of fully developed eggs.
2. Each egg releases a single larva.
3. These larvae migrate to the large intestine especially the cecum and colon where they attach superficially to the mucosa. Many are found down at the base of intestinal crypts.
4. The larvae reach adulthood within 3 to 4 weeks and infection generally lasts for one to two months.
5. After fertilization, the gravid female worm migrates to the anus and emerges at night to extrude the eggs on the perianal region and on perianal skin.
6. Each female may deposit upto 11,000 to 15,000 eggs before she dies.
7. Eggs have a sticky albuminous covering and adhere to the skin, clothing, hair and bedding.

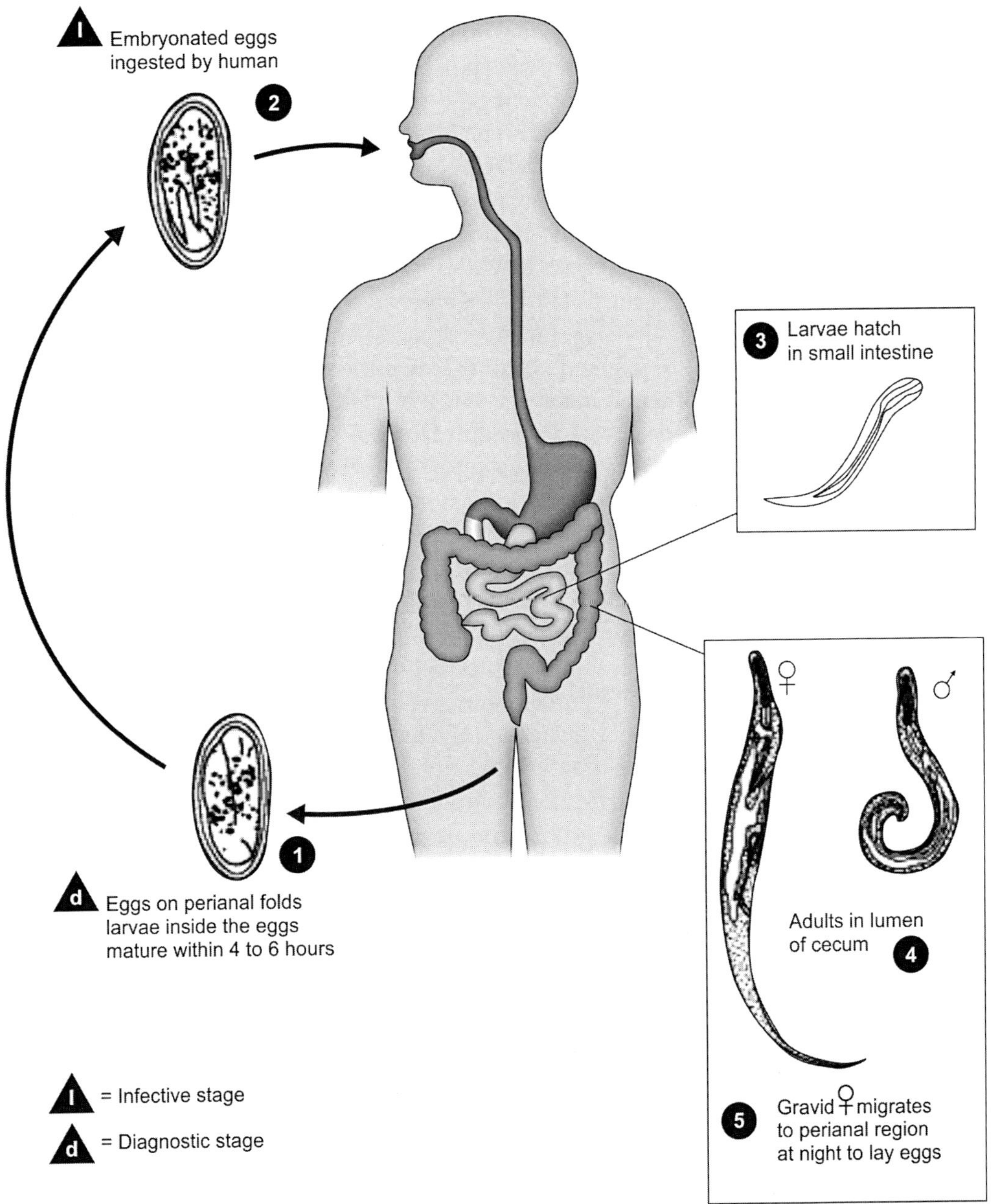

Fig. 23.17: Life cycle of *Enterobius vermicularis*

8. They become infective to humans within 4 to 6 hours
9. Occasionally the female worm may enter vagina, fallopian tubes, uterus and peritoneal cavity during its migration.
10. Such migrations are rare but can cause severe complications.

11. To some extent, the eggs deposited on the perineal region may hatch prematurely and the released larvae may re-enter the intestinal tract of the host (Retroinfection) through the anus. When this occurs, the life cycle may be lengthened considerably.

The intense pruritus produced by the migrating females as well as eggs deposited by them results in scratching of the affected area. As a result, the eggs are transferred to the fingertips and reinfection follows when the finger or the food contaminated by the fingers is placed in the mouth. The matured eggs may also reach the intestinal tract by indirect routes. The eggs adhere to the clothing or bed linen. The eggs are very light in weight and can be dispersed easily that results in widespread in bedrooms and houses. Hence, accidental transmission can occur to family members from these inanimate sources. The eggs remain viable for several weeks under cool moist environmental conditions. If the environmental conditions are dry and warm (>25°C), the eggs perish within one to two days. The parasite has no other animal reservoirs and man is the only source of infection. Hence, good personal hygiene is very important factor in the prevention of infection due to *E. vermicularis*.

Majority of *E. vermicularis* infections are asymptomatic. The most common clinical presentation is intense itching in the perianal region. Infected children may show irritability, enuresis and weight loss. Pinworm infection is not associated with marked eosinophilia or elevated serum IgE levels. In young girls and young women, the worm can cause vaginitis. Rarely the worms enter the peritoneal cavity either from the intestines or through the migration from the female reproductive tract. Dead worms or eggs may be identified in the granulomata in several organs (Fig. 23.18).

Pinworms are easily removed from the infected host by antihelminthic drugs like piperazine citrate and treatment is to be continued for 7 days. Pyrententel pamoate is effective (10 mg/kg wt) as a single dose, similar to that of mebendazole (100 mg) or albendazole (400 mg). Use of mebendazole or albendazole is advantageous when mixed infections are suspected or diagnosed.

Though the treatment is effective, reinfection occurs readily unless contact with the eggs is prevented. Personal hygiene specially cleaning the nail beds, heavily infected areas such a bedrooms, linen are cleaned scrupulously and kept dust free. The bed linen and night clothing are washed frequently. However, elimination of contact with these

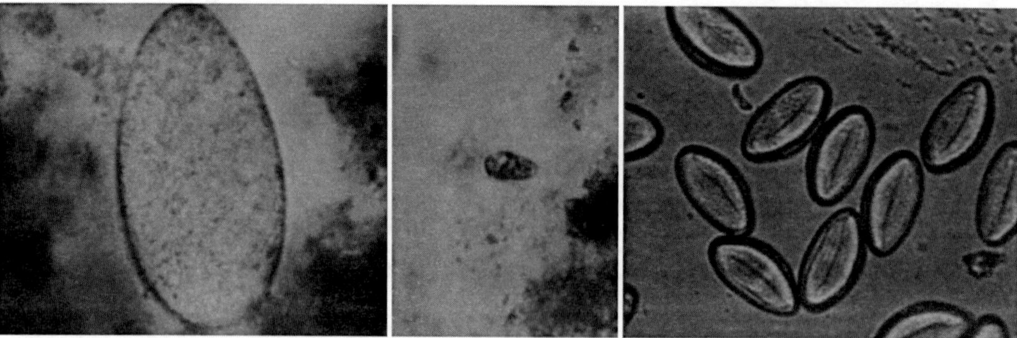

Fig. 23.18: Ova of liver fluke and pinworm (*Enterobius vermicularis*) (*For color version, see Plate 10*)

recommended procedures is very difficult and these procedures should be combined with repeated chemotherapy to remove the adult worms.

ASCARIS LUMBRICOIDES (ROUNDWORM)

With an estimated figure of 250 million people infected human infections due to *Ascaris lumbricoides* (*A. lumbricoides* or roundworm) is distributed worldwide. Several early records such as Egyptian papyri of 1500 BC, the Chinese descriptions of 2nd and 3rd century BC, the works of Hippocrates in 5th Century BC, and the texts of Arabic and Roman physicians describe the existence of this parasitic worm. Eggs of *A. lumbricoides* have been recovered from the human remains of 800 BC. This multicellular parasite was listed by Linnaeus and its name remained unchanged since 1758. The complete life cycle of the worm was described in 1922.

Freshly recovered adult male or female worms are pinkish cream in color and measure 20 to 30 cms in length. Male worms are shorter than female worms and each male worm has a curved posterior tail that accommodates the copulatory apparatus. The mouth of the adult worm is surrounded by three well-developed lips, rows of small teeth (known as denticles of Sprent) on the lips. The body is covered by cuticle with transverse striations. The female worm possesses a didelphic uterus and vulva in the anterior half of the body. The cuticle of *A. lumbricoides* is mainly composed of collagen stabilized by disulfide bonds that become more complex with each moulting. The cuticle of third and fourth larval stage contains proteins that are extractable with 2-mercaptoethanol. These proteins are easily digested by the bacterial collagenases. The collagen present in the second stage larva is not extractable with 2-mercaptoethanol and is resistant to digestion by bacterial collagenases. These observed differences may be a part of adaptation to survive outside the host, for infection process, or for both.

The eggs of *A. lumbricoides* excreted in human feces are seen in two general forms; unfertilized and fertilized eggs. The eggs possess a cortical layer. The eggs are yellowish brown in color because they are bile-stained. The fertilized egg measures 50 to 70 × 40 to 50 μm in size, oval or round in shape. The egg has an inner lipid layer responsible for structural strength and an outer vitelline layer. The inner layer contains a lipoprotein called ascaroside, which protects the egg from the disinfectant action of chemicals like formaldehyde. The outer surface of the fertilized eggs has an uneven deposit of mucopolysaccharides. These mucopolysaccharides have an adhesive property and this compound is acquired by the eggs while passing through the uterus (Fig. 23.19).

Life Cycle (Fig. 23.20)

1. The adult worms live unattached in the lumen of the small intestine of the host.
2. When the worms attain the sexual maturity, copulation occurs and soon after the female begins to lay eggs. The daily egg production per female is phenomenal averaging about 20,000. The eggs are excreted along with the feces.
3. The first larval stage develops within the egg and undergoes moulting.

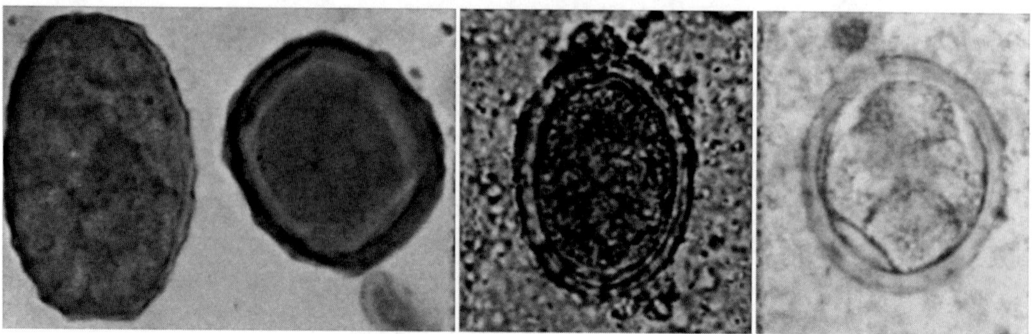

Fig. 23.19: Ova of the roundworm (*Ascaris lumbricoides*) (*For color version, see Plate 11*)

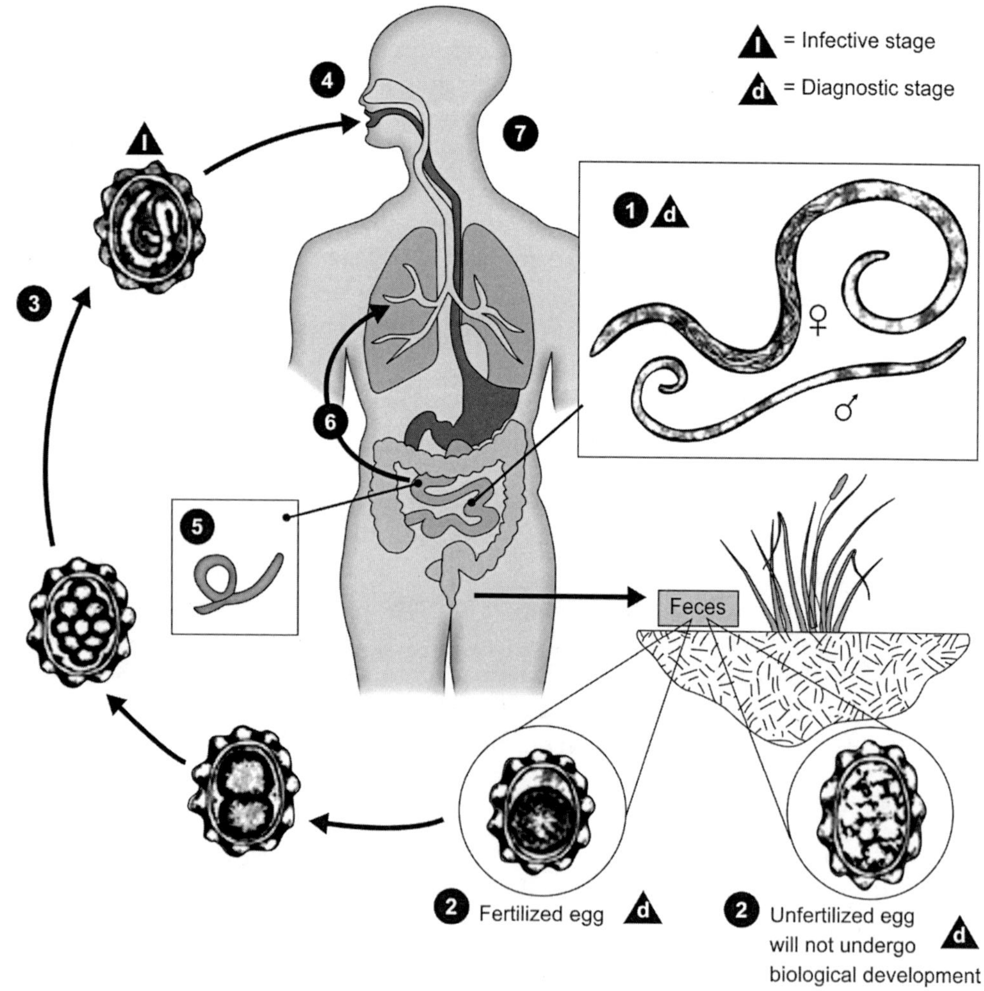

= Infective stage

= Diagnostic stage

4

7

3

1

6

5

Feces

2 Fertilized egg

2 Unfertilized egg will not undergo biological development

Fig. 23.20: Life cycle of *Ascaris lumbricoides*

4. The host infected when the fertilized eggs are ingested along with the contaminated food. Water, however, is not thought to be important source of infection.
5. Under favorable conditions of temperature, moisture and shady areas, the eggs develop into larvae.
6. The eggs when ingested by the host results in infection.
7. The eggs hatch in the duodenum, the emerging larvae are second stage larvae, and they have typical filariform appearance and measure 250 × 14 μm in size.
8. The larvae penetrate the duodenal wall enter circulatory system and carried to the right side heart and from there, they reach lungs. The second and third moulting occurs in the lungs.
9. The larvae filtered from the lung capillaries and later penetrate into the lungs.
10. After about two weeks of development in the lungs, the larvae migrate up the respiratory tract, to the epiglottis. From there, they are swallowed into the stomach.
11. The fourth moulting takes place in the intestine and the larvae develop rapidly into adult forms.
12. It is assumed that the whole life cycle takes at least 65 days to complete before the eggs are first detected in the feces.

Although there is no doubt that transmission mainly occurs due to ingestion of fertilized eggs, other routes of transmission may also exist. The larvae occasionally may pass through the placenta. There is even slight chance that infection may be established inadvertently through organ transplant surgery.

A. lumbricoides may cause both acute and chronic infection. The acute form may occur either due to larval migration or due to allergic responses or complications involving adult worms. The clinical manifestations of ascariasis are summarized in Table 23.13.

Only supportive treatment is required during the lung migration phase of the infection. Intestinal obstruction due to adult worms may require intubation, surgery and drainage. When adults are in ectopic sites due to abnormal migration, surgery is indicated if they produce complications. Saline enema may be useful in removing the worms from the large intestines during therapy. Many drugs are reasonably effective in treating intestinal ascariasis. Pyrantel Pamoate or mebendazole is commonly used for treatment. It must be kept in mind that when ascariasis coexists with other helminthic infections of the intestine, it is important to treat ascariasis first, otherwise ascarids become irritated and migrate to ectopic sites.

The prevalence and intensity of this helminthic infection cannot be reduced to a significant level without reduction in poverty and improvement in sanitation, living conditions and safe water supplies. There are compelling reasons for targeting antihelminthic treatment against particular groups in endemic areas. Children attending the primary school are the best-targeted group for such mass treatment. Whether control measures are to be implemented or not, depends upon the needs and resources of the people involved. A wide range of control strategies are now available and some progress against intestinal worm infections can be made if the local people are motivated and helped to organize and control their community health needs.

Table 23.13: Clinical manifestations of ascariasis

Stage	Event	Clinical features	Outcome
Larval migration	Migration of larvae through liver and lungs	Pneumonitis, asthma, dyspnea, cough, substernal pain	Decrease food intake
Maturation and oviposition	Presence of juvenile and adult worms in the intestines	Abdominal pain, abdominal distension, colic, nausea, vomiting, Intermittent diarrhea, anorexia, restlessness, anal itching, enterocolitis, disordered small bowel pattern and abnormalities of jejunal mucosa	Decreased food intake, increased nutrition loss, malabsorption of proteins, fats, xylose and lactose intolerance
Allergic reactions	Exposure to ascaris allergens at any stage of the life cycle	Hypersensitivity reactions	Decreased food intake and increased nutritional loss
Complications	Migration or aggregation of adult worms in the intestines	Intestinal obstruction, intussusceptions, volvulus, invasion of bile duct with obstruction, gallstones, acute pancreatitis, peritonitis, upper respiratory tract obstruction	Life-threatening illness which decrease the food intake and increase the nutritional requirements due to diarrhea

TRICHURIS TRICHIURA (*T. TRICHIURA* OR WHIPWORM)

Calandrucci in 1886 swallowed the eggs of *T. trichiura* after confirming that he was free from the infection due to this nematode during the past six months and passed the eggs of this nematode after 27 days. These results were published by Grassi in 1887. *T. trichiura* is commonly known as whipworm as it resembles the buggy whip. The anterior end is long and slender, whereas the posterior end is more robust, shorter and broader. Male worms are shorter than the female worms. Female worm measures upto 5 cm in length. The male worm possesses a curved tail. The fertilized eggs are barrel shaped, measure 50 × 20 µm in size, golden brown in color due to bile staining and they have transparent prominences called polar plugs at each end. The eggs float in the saturated solution of common salt or 33% solution of zinc sulfate (Fig. 23.21).

Life Cycle (Fig. 23.22)

1. The infection is acquired by the ingestion of fertilized eggs along with contaminated food and water.
   a. The incubation period varies between 1-3 months and the adult worm may persist in the host upto 6 years.
   b. The ingested fertilized eggs hatch in the small intestines. Some studies indicate that the free larvae (2nd stage) enter nearby intestinal crypts and penetrate into glands and stroma.

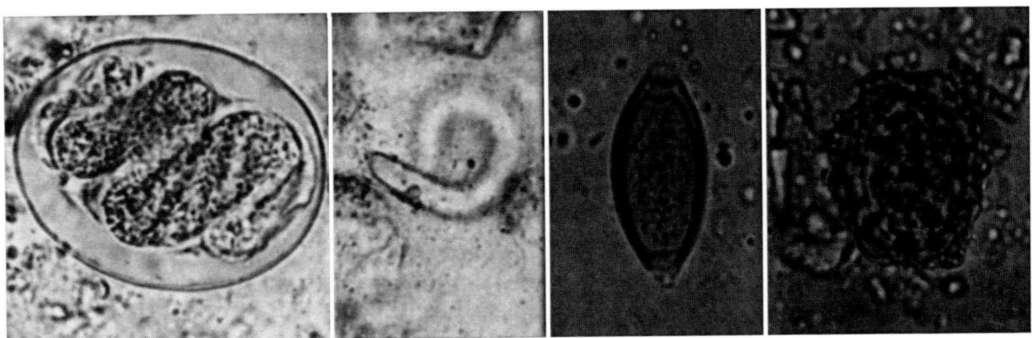

Fig. 23.21: Hookworm embryo and ova of the whipworm (*Trichuris trichiura*)
(*For color version, see Plate 11*)

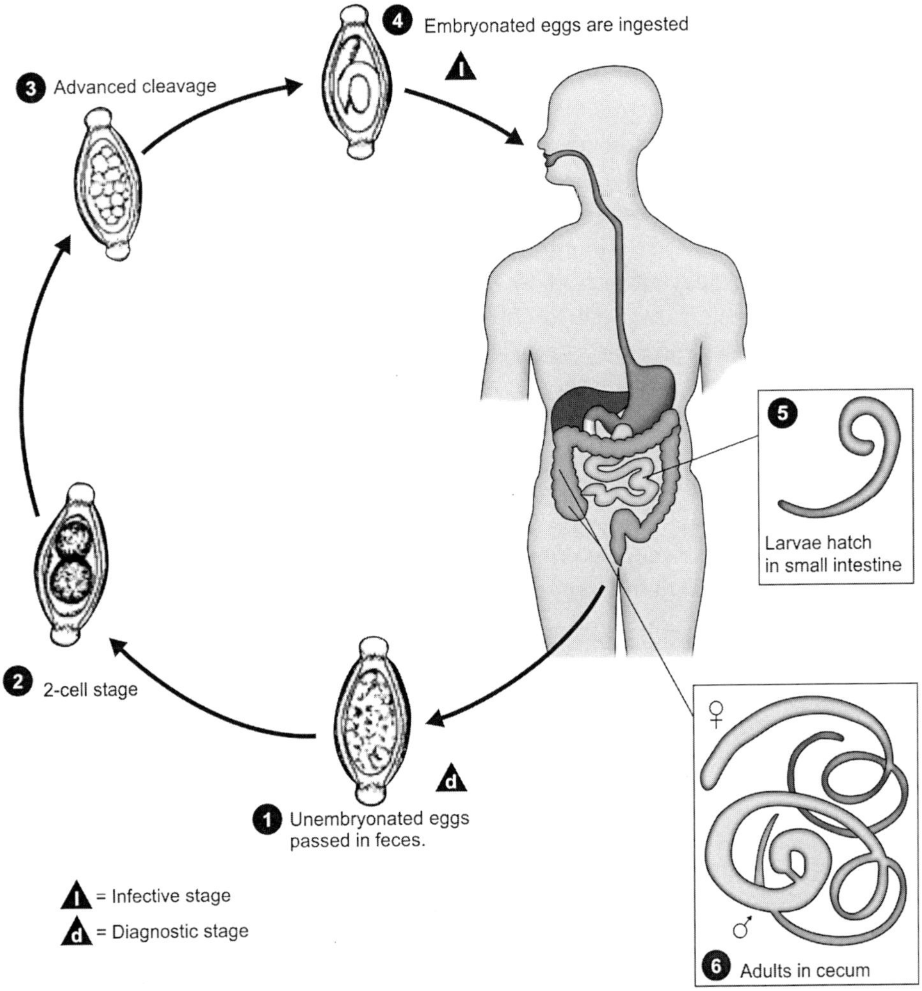

Fig. 23.22: Life cycle of *Trichuris trichiura*

2. They re-enter the lumen of the small intestines from these sites after about 10 days and migrate to large intestines where the anterior end of the developing adult is sewn into the mucosa of the large intestine, cecum or appendix.
   a. The posterior end of the adult worm hangs freely into the lumen of the intestine.
   b. The adult male and female worms after attaining sexual maturity copulate and the gravid female releases 2000 to 6000 fertilized eggs per day.
   c. These eggs are excreted along with the feces of the infected person and at that stage they are still underdeveloped (noninfectious).
   d. Under favorable conditions such as warm temperature, moisture, sandy humus soil and shady area, the eggs develop and become infective within 3 to 6 weeks.
   e. The eggs of *T. trichiura* are not as resistant as that of *A. lumbricoides,* and their survival is considered to be relatively for a brief period.
   f. Some studies showed that the freed larvae in the intestine migrate directly or hatch directly in the cecum without the tissue phase in the small intestine.
3. There is some controversy about the exact place of the intestinal penetration by the larvae, or whether the larvae migrate along the intestinal tissues to reach large intestines.
4. *T. trichiura* must complete the series of four moults before the adult worms are intimately associated with the wall of large intestine.

Infections due to *T. trichiura* are more common in areas that have high humidity, warm temperature and soil that has good holding capacity. Dooryard pollution and poor sanitation may cause heavy infection. Infection may coexist with amoebiasis, ascariasis and hookworm infections. Malnourished children are severely infected. No animal reservoir exists except man. Mebendazole is considered as the drug of choice, but it is not effective in all cases. It is suggested that light and asymptomatic cases need not be treated.

The general principles applicable to all helminthic worm infections also hold good for the control and prevention of trichuriasis. Schools serve as gathering point for drug delivery and administration, which can be undertaken by the teachers and schools, are the focus for education in the community so that health education can be reinforced. Most importantly children are more vulnerable to much morbidity as well as impairments in their growth and general development. Treatment is targeted to reduce the intensity in the community, not seeking eradication.

ANCYLOSTOMA DUODENALE (A. DUODENALE), NECATOR AMERICANUS (N. AMERICANUS, HOOKWORM)

Two genera of ancylostomitids (commonly known as 'Hookworm') occur in humans mainly in tropical areas. *Ancylostoma* species are intestinal nematodes infective to humans during the larval stage. Human hookworm infections are caused by *A. duodenale* and *N. americanus* species. The former is originated in Asia and the latter in Africa, has been associated with humans for over 5000 years. Hookworms reached America before fifth century BC, and the larvae have been identified in coprolites dating from this period. Hookworm disease is known since the time of earliest records such as Egyptian papyrus of 1500 BC. Hippocrates and Avicenna gave accurate description of the disease. The adult *A. duodenale* worm was first recognized by Angelo Dubini in 1843. Arthur Looss discovered that humans become infected through the skin and he himself was accidentally infected. The major contributions made in 20th century about this parasite include the determination of blood loss that leads to anemia and the valiant efforts of the Rockefeller Foundation to control the disease. This activity resulted in establishment of several schools of public health and the creation of World Health Organization (WHO).

Four species are involved in human infections; two of these, *A. duodenale* and *N. americanus* are true human parasites and the other two, *A. brasilense* and *A. caninum* are the parasites of cats and dogs. The latter two species produce dermatitis (Cutaneous larva migrans or creeping eruption) in humans after the penetration of the skin by the filariform larvae.

When observed in human feces, the eggs of both *A. duodenale* and *N. americanus* are indistinguishable and are oval with thin shell. The egg measures about 60 × 40 µm in size color less, not bile stained and floats in saturated solution of common salt or 33% zinc sulfate solution. The fertilized egg shows four blastomeres. With microscopic examination of eggs in the fecal specimens alone, it is not possible to differentiate the two species. The first stage larvae that escape from egg measures 200 µm in length. They feed on organic debris. The resulting second stage larvae are about 500 µm in length. After another moult, the infectious third stage larvae measure 500 to 700 µm in length. *A. duodenale* is generally longer than *N. americanus*. The adult male worm is shorter than female worm. *A. duodenale* is stronger and sturdy than *N. americanus* (Fig. 23.23). The species are identified by the morphology of the buccal capsule. The term 'Hookworm' derives from the prominent curve to the anterior end of the specimen of *N. americanus*. The male worm possesses umbrella-like coupulatory bursa.

Life Cycle (Fig. 23.24)

1. Life cycles of various hookworms are similar. The adult worms are attached to the mucosa of the upper levels of small intestines with the head anchored securely to the mucosa of intestines. The villous is drawn into the mouth of the worm and the blood from the host's capillaries is sucked.
2. After fertilization, the female worm lays eggs, which are passed in the feces in an underdeveloped state.
3. Under favorable conditions, the eggs develop in 1 to 2 days and the free-living larval stages (Rhabditi form larvae) are released.
   a. These larvae feed on bacteria and detritus in the feces and soil and moult in turn to form third stage larvae. They eventually metamorphose into infective forms (Filiariform larvae). Filariform larvae do not feed and can survive upto two weeks.
4. These larvae when come into contact with human skin, they penetrate the skin. The penetration requires human essential fatty acids like linoleate, influenced by the secretion of eicosanoid compounds by the larvae. The T cell and B cell responses are probably modulated by eicosanoids during skin penetration.

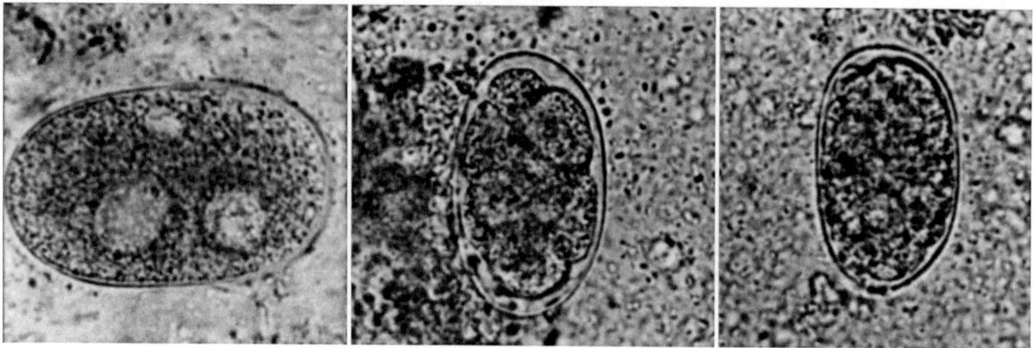

Fig. 23.23: Ova of the hookworm with embryo in different stages (*For color version, see Plate 11*)

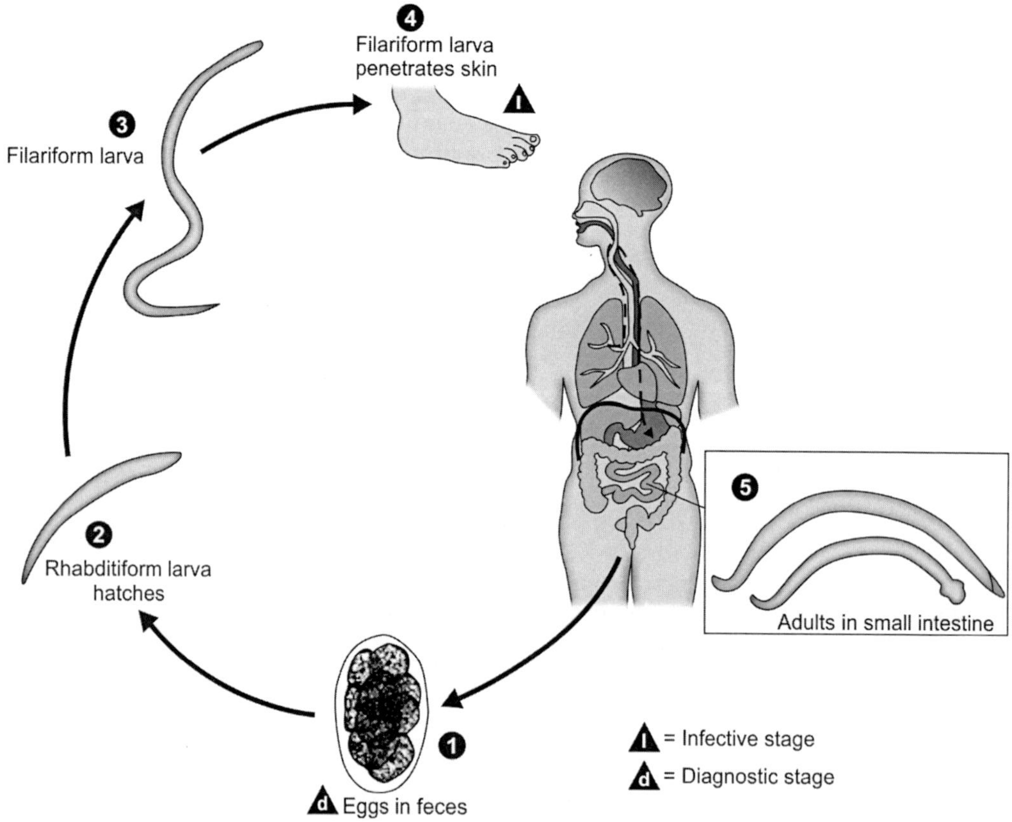

4 Filariform larva penetrates skin

3 Filariform larva

2 Rhabditiform larva hatches

5 Adults in small intestine

1 Eggs in feces

= Infective stage

= Diagnostic stage

Fig. 23.24: Life cycle of *Ancylostoma duodenale* (Hook worm)

5. After many hours following the penetration, they enter the cutaneous blood vessels and are carried to the right side of the heart and then to lungs. After a few days, they penetrate the pulmonary capillaries and reach the alveoli, ascend the respiratory tract to the epiglottis, and once they have been swallowed, descend to upper portion of the small intestine where they develop and grow in to sexually mature adults. The

incubation period is about six months and the adult worms in humans may survive for 10 to 15 years. However, most of them may die within 1 to 4 years.

6. Recent studies confirm that transmammary infection is also possible for *A. duodenale*.

Under favorable conditions, 80% of the population may be infected. Sandy, loamy soil with well-defined crumb structure, which is well aerated, is favorable for the development of larvae and for vertical migration. In rural gangetic Bengal, prevalence is high but only a few cases with overt disease are seen.

Blood loss from the intestinal wall constitutes greatest damage from hookworm infection. The blood loss unless well compensated, results in macrocytic-hypochromic anemia. Moderate blood decompensation causes anemia, palpitations of heart, and lassitude. Common signs and symptoms of chronic hookworm disease are anemia, epigastric burning, flatulence, sallow skin, tender abdomen, irritability, alternating diarrhea and constipation, dry skin, blurred vision finally leading to marked physical weakness. This accounts for the early term lazy disease. Cardiomegaly and cardiac symptoms are evident in many cases. Physical stunting (including sexual) is characteristic in children and many of them show significant mental retardation.

Cutaneous larva migrans (CLM), generally referred to as creeping eruption is primarily due to the filariform larvae of dog and cat hookworms (*A. caninum* and *A. catis*), penetrating the human skin and subcutaneous tissues. It is also caused by hookworm larvae of other human hookworms like *Uncinaria* and *Bunostomum,* parasites of domestic animals. These hookworms are unable to mature in humans but the larvae are capable of living for many years in the subcutaneous tissues. Cutaneous larva migrans is worldwide, wherever cats and dogs are domesticated. It is commonly seen in areas where the climate is warm and moist. The life cycles of these worms are same as that of the human hookworms. The larvae, though capable of penetrating the skin of humans, cannot mature to the adult stage.

Migrating larvae produce an intensely pruritic eruptions along with papules and vesicles. After a few days, each larva develops a serpigenous tunnel in the epidermis as it proceeds at the rate of a few millimeters per day. This results in edema and a raised inflammatory tract with a crusty opening that is very characteristic. There is also cellular infiltration with predominance of eosinophils. After a period of several weeks or months, the skin is extensively involved. Some individuals may show systemic manifestations. The intense pruritus leads to scratching and that exposes the lesions to secondary bacterial infections. In hookworm infection, the cutaneous variety is more common. Larva migrans occurs due to invasion of the skin of humans by the third stage larvae. The clinical condition is self-limiting. Repeated infections may be necessary with some species to establish hypersensitivity before the skin lesions develop.

Hookworm infection may be difficult to eradicate because reinfection usually occurs. Mebendazole and Pyrentel Pamoate are useful in treating the heavy infections. Iron supplements are required in those who are severely anemic or malnourished. Iron deficiency is corrected before the treatment is started.

Significant reduction in the disease due to all these soil-transmitted nematodes will not occur until poverty is reduced and the living conditions are improved. Antihelminthic treatment against targeted population like schoolchildren, health education, involvement of community, judicious use of available resources may help in reducing the infection and some progress against intestinal worms can be made if local people are helped to identify their health needs and organize their community health affairs.

STRONGYLOIDES STERCORALIS

Normand in 1876, observed the nematodes of the genus *Strongyloides* in the fecal specimens of French troops in Cochin-China. Autopsy conducted on patients with overwhelming infection revealed morphologically distinct worms in the intestinal mucosa. Bavay, in the same year, named the intestinal forms as *Anguillula intestinalis* and the fecal forms as *Anguillula stercoralis.* Soon it was recognized that both are different stages of development of the same parasite. The studies of Fuelleborn in 1914, and that of Nishigiri in 1924 confirmed the existence of an auto-infective cycle and the first stage larvae could indeed develop into mature filariform larvae and invade the colonic mucosa, thus initiating the development of adult worms in the same host. The genus *Strongyloides* belongs to the phylum *Nematoda* and it is placed in the class *Phasmida* (Nematodes containing phasmids or caudal chemoreceptors). The genus has two species; *Strongyloides stercoralis (S. stercoralis)* and *Strongyloides fuelleborni (S. fuelleborni).*

The female worms are small, measuring about 2 to 3 mm × 30 to 50 μm in size. The anterior portion of the worm contains the esophagus and it is thicker. The triradiate pharynx has two subventral and one dorsal gland. The worms reside in the mucosa of intestine and depot their secretions from the glands into the lumen of the intestine. The reproductive system comprises of vulva placed in the midline, paired uteri leading posteriorly and anteriorly from vagina. The ovaries in *S. stercoralis* are aligned linearly and in *S. fuelleborni,* they are spirally wound.

The first stage rhabditiform larvae measure 250 × 15 μm in size and they have a muscular esophagus that occupies anterior third of the body. The buccal cavity is small compared to other nematodes (Fig. 23.25).

The third stage filariform larvae are longer and thin with paired alae on both sides of the larva that offer more stability during movement along the ground. The mouth is small and closed indicating that probably filariform larvae do not feed. Electron microscopy revealed that these larvae possess amphidial neurons, which are highly specialized organs through which the larvae sense the environmental stimuli.

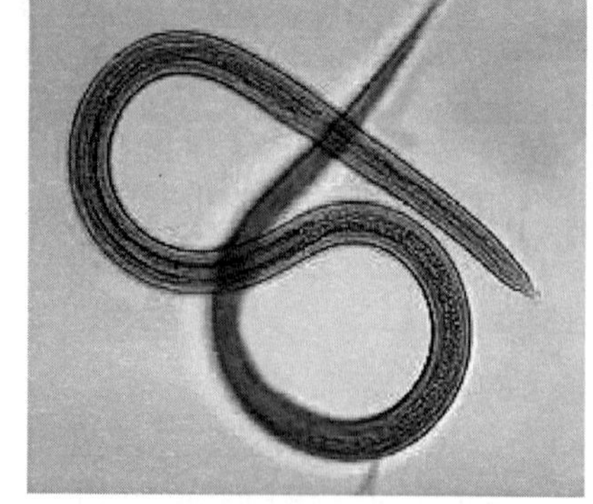

Fig. 23.25: *Strongyloides stercoralis*

Life Cycle (Fig. 23.26)

1. The female worm after fertilization deposits the eggs within the intestinal mucosa and they usually hatch before reaching the intestinal lumen. As a result, it is rare to find the eggs in the fecal specimens.

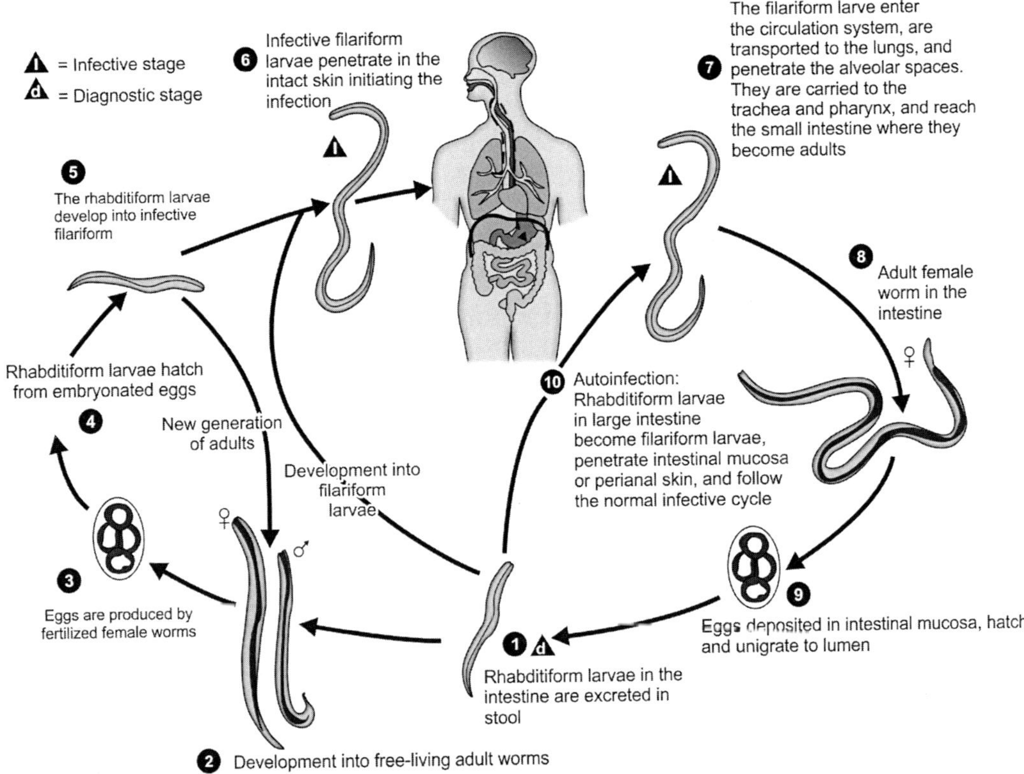

Fig. 23.26: Life cycle of *Strongyloides stercoralis*

2. The released larvae from the fertilized eggs are known as Rhabditiform larvae. These are smaller with short esophagus, which ends in dilated bulb-like structure. These larvae take any of the following courses.
3. They are excreted in the feces and in suitable humid soil; these Rhabditiform larvae undergo maturation after moulting three times. The adult worm leads an independent life in the environment.
4. Sometimes, the released Rhabditiform larvae undergo maturation rapidly to become male or female worms, which after fertilization give rise to second generation of Rhabditiform larvae which later develop independently.
5. Under adverse conditions, the Rhabditiform larvae metamorphose into filariform larvae (These are longer than Rhabditiform larvae and possess short mouth and cylindrical esophagus). These are the infective forms.
6. These filariform larvae are formed in the intestine, from where they pierce the mucosa, through venous circulation carried to right side of the heart, enter pulmonary alveoli, travel through bronchioles, bronchi and trachea, are swallowed when they enter pharynx, and finally reach the intestine. This is known as endoautoinfection.

7. Sometimes these filariform larvae derived by the metamorphosis of Rhabditiform larvae are excreted in the feces and while passing they penetrate the perianal skin and undergo the extraintestinal migration as described above and reach finally the intestine after maturation. This is known as exoautoinfection.
8. The last course that the Rhabditiform larvae might take is that, either they are liberated through the feces and undergo metamorphosis in the soil in to filariform larvae, or the filariform larvae that are formed within the intestine itself are passed in the feces. These infective forms pierce the skin of the person walking bare-footed, in moist soil and from there they follow the usual course of extraintestinal migration, attain maturity before they reach the usual habitat, the small intestines.

Strongyloidiasis is prevalent both in temperate and tropical areas because of its remarkable ability to adapt its life cycle and development to suit the environmental conditions. Internal autoinfection is responsible for maintenance of infection within the host for many years. All infected people are at risk of hyperinfection and disseminated disease, and identification of individuals who acquired infection in the past is of clinical significance. *Strongyloides* hyperinfection is frequently seen in those with immune defects and underlying diseases like malignancy, autoimmune diseases, severe mal nutrition, steroid therapy and immunosupression in transplant patients. Coinfections like HIV and HTLV-1 may be associated with severe strongyloidiasis. The infection is predominantly transmitted by entry through the skin from the contaminated soil. Infection is common in close communities, in areas with poor sanitation in both urban and rural areas.

Strongyloidiasis can occur as asymptomatic infection, intestinal disease and hyperinfection with or without dissemination. Symptoms of the disease appear to be dependent on worm load, immune status of the host and developmental tendencies of the parasite. In chronic infections, the egg output is considerably less but remains constant. Accordingly very few larvae cause internal autoinfection. The reverse process is true with hyperinfection.

Chronic infection is usually asymptomatic. When symptoms do occur they usually involve the gastrointestinal tract, causing abdominal pain, diarrhea alternating with constipation and distension of the abdomen. Children may develop malabsorption syndrome and stunting of the growth. Skin penetration by autoinfective filariform larvae may produce serpigenous pruritic eruptions around the perianal region. The pathognomonic rash progresses for some period and subsides over a period of hours. The most serious clinical manifestation of strongyloidiasis is hyperinfection due to dramatic increase in the number of parasites within the host leading to dissemination. Hyperinfection is common in people with underlying diseases, immunosuppressive therapy, and steroid usage in some hematological malignant conditions. Patients with hyperinfection may develop paralytic ileus, gastrointestinal bleeding or perforation. Migration of increased numbers of larvae in the lungs may result in pneumonic consolidation, wheezing, dyspnea and other complications of respiratory tract. During hyper-infection, the filariform larvae are recovered from various tissue biopsies like lymph node, liver and rarely from central nervous system.

Thiabendazole is the drug of choice for chronic strongyloidiasis. The drug is administered orally at dose of 2 mg/kg two times daily for two days. The drug offers parasitological cure rate 60 to 100 percent in children, although very limited studies are available. Severe side effects like nausea, dizziness and neuropsychiatric symptoms may result in noncompliance by the patients.

Ivermectin, a broad-spectrum antihelminthic drug is also equally effective in the treatment of chronic strongyloidiasis. The drug is given as single dose and it is associated with lesser side effects.

Patients who are on treatment for chronic strongyloidiasis should be followed with periodic fecal examinations for larvae. The serum eosinophil counts should return to normal in 2 to 3 months. Follow-up of patients with serological test by ELISA is useful in monitoring long-term treatment especially in patients with an underling immune defect or immunosuppression.

Successful treatment of hyperinfection due to *S. stercoralis* depends upon prompt diagnosis and early initiation of therapy with thiabendazole at a dose of 25 mg/kg wt, twice a day and it should be continued indefinitely pending both clinical response and eradication of larvae from all body sites and body fluids. Secondary bacterial infections should be treated aggressively with suitable antibiotics based on laboratory culture and sensitivity reports.

Control measures in an endemic area require effective disposal of human excreta. Strict aseptic conditions are maintained while handling the specimens from laboratory animals.

TRICHINELLA SPIRALIS

The nematode *Trichinella spiralis* is the causative agent of trichinosis (also known as Trichinellosis or Trichina infection). The infection is acquired by consumption of raw or under cooked pork. Foster (1965) believed that trichinellosis is one of the most interesting parasitic infection and more likely to be responsible for the Mosaic and Mohammedan traditions of avoiding pork than the possibility of tapeworm infection. Earlier, people like Aristotle and Hippocrates recognized association of the infection with pigs. Nevertheless, the encysted larvae in the muscles were not seen until 1822 and even then, their presence was not attributed to the infection in humans. In 1835 James Paget, a medical student at St. Bartholomew's Hospital in London discovered the worm in humans. The discovery created interest among well-known parasitologists and it was Owen in 1835, presented a definite report but played down Paget's role in the discovery of the parasite. The larval stage in human muscles was not recognized although French and German scientists suspected in the 1840s. Rudolph Virchow and Friedrich Zenker discovered the adult worm and it was Friedrich Zenker, who recognized the clinical significance of the infection.

Both female and male worms are recognized by their morphology. The female measures 3 mm in length and 50 µm in breadth. The male worm is almost half the size of female (1.5 mm × 30 µm). At the tail end, the male has a set of reproductive organs called claspers. Claspers are seen easily and the male uses them to hold the female worm during mating.

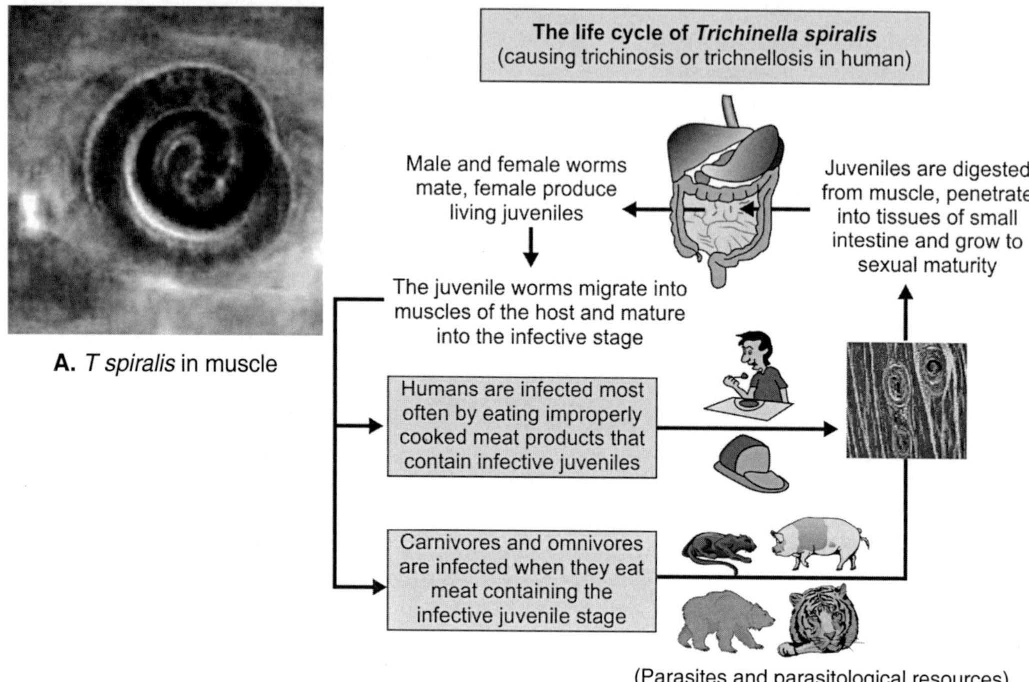

A. *T spiralis* in muscle

B

Fig. 23.27: *Trichinella spiralis*

The newborn larva measures 80 × 7 to 8 µm in size and it has a retractable stylet in the esophagus. The infective muscle larva measures 1 mm × 36 µm (Fig. 23.27).

1. Infection occurs due to ingestion of muscle tissue containing larvae in their nurse cells (modified skeletal muscle cell).
2. The ingested larvae are released in the stomach due to the action of digestive enzymes and are transported to the upper third of the small intestine.
3. The larvae penetrate the epithelium, undergo four moultings within 30 hours, and develop into adult forms.
4. The female after fertilization and after 5 days incubation starts depositing the larvae continuously for five days. A single female releases upto 1000 larvae. The intestinal infection lasts upto 2 to 3 weeks and ultimately the adult worms are expelled by the immune mechanism of the host. It appears that inflammatory responses play key role in expelling the worms from the intestine.
5. The newborn larvae enter the lamina propria and from there penetrate the lymphatics and reach the general circulation. The larvae are distributed to all tissues.
6. Larvae emerge from the capillaries and penetrate the cells. Except the muscle cells all other cells die after the penetration of the larvae.
   a. Skeletal muscle fibers provide proper conditions to support the growth and development of the larvae. Within 20 days after entering into the muscle tissue, the larvae alter their environment and create the nurse cell.

b. The mechanism of formation of nurse cell is not known. It appears that worm interacts directly with the genome of the host through some specialized secretions, which result in symbiotic relationship.
c. The larvae can survive in the nurse cells for months to years. However, most of them are either calcify or die. Larvae that enter tissues other than muscle cannot induce nurse cell and they either re-enter the circulation or die.

Trichinellosis is often misdiagnosed and mistaken for many other non-related clinical syndromes. Patients suffer many effects related to the damage of the intestinal epithelium, intense mucosal inflammation due to newborn larvae and the antigen-antibody complexes formed also contribute to the intestinal disease experienced by the patients. Larvae penetrating the central nervous system or the cardiac muscle produce serious disease. Myocarditis is some times severe enough to cause death. In skeletal muscle, the parasite-secreted proteins and antigens induce progressive infiltration with inflammatory cells. Myositis and tissue edema occurs within 14 days after the penetration of the tissues by the larvae. The pathological changes are directly proportional to the number of larvae shed in the intestines.

Early intestinal infection is manifested as abdominal pain, diarrhea and vomiting. The invasion of tissues by the newborn larvae results in fever, myalgias, periorbital edema. Hemorrhages in the nail beds, sclera of the eye and in the mucous membranes may be seen. Edema leads to muscle tenderness, photophobia. Progressive infection is more serious in nature. Myocarditis is seen in about 20% of the infected patients along with ECG changes. Dyspnea is another complication of myositis. Neurological symptoms and signs vary greatly. There is no evidence for any long-term sequelae due to *Trichinella spiralis* infection. Nevertheless, as the time progresses numerous nurse cells calcify resulting in the death of the larvae inside them.

Unfortunately, chemotherapy is of little use in treating trichinellosis. The adult worms are removed from the intestines by treating with thiabendazole or mebendazole to reduce the number of newborn larvae that reach muscle tissue or other tissue but by the time the diagnosis is made, majority of larvae have been produced. Experimental studies showed that the antihelminthic drugs also reduce the worm burden in muscle tissue but their efficacy in humans is doubtful. Even if they are effective, it is of little clinical significance because the pathological effects of the infection is largely due to the migrating larvae that are unaffected by the treatment.

Cooking of all pork products at 59°C for 10 minutes or freezing them at –20°C for three days to destroy the larvae. Inspection of slaughtered pigs may reduce the prevalence of infection as seen in some countries of European Union. Prevention of outbreaks due to consumption of meat of game animals is more difficult because strains of *Trichinella* spp. infecting wild animals are more resistant to freezing. Strict herbivores are not infected with *Trichinella* spp., usually. Nevertheless, they may acquire infection by accidental ingestion of the infected carcass.

FILARIAL NEMATODES

The filarial nematodes are the major group of tissue nematodes. Eight species of these nematodes are of human importance and they share a number of morphological features. The first three species namely, *Wuchereria bancrofti, Brugia malayi* and *Brugia timori* are known as lymphatic filariae. The other species, *Onchocerca volvulus* is associated with dermal and ocular diseases. The rest of the four species; *Loa loa, Mansonella ozzardi, Mansonella perstans* and *Mansonella streptocerca* are rather less well known and also appears to be less important as causative agents of human disease.

The unique pathology of lymphatic filariasis due to lymphatic filariae infection especially the gross enlargement of limbs popularly known as elephantiasis has been known to our ancestors. The description of the disease is recorded in the ancient medical literature of China, Japan, India and Persia. In the Western countries, it was known as elephantiasis arabicum. The microfilarial stage of these nematodes was first demonstrated in the hydrocele fluid of patients of Cuba in 1863. Wucherer found microfilariae in the urine of a patient in 1866 and later they were demonstrated in the blood by Lewis in 1872. Bancrofti in 1877 found the adult worm in the abscess of a Chinese patient in Brisbane. Cobbold in 1877 proposed the name for the nematode as *Filaria bancrofti,* which was later changed to *Wuchereria bancrofti* in 1878.

The discovery of the life cycle by Patrick Manson in 1877 is one of the most significant contributions to parasitology and tropical medicine, the implications of which reached beyond helminthology into diverse areas like malaria and Arboviruses. Patrick Manson while working in Amoy in China found microfilariae in the blood of dogs and humans; he suspected that these parasites in the blood might be transmitted by blood sucking insects. In order to confirm his suspicion he fed the mosquitoes on the blood of his gardener harboring these parasites, and subsequently detected the larval stages in the mosquitoes. However, Manson thought that the parasites from mosquitoes escaped into water and humans acquired infection through contaminated water. The actual mode of transmission was established by the Australian Parasitologist, Thomas Bancroft and that was confirmed by one of the Manson's assistant, George Carmichael Low in 1900. The lecture theater of the Royal Society of Tropical Medicine and Hygiene in London is named after Low. Further studies identified *Culex fatigans* and *Culex quinquefasciatus* as an important vectors species responsible for transmission of the disease filariasis.

Filarial nematodes belong to phylum *Nematoda,* class Secernentea and superfamily *Filarioidea.* These nematodes are long, smooth, and cylindrical with simple head and the mouthparts lack lips. The buccal cavity is small. The females measure 80-100 × 0.25-0.30 mm in size. The mouth leads to oesophagus, which has muscular region at the anterior end and glandular region at the posterior end. The tail of the male possesses perianal papillae and copulatory spicules. The vulva of the female is located anteriorly which opens through vagina into long, coiled, bifurcated uterus that runs the length of the body. The females are ovoviviparous or viviparous. The uterus contains microfilariae-embryos that develop within thin shells that in some species retained as sheath. Adult worms are rarely seen as intact, sometimes only in histological sections. The microfilariae on the contrary, appear in blood and are easily seen in the peripheral blood smears.

Microfilariae are relatively undifferentiated. Their size varies with species. The body contains a number of nuclei that may or may not reach the tip of the parasite. Because of their host specificity, the biology and the metabolism of filarial nematodes are not well understood. The closely related species *Brugia pahangi,* which can be maintained in cats, has been used to study the pathophysiology of filarial infection and our knowledge of the biology of lymphatic filariae has come from this animal model.

The microfilariae circulating in the peripheral blood are ingested by the insect vectors during their blood meal (Fig. 23.28).

The ingested microfilariae reach the midgut of the insect and the sheathed microfilariae lose their sheath. The larvae then penetrate the midgut wall and migrate in to the hemocoel of the insect. Thereafter they penetrate the thoracic flight muscles where they first develop into short thick 'sausage' forms and within two weeks they grow, undergo two moults to become filariform infective third stage larvae.

The infective filariform larvae that measure 1 mm in size, migrate out of the muscles of the insect vector and reach ultimately the proboscis and remain there coiled up. When the infected vector bites another host, these larvae enter the lymphatics. The third stage larvae finally reach the lymph node.

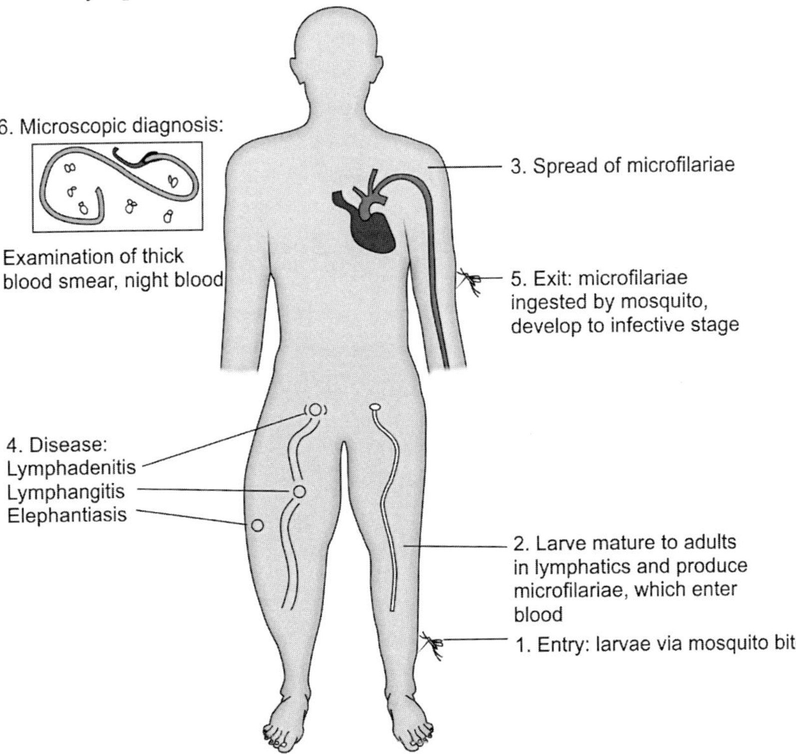

Fig. 23.28: Filarial nematodes

After three weeks they moult and mature to become adult worms. Details of the development of human filarial larvae are largely unknown. Some of the adult worms die after maturation but those that survive may live for years. The female liberates microfilariae throughout the rest of its life. The time taken for the appearance of microfilariae in the blood of infected humans is about 12 months for *W. bancrofti* and it may be less for other species. The microfilariae are colorless, transparent and actively motile even within the sheath. The released microfilariae are capable of surviving for many months.

The most interesting characteristic of lymphatic filarial worms is that the microfilariae show marked periodicity in their appearance in the peripheral blood. Manson demonstrated that the microfilariae of *W. bancrofti* appeared for about 1 to 2 hours before and after midnight and thereafter they disappear from the peripheral blood for the rest of the 24-hour period. This is classically known as nocturnal periodicity and is true of *W. bancrofti* throughout its geographical range such as Asia, Africa, Australia and South America. However, in Pacific areas nonperiodic or slightly diurnally periodic forms are present. In this type, the microfilariae are present more or less constantly throughout the 24-hour period. In South East Asia, subperiodic form of *W. bancrofti* is present. These microfilariae are present throughout 24-hour period but the numbers are elevated at night. Microfilariae with nocturnal periodicity are common in coastal regions, open swamps and rice fields of India, Sri Lanka, Thailand, and Malaysia and are transmitted by anophiline mosquitoes as well as by *Mansonia* and *Aedes* species of mosquitoes. The sub periodic forms are highly infective to Mansonia species than anopheline mosquitoes. Sometimes the periodic form of microfilariae may shed the sheath during the preparation of smears and this can be useful for diagnosis. The periodicity of other filarial species varies. Several reasons have been suggested for the periodicity of these microfilariae such as (a) relaxation of host's body during sleep, (b) may be due to assort of response to the changes of CO_2 and O_2 in blood, and (c) the feeding habits of the insect vector.

Mosquitoes belonging to the genera *Culex, Anopheles* and *Mansonia* transmit the filarial worms of human importance, *W. bancrofti, B. malayi* and *B. timori. Culicoides* midges transmit the *Mansonella* species of filarial worms and *Chrysops* transmit *Loa loa.* Only adult female mosquitoes feed on human blood. *Culex quinquefasciatus* is the most important vector of periodic *W. bancrofti* and it is responsible for more than 50% of the cases of lymphatic filariasis. Drains and cesspits are the most common places of breeding of *Culex* mosquito (Table 23.14).

Lymphatic filariasis rather follows variable course in individuals but a general pattern can be seen when populations are considered. Asymptomatic, amicrofilaremic patients are negative for symptoms and microfilariae in the blood but are immunologically reactive. They can be positive for detectable antigenemia indicating a subclinical infection. This may be due to the fact that these individuals are not exposed sufficiently to the infection to manifest clinically or cleared the infection without any symptoms (Immune individuals). They may be harboring developing worms of one sex or unfertilized female worms (Table 23.15).

Table 23.14: Differentiation of *W. bancrofti* and *B. malayi*

Character	*W. bancrofti*	*B. malayi*
General appearance	Graceful sweeping curves	Wrinkled with secondary curves
Length	Longer	Shorter
Free cephalic space	As long as broad	Nearly twice long as broad
Excretory pore	Not prominent	Prominent
Caudal end	Uniformly tapering	Kinkled
Nuclear column	No terminal nuclei	Two terminal nuclei present

Table 23.15: Characteristic features of microfilariae

Species	Microfilarial sheath	Vector	Habitat of microfilaria
W. bancrofti	+	*C. fatigans*	Blood circulation
B. malayi	+	*Mansonoides*	Blood circulation
Loa loa	+	*Chrysops*	Blood circulation
S. perstans	–	*Culicicoides*	Blood circulation
M. ozzardi	=	*Culicicoides*	Blood circulation
O. volvulus	=	*Simuliidae*	Skin

Asymptomatic but microfilaremic patients do not have any clinical disease. They show lowered parasitic specific IgE response and large amounts of IgG4 type of antibody that acts as a locking antibody.

Some individuals develop atypical hypersensitivity responses and show wide variety of clinical symptoms such as fever, chills, malaise, vomiting, Adenolymphangitis involving mostly lower limbs, groins, genitals and breasts in females. Cute attacks never occur at more than one site at the same time. Adenolymphangitis attacks commonly occur in patients with chronic filarial disease more frequently with lymph edema than hydrocele. The attack lasts for 3 to 5 days but may persist upto 15 days. The frequency of attacks is one to three years.

Chronic manifestations affect male genitals and limbs of both sexes. Most of these patients with chronic disease are microfilaremic. The severity of these chronic manifestations tends to increase with age. The manifestations are due to lymphatic obstruction and fibrosis. Genital manifestations include hydrocele, lymphangitis, funiculitis, chronic epididymitis and lymph scrotum.

Approximately 11% of population at risk develop lymphedema and it commonly seen affecting the lower limbs and rarely other organs. Lymphedema is graded as follows:

Grade I: Reversible edema on elevation of the affected limbs

Grade II: Not reversible spontaneously. The skin is not thickened

Grade III: Not reversible spontaneously. The skin is thickened

Grade IV: Not spontaneously, reversible and the skin is thickened with warty papillomatous growth.

Hydrocele is the collection of straw-colored fluid (sometimes milky in nature due to chyle). Occasionally microfilariae can be detected in the hydrocele fluid.

Elephantiasis is due to persistent fibrotic changes.

Chyluria or milky urine is due to admixture of urine and chyle because of blockage of retroperitoneal lymph nodes below cisterna chyle. Microfilariae may or may not be found in chyluria.

Allergic manifestations of filariasis comprise of nocturnal paroxysmal cough, prominent bronchoalveolar markings in X-ray film, elevated ESR and impaired lung function. These manifestations are rarely seen in children. It may also manifest as tropical eosinophilia with hypereosinophilia along with high titers of antifilarial antibodies of IgE class directed against microfilariae.

The other clinical manifestations include filarial arthritis that may be seen in endemic areas as monoarthritis especially knee joint.

Diethylcarbamazine (DEC) is the drug of choice that was discovered in 1946. Asymptomatic infected patients (Microfilaria carriers and antigen positive group) are treated with DEC at dose 6 mg/kg body weight in divided doses after meals for 12 days. Ivermectin 400 µg/kg body weight every three months for 12 months is another choice. Ivermectin can be combined with DEC. DEC can also be given in combination with albendazole. Acute manifestations can be treated with benzathine penicillin G, 1200000 units every month along with antipyretics, anti-inflammatory agents. Rest and immobilization of the affected limb, surgical drainage of the abscess followed by standard regimen of DEC are recommended for relieving the symptoms of acute manifestation of filariasis. Surgical drainage of the hydrocele is followed by monthly courses of DEC 10 mg/kg body weight for three weeks for a period of six months. For patients with lymphedema, physiotherapy, massage, pressure bandage thermotherapy and pneumocompression are recommended. Immersing the affected limb in warm water increases circulation and this should be combined with standard DEC therapy for 12 months. Surgical intervention, drainage, lymphangioplasty, lymph-vein anastomosis and lymph node venous shunt are useful. DEC is capable of killing both adult worms and microfilariae of *Loa loa* but care should be taken to avoid complications. If there is heavy microfilaremia very low doses of the drug is given initially.

DRACUNCULUS MEDINENSIS (GUINEA WORM)

Dracunculus medinensis is the causative agent of dracunculiasis and it is the largest nematode whose description has been mentioned in "Bible". The nematode was known as 'fiery serpent' to people of Israel in the region of Red Sea between 1300–1234 BC. The 2nd century papyri from Egypt recorded this parasite. Writings from Mesopotamia in the 7th century BC, records by Greek, Roman and Arabic physicians mention about this worm. Thomas Herbert in 1643 recognized the presence of this worm in the leg of the infected person. Huyghen van Linschoten, a Dutch navigator recorded that the transmission was through drinking water. Russian scientist, Aleksej Fedchenko, who suspected the water flea as the transmitting agent, described the actual life cycle. Robert Leiper in 1905 and

Dynsehvar Turkhud finally described the complete life cycle of the parasite that helped in controlling the infection and now progressing toward eradication.

The mature female worm (Guinea worm) is the longest nematode that infects humans. It measures 100 to 500 cm in length and 1.0 to 2.0 mm in width. A quadrangular cuticularized plate and an internal circle of four double papillae surround the mouth that has a triangular opening. The vulva opens halfway down the body. The uterus has an anterior and a posterior branch. The gravid uterus is filled with 1 to 3 million larvae and occupies entire pseudocoel (body cavity). The parasite is viviparous. Male worms are smaller, measuring 15 to 40 × 0.4 mm in size. The tail has four pairs of preanal and 4 to 6 pairs of post anal papillae. The gubernaculum measures about 117 μm in size and the subequal spicules are 490 to 750 μm in length. The males die in the tissues before the female matures and are rarely seen in human tissues.

The female worm matures in the human body within one year and migrates to surface of the skin. It initiates the formation of a blister at site, which breaks open leaving an ulcer. About 5 cm portion of the gravid female is extruded through the ulcer, particularly after immersion in the water. The female worm discharges many thousands of larvae into the water where they can survive only for a few days unless taken up by the fresh water crustacean, *Cyclops*. The larvae moult two times in the body of *Cyclops* in about two weeks. The infected *Cyclops*, when ingested along the drinking water, the larvae is released by the action of digestive juices in the stomach of the host. The larvae penetrate the intestinal wall and settle down in the connective tissues where the males and females mate after maturation. The cycle is thus repeated.

Guinea worms have been wound out on sticks since ancient times (mentioned in Rig Veda of about 1350 BC). Regular winding out of the worm on a small stick, combined with application of acriflavine cream results in complete expulsion of the worm without loss of mobility provided there are no complications due to secondary bacterial infection. Sometimes the worms can be removed even before they emerge from the ulcer while there is no tissue reaction against them. The chemotherapy should be started as soon as the worm is emerged. However, there is no evidence that any chemotherapeutic agent has a direct action on the worm. Many compounds like thiabendazole, niridazole, metronidazole, mebendazole and albendazole have been used to hasten the expulsion of the worm and these drugs may act as anti-inflammatory agents. Ivermectin has no effect on pre-emergent worms.

The eradication of dracunculiasis was adopted as a part of the clean drinking water supply and sanitation decade (1981–1990). The disease is likely to be eliminated from Asia in the near future with no cases from Pakistan and only handful of cases from India.

CESTODES

The cestodes or tapeworms occur in wide variety of vertebrates. These worms are classified under the phylum Platyhelminthes. The worms belonging to this phylum, fall under three classes; ***Monogenea, Cestoidea*** and ***Trematoda***. Cestodes are closely related to the

Monogeneans from which these are likely to have been derived during evolution. The taxonomical classification of cestodes is very complex.

Human adult tapeworms are flat dorsoventrally with length ranging from a few centimeters to several meters. They are white or grayish to yellow in color. Calcareous corpuscles are present in the tissue filling the spaces between the internal organs of the parasite. The tapeworms found in the small intestines of humans are adult worms in different developmental stages. The adult worm has a head (scolex), a neck (the growth region) which continues in a series of proglottids (segments) which together form strobila. The scolex has either four round muscular suckers (Acetabulum) in tapeworms belonging to Cyclophillidea or two elongated grooves (bothria or lips) in Pseudophillidea. Some species possess small hooks on the scolex that can be inserted into the intestinal epithelium and thus they help the worm in maintaining the position in the gut. The hooks are often situated in one or two circles on a retractable rostellum between the suckers at the anterior end of the scolex. The width of the worm increases from the narrow end of the neck and folds of the body wall are at regular intervals along the length of the worm. This arrangement gives the worm segmented appearance. The body wall or the tegument is a living structure which can absorb the nutrients and also can inhibit the host's enzymes from digesting the worm. The adult worm has an outer circular layer and inner longitudinal layer of muscles that allow the worm to move. The nervous system is primitive and consists of brain-like structure in the scolex comprising of central and lateral and rostellar ganglia that are connected by central nerve ring. Lateral and longitudinal nerves run from the nerve ring all the way back to the posterior end of the worm. The longitudinal nerves are connected by transverse commissures. Connections are also seen to the inner organs and sensory organs in the body wall. The excretory system consists of lateral canal on each side and is connected to the scolex. The dorsal and ventral canals are interconnected by transverse canal in the posterior part of the each proglottid. The terminal cells of the excretory canals are called flame cells. Ultrafiltration takes place at the basal lamina through the gaps in the lattice-like system.

The tapeworms are hermaphrodites, and the both male and female reproductive organs are differentiated progressively from the anterior region. Each matured proglottid contains both the types of reproductive organs. Copulation takes place and the fertilized eggs are formed. When the eggs are matured and contain the first stage larvae the proglottid is considered as gravid. Male reproductive system consists of a few large or many small testes from which the spermatozoa are passed through vasa efferentia to a common vas deferens. From there they enter the seminal vesicle and finally reach the long protrusible cirrus, which is surrounded by cirrus sac. The female reproductive system comprises of single bilobed ovary, an ootype, where the egg composition and its wall formation starts, a vagina leading to a common genital pore. The vitelline glands are either compact or dispersed from which the vitelline cells are brought to the ootype to participate in the formation of capsule (Egg shell). In Cyclophillides the capsule is absent or partly developed and the embryophore forms the shell. In *Hymenolepis nana,* the cyclophllide tapeworm, only one vitelline gland cell takes part in the egg formation. The fertilized eggs are passed into the uterus which may or may not extend upto common genital pore. In species like *D.latum* the eggs are operculated.

Life Cycle

The beef tapeworm, *Taenia saginata* is about 4 to 6 meters or even more in length and has 1000 to 2000 proglottids. The genital pore is placed laterally in the proglottid but irregularly alternates from one side to the other. The scolex has four suckers but no hooks. If the number of the beef tapeworms are more in a given host, the number of proglottids in each worm is decreased which is atypical example of effect of overcrowding. In such situations the parasitic worms not only interfere with each other and compete for space and food but also they influence the immune responses of the host, affecting the growth of the parasite (Fig. 23.29).

1. In the life cycle humans are the only final hosts, and the infection is acquired by the ingestion of raw or undercooked meat containing the cysticercus stage of the worm in a host's capsule.
2. When the cystecercus or bladder worm (previously named separately as *Cysticercus bovis*) reaches the stomach, the proteolytic enzymes denature the capsule. In the small intestines the cysticerci are stimulated to evaginate.

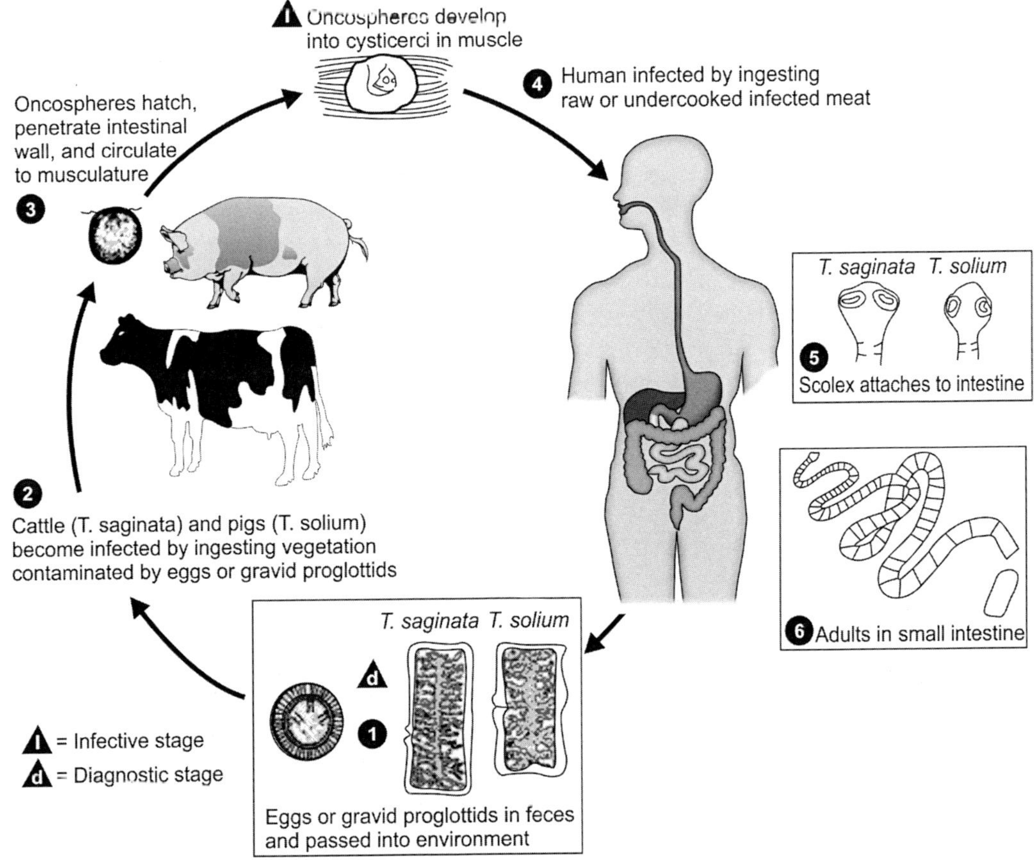

Fig. 23.29: Life cyle of *Taenia*

3. The scolex with the help of suckers attaches to the intestinal mucosa and begins to develop into matured adult tapeworm.
4. The development process may take about 10 to 14 weeks before the worm attains maturity. The gravid proglottids contain upto 80,000 matured eggs each, and on an average 6 to 9 gravid proglottids are expelled each day. Thus, the average output by single worm may be as high as 600,000 eggs per day.
5. Meat from the domestic animals is the main source of infection. However, water buffaloes, llamas in South America and Reindeer in North hemisphere also act as intermediate hosts.
6. The intermediate hosts acquire the infection by consuming the matured eggs or gravid proglottids filled with eggs while grazing in the fields. The proglottids that are expelled after maturation are quite mobile and during the migration most eggs leave the gravid proglottids.
7. The eggs hatch in the small intestines, and the free oncosphere or the six-hooked hexacanth larvae penetrate the gut wall and reach the muscles through the blood circulation.
8. Within the intramuscular connective tissue they develop into cysticerci. These cysticerci mature within 10 to 15 weeks and become grayish white bladder-like structures measuring about 5 to 9 mm in size. And contain an opaque invaginated scolex and neck (Fig. 23.30).
   a. The pork tapeworm or *Taenia solium* is worldwide in distribution except among Muslims and Jews who do not eat pork or where strict veterinary inspection and treatment of human cases eradicated the infection.
   b. The matured worm measures about 2 to 4 meters in length or even more and contains 800 to 1000 proglottids. The scolex has four suckers and as mall rostellum with a double row of 40 to 50 small hooks.
   c. Humans can act not only as final hosts but also as intermediate hosts for the worm which is more serious. The source of infection for humans is the raw or undercooked pork from domestic pigs containing the cysticercus stage (previously named as separate species as *Cysticercus cellulosa*).

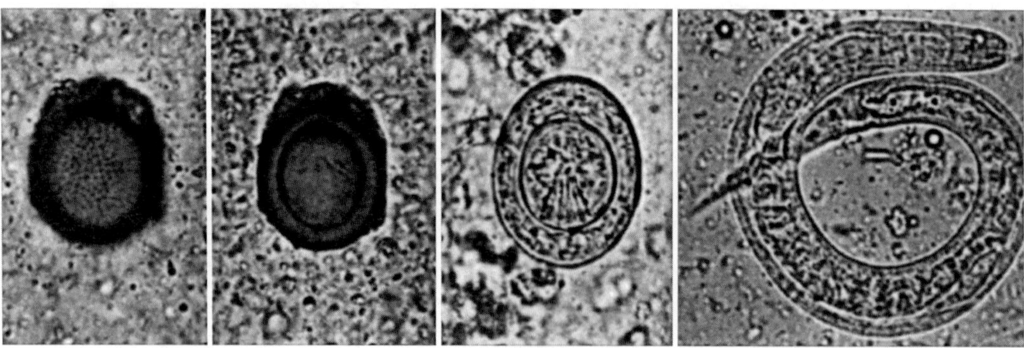

Fig. 23.30: Ova of tapeworm (*Taenia solium*, *T. saginata* and *Hymenolepis nana*)
(*For color version, see Plate 12*)

d. The cysticerci reach the stomach and are digested by the enzymes and in the intestines the stimulated cysticerci evaginate. The evaginated cysticerci with the help of the scolex attach to the intestinal epithelium of the host and subsequently develop into adult worms.
e. The matured proglottids contain about 40,000 eggs. The proglottids of *Taenia solium* are sluggish in motility and are easily consumed by pigs.

The dwarf tapeworm or *Hymenolepis nana* not only infects the humans but also rodents like rats or mice. Some authors consider the rodent tapeworm as a special strain (*H. nana var fraterna*) but cross-reactions in both the directions are known, indicating that *H. nana* infection is a zoonosis where the infection is maintained in the rodents and the humans are the accidental hosts. Stoll in 1917 estimated that approximately 20 million people are infected and this number has probably increased since then. The adult worm is small measuring about 4 to 5 cm in length. The scolex has cup-shaped suckers and a retractably prominent and movable rostellum with a ring of small hooks.

i. *Hymenolepis nana* has an indirect life cycle and the intermediate host is an insect. The worm is also capable of using the final host for development directly from the eggs containing oncosphere larvae.
ii. The intermediate host is a beetle such as *Tribolium* or *Tenebrio* species or fleas such as *Pulex irritans, Xenopsylla cheopis, Ctenocephalides canis* and moths.
iii. The indirect life cycle begins with the uptake of infective form of *H. nana* eggs by one of the insects or their larvae.
iv. The egg shells are crushed and the enzymes in the gut stimulate the oncosphere to free itself from the enclosed membrane. The released oncosphere penetrates the gut of the host with the help of the hooks and glandular secretions.
v. In the body cavity of the insect vector, the oncosphere transforms into a second larval stage called cysticercoid that infects the final host.
vi. When the infected insects are ingested (especially by children), the bile salts stimulate the cysticercoid to evaginate which ultimately develops into adult worm within 3 to 4 weeks.
vii. The direct life cycle takes place when the infective eggs are ingested. In the lumen of the small intestines the released oncosphere penetrates the intestinal villi and develops into cysticercoid stage within four days.
viii. Thereafter, the villi rupture and the cysticercoid larvae are liberated into the lumen of the intestines where it develops into an adult worm. I cases of heavy infection the eggs may hatch in the intestine itself resulting in autoinfection.

Generally intestinal tapeworms are considered to be less pathogenic and cause no or very minimal symptoms. However, they compete for the nutrients with the host and utilize the food consumed by the host. In cases of malnutrition, tapeworm infection may have deleterious effect on the infected person. The large tapeworms may disturb the intestinal motility. Patients may experience abdominal discomfort, nausea, weakness, loss of weight, increased appetite, headache, constipation, diarrhea, dizziness, pruritus ani, excitation, vomiting and anorexia. Nausea and the abdominal pain may be explained as the result of extension or spasm of the intestines due to the movement of the worm. The mechanisms responsible for other symptoms are obscure.

Niclosamide or praziquantel are the drugs of choice for treating taeniasis. Because internal autoinfection is a possibility, nausea and vomiting are controlled during the treatment because they could lead to backwash of the eggs and possible autoinfection, a purge be done after treatment to prevent reverse peristalsis.

LARVAE OF THE CESTODES OF HUMAN IMPORTANCE

The larval stages of the tapeworms of the class Cestoda and the subclass Eucestoda resemble vesicular bladder in shape and these larval stages can parasitize humans. The most common and important larval stages that infect humans are the larvae of *T. solium, Echinococcus granulosus* (*E. granulosus* or dog tape worm), *Echinococcus multilocularis* (*E. multilocularis*), *Echinococcus vogeli* (*E. vogeli*). The metacestode of *T. solium* is known as cysticercus and that of *Echinococcus* is hydatid cyst. The diseases caused by these larval forms are known as cysticercosis and depending upon the location of the larval form different names like neurocysticercosis, ophthalmocysticercosis and muscular cysticercosis are used. In the case of hydatid cyst there are three types of echinococcosis; cystic echinococcosis due to *E. granulosus,* alveolar echinococcosis due to *E. multilocularis* and polycystic echinococcosis due to *E. vogeli.* Cystic echinococcosis is more common among the three types and alveolar echinococcosis is more aggressive. The polycystic echinococcosis due to *E. vogeli* is rare.

Human cysticercosis is a public health problem and the infection is due to deposition of hexacanth larvae liberated from the oncosphere in the intestine which penetrates the intestinal mucosa and lodges in various organs through bloodstream. It is clearly associated with poor sanitation and lack of health education.

The fertilized eggs are released from the definitive host quickly become embryonated and infective to a suitable host. When the eggs are ingested by the intermediate host the external coat is digested and the oncosphere is liberated in the small intestines. This liberated and activated oncosphere is mobile and penetrates the intestinal mucosa to reach the lamina propria within 3 to 120 minutes after hatching. The penetration is probably assisted by the secretions of the penetration glands or it may be purely mechanical involving the hooks and the body movement. The penetrated larvae are carried by the bloodstream to the tissues where they are deposited and in the tissues they develop into metacestode specifically named as cysticercus for *T. solium* larvae and hydatid cyst for the larvae of the *Echinococcus* species. The cysticerci measure 0.3 mm in size and they can be seen in liver, brain and the skeletal muscles of the intermediate host, the pig within six days after the infection. After a period of 60 to 70 days fully developed cysticerci with scolices are seen and they reach a size of 6 to 9 mm. With further development the cysticerci increase in size and measure 8 to 15 mm within 2 to 3 months. The term cysticercus means bladder tail and the name *Cysticercus cellulosae* is given because of its tendency to develop in connective tissues.

There are two types of cystecirci namely cellulosae that is space occupying and are small, spherical, white or yellowish gray vesicles measuring 0.5 to 1.5 mm in size with translucent bladder wall through which the scolex can be seen as a small solid eccentric granule. This stage usually does not grow further and they are well separated from the host's tissue by a thin collagenous capsule, within which it remains alive. The second variety is racimose type that is large, round or lobulated bladder surrounded by a delicate cell wall and resembles a cluster of grapes. The size of racimose type may be 10 cm or even 20 cm and contains about 60 mL of fluid. The scolex is not visible and sometimes only detailed histological studies reveal its remaining. Neuropathological studies on infected human brain suggest that larvae lodged in spacious areas are able to grow further and transform into racimose cysticerci. Alternatively the growth of cysticerci might be controlled by the immune responses of the host and *in vitro* studies showed that the presence of inflammatory capsule that surrounds the cysticerci inhibits the evagination of the scolex.

Neurocysticercosis shows great diversity in both signs and symptoms. It is a complex disease and the major manifestations depend upon the number, location and the type of the parasite lodged and the intensity of the inflammatory response. Seizures are more common in about 70% of cases and late on set of epilepsy is strongly associated with cysticercosis. Seizures due to calcified cysticerci in parenchyma or single cellulose type of cysticercosis are usually mild compared to others who have hydrocephalus as a result of meningeal arachnoiditis which is often fatal.

Racimose type of cysticerci is known to produce intense inflammatory response and produce more severe mass effects. If the parasite is in contact with meninges, inflammation is progressive and that may result in scar tissue proliferation producing mechanical obstruction to cerebrospinal fluid circulation. As a result there is an intracranial hypertension due to hydrocephalus. Acute stage of the disease produces intracranial hypertension, ependymitis or arachnoiditis. Idiopathic epilepsy, multiple space occupying intracranial lesions, chronic meningitis, other bacterial or parasitic infections, primary or secondary malignancies affecting the CNS can mimic neurocysticercosis. Similarly clinical heterogeneity is also common with ophthalmic cysticercosis. Cysticerci in subcutaneous tissue and muscles are usually asymptomatic and well-tolerated because they are less in number. Pseudomuscular hypertrophy may be seen, if there are many cysts in the muscles.

The life cycle of *Echinococcus granulosus* was first demonstrated by Carlvon Siebold in 1853 by infecting the dogs hydatid cysts from sheep. He named the adult worms which were seen in sheep after 27 days following the infection as *Taenia echinococcus*. Further experiments by Leuckart in 1867 and by Naunyn in 1863 confirmed that the hydatid cysts of human origin undergo same development as that of animal origin. Naunyn concluded that the Echinococcus from man is the bladder stage of the ***Taenia echinococcus*** which was later changed to ***Echinococcus granulosus***.

Echinococcus granulosus or dog tapeworm measures only a few millimeters with 2 to 5 segments. The scolex has four suckers and rostellum with double crown of hooks. Eggs are spherical, 20 to 50 μm in size. Under the microscope they show radial appearance and bear the embryophore that surrounds the embryo, the oncosphere. The embryophore is formed by contiguous blocks. The eggs of *E. granulosus* are morphologically indistinguishable from other taenia eggs.

The gravid proglottid liberates the embryonated eggs that are ingested by the intermediate host.

In the small intestine of the intermediate host, the oncosphere is liberated due to digestion of the cementing substance that forms the embryophore blocks.

The liberated oncosphere is mobile and penetrates the intestinal mucosa and through *blood stream* it reaches the tissue where they settle and develop. Several *in vivo* and *in vitro* studies showed that the oncosphere of *E. granulosus* rapidly undergoes a series of reorganizational events during the first two weeks involving cellular infiltration, degeneration of the hooks, muscular atrophy, vesicularization with central cavity formation and development of both laminated and germinal layers.

The time required for the formation of protoscolices inside the cysts in humans is not known.

Each hydatid cyst (bladder worm stage of *E. granulosus*) contains multiple protoscolices formed by asexual budding from the bladder's germinal layer. Completely developed cyst of *E. granulosus* is typically unilocular, subspherical with fluid in the cyst. The cyst consists of an inner nucleated germinal layer supported by an external tough, elastic laminated layer of variable thickness surrounded by a host-derived fibrous adventitial layer. Asexual reproduction occurs in the germinal layer and the formation of brood capsule is entirely endogenous. In each capsule several scolices and protoscolices can be seen. Rarely the cysts may coalesce and form clusters of cysts of variable size. In humans, the hydatid cyst grows slowly and may attain a size of several liters and contains thousands of protoscolices. With time internal septae and daughter cysts are formed within the primary cyst disrupting the unilocular pattern.

The metacestodes of *E. multilocularis* are more complex and develop quite differently from that of *E. granulosus*. The size of the worm varies from 1 to 20 mm, but the metacestodes vary from minor foci to a very large area of infiltration. The metacestode is multivesicular and has no limited host-parasite barrier. The larval mass is usually semisolid matrix rather than fluid and it is formed by multiple small vesicles embedded in a large stroma of connective tissue. The metacestode consists of a network of filamentous solid cellular protoscolices of the germinal layer which are responsible for infiltrating growth, transforming into tube-like and cystic structure where proliferation occurs endogenously as well as exogenously. Alveolar cysts of echinococcus may metastasize due to the detachment of the germinal cells from the infiltrating cellular protrusions and their subsequent distribution through the lymph and blood to the other tissue. In humans the larval mass of *E.multilocularis* may mimic malignancy because of continuous proliferation by exogenous budding and invasion of the neighboring tissue. Protoscolices are rarely seen in human infection.

TREMATODES

The trematodes are flukes or flat-worms resembling leaf-like and they initially evolved as parasites of molluscs and all species of trematodes still retain the molluscan element in their life cycle. Trematodes are subdivided into two groups: (a) *Digenea* and (b) *Aspidogastrea*. Only those flukes that belong to the subclass Digenea are of human importance. These are easily recognized by their suckers which are two in number and they serve as attachment organs. They have a single set of reproductive organs and a functional gut. They are endoparasites and are seen in the gut, liver, bile duct, lungs and in the bloodstream. The important trematodes that affect humans belong to the following genera: (a) *Schistosoma,* (b) *Faciola,* and (c) *Paragonimus.*

SCHISTOSOMA

The trematodes of the genus *Schistosoma* are the causative agents of human schistosomiasis or bilharziasis that affects between 200-300 million people. Urinary schistosomiasis is caused by *Schistosoma haematobium* (*S. haematobium*), is characterized by the presence of blood in the urine. The disease was known to Egyptians. Theodor Bilharz in 1851 described *S. haematobium* for the first time and the popular name for all forms of schistosomiasis is now 'Bilharzia' is named in honor of his discovery. It took quite a long time to find the intermediate host for these flukes. Finally in 1915, Robert Leiper succeeded in demonstrating the complete life cycle of this parasite.

In contrast to urinary schistosomiasis our knowledge on intestinal schistosomiasis caused by *Schistosoma mansoni* (*S. mansoni*) is relatively of recent origin. Patrick Manson in 1902 suggested that there were two species of *Schistosoma* in humans (which was also suggested by earlier workers). However, Manson's conclusions were not accepted universally at the beginning but the work of Robert Leiper in 1915 firmly established the existence of *S. mansoni* as a separate species. Katayama disease due to *Schistosoma japonicum* was recognized by Akira Fujinami, a Japanese parasitologist in 1847 and the worm itself was discovered by Fujiro Katsurada in 1904. Robert Leiper independently described the life cycle of *S. haematobium*. During 20th century other species of *Schistosoma, Schistosoma intercalatum* and *Schistosoma mekongi* were discovered along with control measures and effective drugs for treatment. Currently detailed studies on schistosomiasis are providing a hope for an effective vaccine against this important complex disease.

The human schistosomes or blood flukes are digenetic trematodes that belong to the super family Schistosomatoidea of the suborder Strigeata. The blood flukes are dioecious, and the adult worms are located in the blood vessels (Fig. 23.31). They lack muscular pharynx and they produce non-operculated eggs. The cercaria possesses bifurcated tail and it invades the final host percutaneously. Four species: (a) *S. haematobium,* (b) *S. mansoni,* (c) *S. mekongi* and (d) *S. japonicum* are the important causative agents of human schistosomiasis.

Life Cycle

The flat worms of the subgroup *Digenea* have a unique life cycle comprising of two asexual generations in the molluscan host and a sexual generation in the vertebrate host (Fig. 23.32).

1. The fertilized eggs are excreted in the feces of the vertebrate host and after hatching, a ciliated larva called miracidium is released.
2. Miracidium penetrates the specific molluscan host where it develops into a sac like parthenogenic adult, the mother sporocyst which subsequently produces daughter sporocysts.

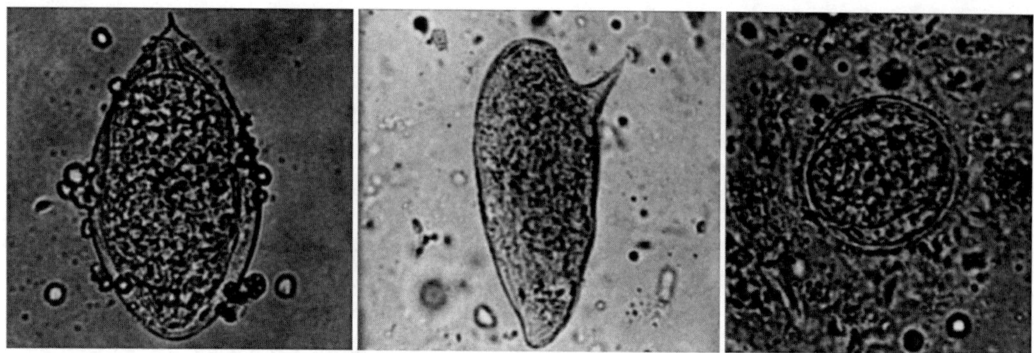

Fig. 23.31: Ova of the blood flukes (*For color version, see Plate 12*)

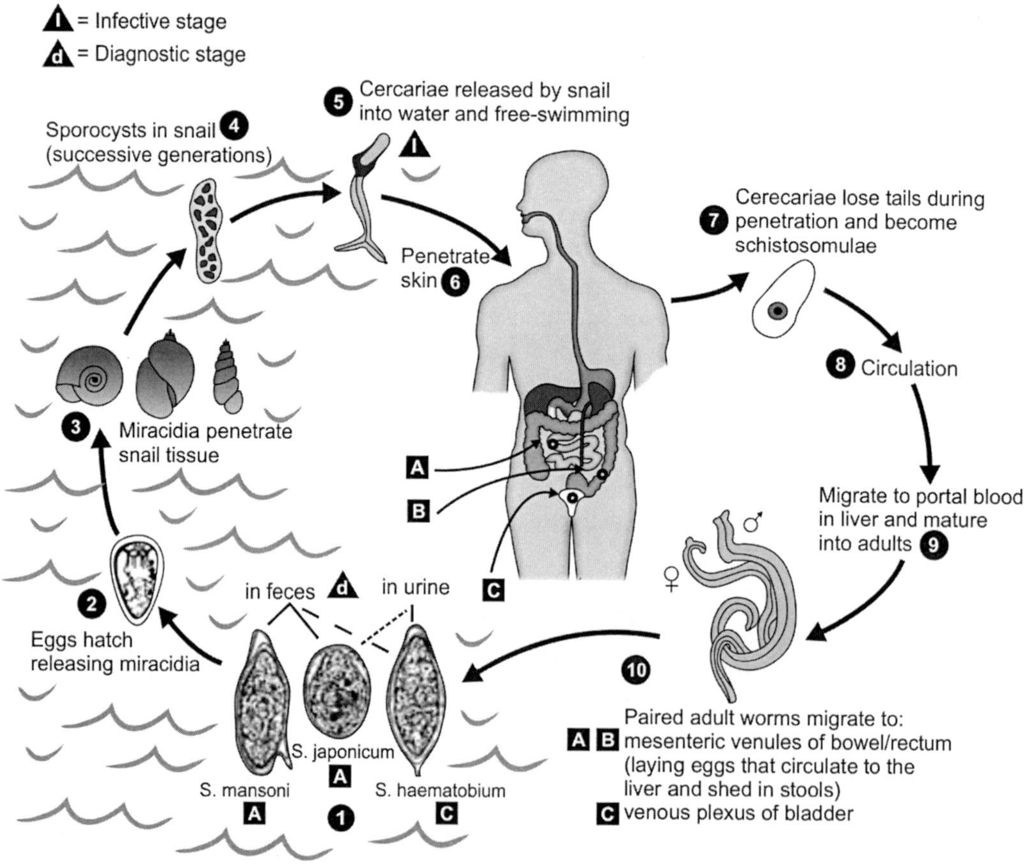

Fig. 23.32: Life cycle of *Schistosoma haematobium*

3. The daughter sporocysts are transferred into rediae with a saclike gut.
4. The rediae undergo a second parthenogenic generation and generate short-lived larvae with a tail and are developed in large numbers. These larvae escape from the molluscs and swim freely or crawl to the next host.

5. Some cercariae penetrate the final vertebrate host directly. But majority of them penetrate or settle upon its food as long-living resting stage called metacercaria.
6. Metacerariae are normally encysted in the invertebrate host or other vertebrate host which acts as intermediate host or upon vegetation.
7. The final vertebrate host becomes infected by feeding on the prey or vegetation containing the encysted metacercariae.
8. Digeneans tend to be very specific in relation to their molluscan host and relatively non-specific to their final vertebrate host.
9. The cercariae measure around 400 µm in length including the forked tail. The surface and the internal structures are essentially similar to the adults of any species of *Schistosoma*.
10. The cercariae infect the definitive host by penetrating through the skin with the help of proteolytic enzymes released by the penetration glands. They lose their tail and transform into the next larval stage, the schistosomulum.
11. After penetration the schistosomula migrate to the lungs through the venous circulation. This migration is essential for development. Schistosomulae recovered from the lungs are more resistant to antibody dependent cell-mediated cytotoxicity.
12. Schistosomulae from the lungs reach the left side of the heart and enter the circulation and finally reach the portal system. Some of them may reach the liver through the diaphragm.
13. Within the intrahepatic portal circulation the schistosomulae develop and after pairing, the worms migrate to the mesenteric veins or vesical plexus where the female lays the eggs.
14. The total period from the penetration by the cercariae and the first appearance of the eggs in the excreta is about 35 days for *S. japonicum* and *S. mansoni*, 75 days for *S. haematobium*.

Clinical manifestations may reflect developmental stages of the parasite and host responses to toxic or antigenic products derived from the parasite or the eggs. Dermatitis may occur due to migration of the cercariae from the skin to lungs with slight exanthema and pruritus. Migration of schistosomulae in the lungs may initiate cough, mild fever and dullness. Anemia is seen in about one fifth of the infected patients. After a latent period of one month the acute sudden onset starts with high fever, rigors known as Katayama fever after the Katayama district in Hiroshima, Japan where Yoshinao Fujii originally described the acute onset of the disease. The onset corresponds to the oviposition by the female worms.

Infection due to *S. mansoni* or *S. japonicum* results in inflammation leading to recurrent daily fever, abdominal pain, tender hepatosplenomegaly and discharge of eggs into the lumen of the intestines produces diarrhea and transient elevation of liver enzymes as well as IgE levels. These symptoms and findings characterize intestinal schistosomiasis.

Chronic infection due to *S. mansoni* or *S. japonicum* produces hepatosplenomegaly and the disease is called hepatosplenic schistosomiasis. Some patients may show polyp or mucosal proliferation of the intestines. The egg granulomas are replaced by fibrosis and periportal fibrosis leads to the development of pipe stem fibrosis. The liver size is decreased and becomes harder due to extensive fibrosis that may eventually lead to cirrhosis of the liver. Massive spleen enlargement, portal hypertension with ascites, hypoalbuminemia, disturbances in abdominal motility, development of esophageal varices is seen in advanced cases. Embolization of cerebral circulatory system due to eggs or heterotropic female worms may cause CNS symptoms like headache, Jacksonian type of epilepsy, parasthesias and diminished vision. Hepatic coma and corpulmonale are the other rare complications of schistosomiasis.

The main complaint of urinary schistosomiasis are pain less hematuria, burning micturition, dysuria and suprapubic discomfort. The bladder wall may be thickened with papillary proliferation that can be reversible with appropriate therapy. In chronic cases complications like hydronephrosis, secondary bacterial infections may result in chronic kidney disease and renal failure. Obstructive uropathy predisposes to urinary calculi and this may result in endogenous formation of carcinogenic N-nitroso compounds. *Schistosoma haematobium* can cause infection of the female reproductive system and female genital schistosomiasis may be an important risk factor for transmission of HIV.

Between 1920–1960 antimony compounds were the only chemotherapeutic agents available for treatment of schistosomiasis. Subsequently there have been great advances in the treatment of this disease due to the discovery of praziquantel which is effective against all species of *Schistosoma*. The precise mechanism of this drug as schistosomicidal drug is not very clear. *S. japonicum* infection treated with Praziquantel, 20 mg/kg body weight three times per day orally at 4 hours intervals results in 80% cure. The side effects at this dosage are usually minimal and self-limiting. Single dose of Praziquantel, 40 mg/kg body weight is effective for treating the infections due to *S. haematobium* and *S. mansoni*.

OPISTHORCHIS, CLONORCHIS, AND FACIOLA (LIVER FLUKES)

The genera *Opisthorchis, Clonorchis* and *Faciola* comprise of food-borne trematodes (known as Flukes) that affect an estimated 70–100 million people all over the world. The disease clonorchiasis is due to *Clonorchis sinensis* and opisthorchiasis is caused by the species of the genus *Opisthorchis*. All the discoveries were based on the observations made on other parasitic flukes such as *Faciola hepatica* infecting the sheep and others of zoological interest. The discovery of a food fish as an intermediate host had a great impact on the control of the infections due to these flukes. *Faciola hepatica* was first referred by de Brie in 1379 in sheep suffering from 'Liver rot', 500 years before the formal description of trematodes that infect humans. *Faciola hepatica* (*F. hepatica*) and *Faciola gigantica* (*F. gigantica*) are the liver flukes of veterinary importance causing huge economic losses of livestock such as sheep, goats and cattle. The two species are morphologically indistinguishable but they have different snail species as intermediate host. Human facioliasis is uncommon but distributed throughout the world.

The liver flukes belong to the phylum Platyhelmenthes, class Trematoda and subclass Digenea. The digenetic trematodes undergo an indirect life cycle with several morphological stages and they have at least one intermediate host. The medically important food-borne flukes were once grouped under the genus *Distoma*. Most food-borne trematodes are zoonotic and can infect a large variety of animals like birds and mammals.

The food-borne flukes are often described as 'leaf-like' and they are elongated, flat bilaterally symmetrical with three body layers. They are devoid of body cavity and the entire body is covered with non-ciliated integument which is a complex living tissue containing invaginations and spines and it is not simply a secreted sheath. The muscles lie below the integument enveloping the body. The worm possesses special structures such as esophagus, suckers that possess radial muscle fibers. At the anterior end, the oral and ventral suckers are situated. The digestive system is incomplete and end blindly without rectum and anus. The flame cells or solenocytes are specialized cells that join with an excretory bladder that has an excretory pore at the posterior end. There is no circulatory system and the nervous system is partially developed. The food-borne trematodes are hermaphrodites. Each individual worm has both male and female reproductive organs. Both *F. hepatica* and *F. gigantica* that infect man possesses shoulders and a conical anterior end. Both the species are morphologically difficult to differentiate but they are genetically different.

Clonorchis sinensis measures upto 20 × 5 mm in size whereas *Opisthorchis* species are smaller than *C. sinensis*. The ventral sucker is smaller than the oral and located within the anterior half of the worm. Similar to *Faciola hepatica* the morphological features of the adult worms cannot be differentiated the species. However, the flame cells pattern in the cercariae is distinct. The number, shape of testicular lobes, their location and the appearance of vitelline glands vary between as well as within the species.

Life Cycle (Fig. 23.33)

i. The life cycles of food-borne trematodes are complex and involve one or two intermediate hosts of which the first one is always a snail. The infective stage of the fluke is metacercariae
ii. Humans are infected with *Clonorchis* or *Opisthorchis* species due to consumption of raw or undercooked fish containing the encysted metacercariae. The metacercariae of *Faciola hepatica* encyst on aquatic plants.
iii. The ingested metacercariae excyst in the duodenum and release the larvae. The excysted larvae migrate through the ampulla of Vater and to the extra hepatic bile ducts to the small intrahepatic ducts where they mature.
iv. Within one month the adult worms start producing the eggs on an average 10,000 eggs per day. The eggs are excreted in the feces. The metacercariae of *Faciola hepatica* excyst in the duodenum and the immature worms migrate through the duodenal wall into the body cavity. They then burrow through the Glisson's capsule and cross hepatic parenchyma to the proximal bile duct and gallbladder where they undergo maturation and become adult worms. The migration takes 6 to 7 weeks. The adult worm begins producing the eggs which are excreted in the feces, 3 to 4 months after ingestion of metacercariae. The adult worm lives for many years ranging from 6 to 30 years with an average period of 10 years.

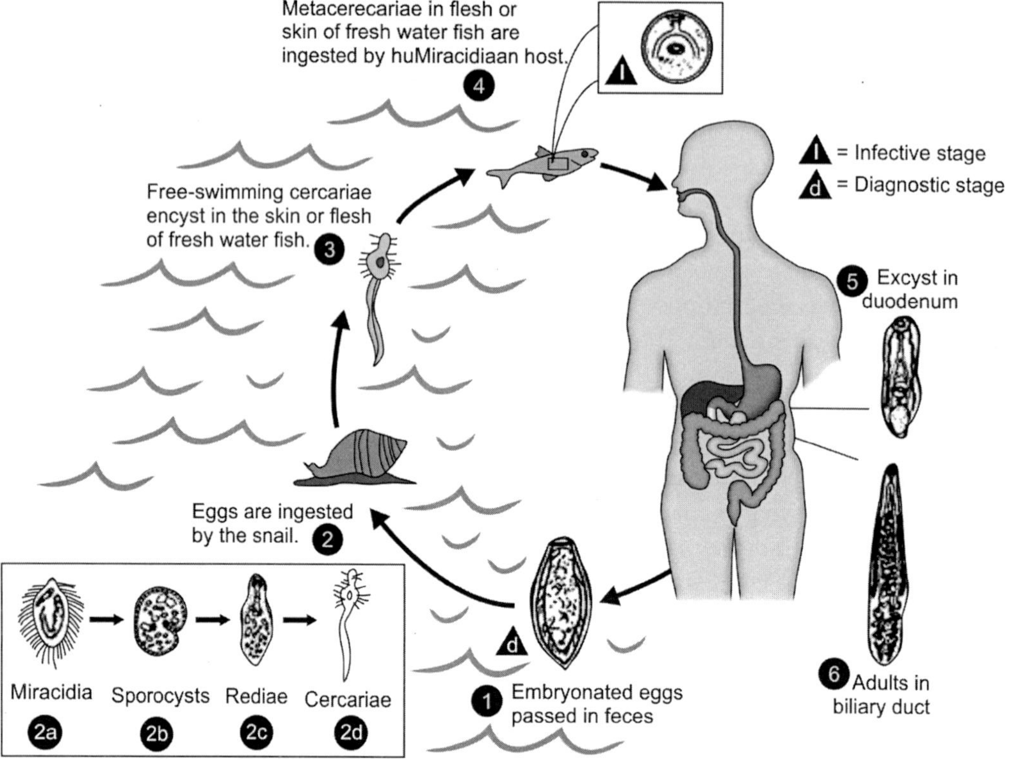

Fig. 23.33: Life cycle of *Opisthorchis*, *Clonorchis*, and *Faciola*

v. Fresh water sources or submerged grass become infected with eggs from the feces of infected patients or the reservoir hosts. The eggs enter appropriate snail host. The miracidia develop and hatch within two weeks and swim freely till they find appropriate snail host of the genus *Lymnaea*.

vi. Inside the snail the miracidia develop into sporocyst, and rediae which undergo parthenogenic reproduction and finally give birth to cercariae.

vii. The cercariae emerge and swim freely to find an appropriate site to become metacercariae. Nearly 100 species of cyprinoid fish serve as second intermediate host for *Clonorchis* and *Opisthorchis* species. The cercariae transform into metacercariae in the second intermediate host. The cercariae of *Faciola hepatica* encyst on green water vegetation. There is no second intermediate host for this fluke.

viii. These life cycles require at least 4 months to complete or may be prolonged due to winter hibernation of the snails. Seasonal variations in transmission, temperature, density of intermediate host, human sanitation, eating behavior govern the life cycle completion and the prevalence of the human infection.

The important clinical manifestation of liver flukes especially *Opisthorchis viverrini* and *Clonorchis sinensis* is extreme susceptibility to bile duct cancer that has very poor prognosis. In endemic areas infection may be asymptomatic or the symptoms are usually nonspecific requiring differentiation from bacterial infections and tuberculosis. The common clinical manifestations are hepatomegaly, abdominal pain, flatulence, dyspepsia weakness and other nonspecific symptoms like nausea, diarrhea, anemia, edema, dizziness, and neuropsychiatric symptoms. Gallbladder stasis, hepatolithiasis, ascending cholangitis, obstructive jaundice, portal hypertension, ascites, gastrointestinal bleeding are the severe complications of liver fluke infection.

Treatment is required to eliminate the long-lived parasite immediately. A single dose of praziquantel at 40 mg/kg body weight for opisthorchiasis and clonorchiasis is used in Korea. *Faciola hepatica* is not sensitive to praziquantel. Drugs currently used are dihydroemetine, bithionol and triclobendazole. Improvement in sanitation interrupts transmission from human excreta to snails and health education prevents people from eating raw or undercooked sea foods. Alternative methods such as freezing or irradiation of fish may be useful. Biological agents to destroy the cercariae and treating the reservoir hosts have been suggested but not widely implemented. Despite successful treatment reinfection can occur and complete success in curing is hampered by difficulty in changing human behavior.

PARAGONIMUS

The genus *Paragonimus* has nine species of which *Paragonimus westermani* is an important lung fluke that is pathogenic to humans. *Paragonimus westermani* (*P. westermani*) was found in the lungs of a patient by Ringer in 1870. Later on several Japanese workers including Roan Nakagawa, Sademu Yokogawa described the complete life cycle in the snail. Interestingly *P. westermani* was first discovered in Bengal Tigers by Kerbert in 1878.

Paragonimus species are roughly half the size of *Faciola* and measure 16 × 8 mm in size, oval in shape and reddish brown in color. The tegument is covered with scale-like spines. The ventral sucker is situated towards the middle of the body and its size is similar to that of the oral sucker present at the anterior end. The parasite has a large excretory bladder. The species that infect the humans can be differentiated by various morphological and life cycle differences in the adult worm. The eggs of *Paragonimus* species are yellowish brown, variable in shape and measure 570 × 55 μm with a flat operculum. When the eggs are laid, they are embryonated.

Life Cycle

1. The metacercariae are the infective forms of the *P. westermani* or lung fluke.
2. The infection is acquired by the ingestion of metacercariae along with raw or undercooked crabs.
3. The larvae of *P. westermani* undergo systemic migration.
4. After ingestion the larvae are released in the duodenum by the action of intestinal juices and enzymes.
5. The larvae penetrate the duodenum and enter the abdominal cavity. They remain in the abdominal wall for some days and then continue their migration through the diaphragm into the pleural cavity and then to lungs.

6. Submerged grass is contaminated with the eggs of *Paragonimus* species. The eggs develop and hatch in water approximately within three weeks and release miracidia.
7. The released miracidia must find and penetrate a permissible species of snail. Inside the snail the miracidia develop into sporocysts and rediae which undergo parthenogenic reproduction to produce cercariae.
8. The cercariae penetrate the gills and muscles of the fresh water mitten crabs or crayfish. Nearly 53 crustacean species serve as intermediate hosts for *Paragonimus* species.
9. The cercariae are transformed into metacercariae in the viscera of the second intermediate host. When these crustacean species are consumed by the definitive host, the metacercariae are released by the action of intestinal juices and enzymes and the cycle is repeated.

Scattered reports especially from Assam have been recorded in India. It is believed that raw crabs have medicinal value. Crabs and crayfish are caught and eaten raw as under roasted form by children and workers of rice fields. Traditional dishes often made from raw crabs or crayfish meat or juice mixed with lemon juice, brine, soya sauce, alcohol or vinegar (drunken crabs).

The inter species differences in migratory behavior, the extent of pulmonary pathology influence the clinical manifestations due to *Paragonimus* infection and the clinical symptoms vary between the species of *Paragonimus* infecting the humans. Many times paragonimiasis is misdiagnosed as tuberculosis. The nonspecific symptoms like diarrhea, abdominal or chest pain, allergic reactions, fever, chills may be present during the migratory phase. Once the worm is established, the common symptoms are cough, dyspnea, hemoptysis, night sweats and general malaise. Up to 50 mL of gelatinous rusty brown sputum containing eggs and traces of blood is expectorated daily by the infected person. Severe infection can lead to pleurisy, rales, clubbing of fingers and pneumothorax. If the parasite lodges in brain or spinal cord which is common in children, severe disease may result. Symptoms include headache, nausea, vomiting, fever and paralysis and other signs and symptoms of CNS develop depending upon the location of the infection. Recovery may be spontaneous but symptoms recur. Migration of the parasite under the skin leads to the formation of migrating swelling containing parasites and eggs. Intestinal paragonimiasis which manifests as multiple granulomatous nodules may be mistaken for abdominal or gastric tumors.

PROCEDURES FOR LABORATORY DIAGNOSIS OF INTESTINAL AND BILIARY PARASITES

Feces, duodenal aspirates or sigmoidoscopic aspirates are routinely preferred specimens from finding the diagnostic stages of the parasites (vegetative forms, ova or cysts). It has been observed that the eggs of the most of the intestinal parasites are uniformly distributed due to the mixing action of the colon because of constant peristaltic movement. However, in situations like schistosomiasis the eggs may be numerous on the surface of the formed fecal specimen. The distribution of protozoan parasites is more variable. There may be a less number of protozoan vegetative forms in the first portion of the evacuated fecal specimen because they are deteriorated easily in the lower colon.

Collection and handling of the Fecal Specimens

Examination of multiple specimens from the same patient is likely to give appropriate identification of intestinal and biliary parasites because some organisms shed the cysts or ova in a variable pattern. In general specimens collected every 2nd or 3rd day for a total of three specimens are usually adequate for diagnosis and identification. From hospitalized patients, one specimen each day for three days is more cost effective and optimal.

A number of substances such as certain antidiarrheal preparations like bismuth, kaolin, antacids, antimicrobials, oils barium, magnesium hydroxide ($Mg(OH)_2$, enemas, soap, irritants, hypertonic saline destroy the trophozoites and distort cysts. So they should be avoided before collecting the specimen. Generally, 5 to 10 days time is required to clear these substances.

Stool specimen containers should be wide-mouthed, water tight and leak-proof with tight fitting lids such as waxed pint-sized icecream cartons or plastic containers. It is advisable that patients should defecate directly into such appropriate well-designed containers. The fecal specimens should not be contaminated with urine as it may inhibit some of the parasites. Toilet paper should not be included in the specimen. Stool specimen should not be retrieved from the toilet bowl as it may contain many free-living protozoa and the water is harmful to the eggs of schistosomes and amoebic trophozoites. Formed stools may be collected on a wax paper (Table 23.16).

Purgation with sodium bisulfate or buffered phosphosoda may be useful for demonstration of trophozoites of *Entamoeba histolytica* or related species and the larvae of *Strongyloides* species. Purgation may be useful if a series of stool samples turn out to be negative for parasitic ova, cysts or trophozoites. Prior arrangements should be made with the laboratory and the specimens are collected during the working hours of the laboratory as far as possible. The specimens should be accompanied with all clinically relevant data of the patient such as duration of the illness, suspected diagnosis and recent travel to endemic areas.

Table 23.16: Laboratory examination for various types of fecal specimens

Types of the specimen	Wet mount	Concentration	Permanent smear
Unpreserved			
a. Formed	+	++	+/–
b. Soft	++	++	++
c. Loose watery	++	+/–	++
Preserved			
Formalin			
a. Formed soft	+	++	–
b. Liquid	++	+/–	–
PVA fixed			
a. Formed	–	–	+/–
b. Liquid/loose	–	–	++

The specimen is may be placed in a fixative before transportation or it may be examined unfixed. It is advisable to use both the methods for optimum diagnosis keeping in mind about the location of the patient, consistency of the specimen, time of the day and the laboratory workload. Soft, loose watery stool specimens are likely to contain trophozoites and therefore they should be examined on priority basis. Formed stools that usually contain cysts, ova or larvae can remain satisfactorily for a number of hours at room temperature or overnight in a refrigerator. Specimens should never be incubated.

Incubation speeds up the deterioration of the organism. Specimens labeled for parasitic examination should never be frozen or thawed.

Use of Fixatives

The commonly used fixatives are 5 to 10 percent buffered formalin or polyvinyl alcohol (PVA). One part of the fecal specimen is added to three parts of the fixative. Unfixed specimens if processed in the laboratory, the smears are prepared immediately and fixed in Schaudinn's fixative. Merthiolate-iodine-formalin is an alternative to formalin fixative. The advantage is that it not only fixes but also stains the parasites. Sodium acetate-formalin is useful for wet mount examination and satisfactory for concentration as well as for permanent staining. This fixative is devoid of mercury, only one vial is sufficient, and it is not toxic. However, permanent stains with this fixative are of inferior quality compared to Schaudinn's or PVA fixative.

Gross Examination

Gross examination should describe the consistency, color, presence of gross abnormalities such as mucus, blood and worms or their segments. The mucus, pus or blood flecks may be examined microscopically for parasites. The adult worms are carefully removed, washed for further examination. Fragments of the worms such as head, segments are to be mounted separately. Worms can be stained by Mayer's paracaramine for 1 to 20 minutes depending on size, destaining in alcohol until the worm is pale pink in color, dehydrating, clearing and mounting in Canada balsam or DPX mount.

Some parasitic infections may require serial histological sections for the identification and in this procedure; orientation is critical which should be done manually. Seeking help from helminth taxonomist is useful for proper identification.

Microscopic Examination

The three principal microscopic examinations performed on stool specimens for the identification of parasites are direct wet mount, wet mount after concentration and permanent stain. Although each procedure contributes to the diagnosis, the yield may be small with certain types of specimens. As a rule, formed stool sample should be subjected to concentration technique. Soft specimens can be examined by wet mount and permanent stain. Wet mount is useful for loose watery diarrhea. If the specimen is sent in a fixative and the consistency is not known, concentration and permanent stain should be performed and other examination may be helpful. Special procedures may be necessary for identification of some specific parasites. Since size is important in the differentiation of parasites accurate, size is determined with a calibrated ocular micrometer.

Direct Wet Mount

Direct wet mounts for fresh unconcentrated feces or for fixed stool samples are most useful for the detection of motile trophozoites of protozoa and motile larvae of *Strongyloides stercoralis*. It is also useful for the detection of protozoan cysts and eggs of the helminths. Wet mount is also useful for the examination of mucus or the blood flecks.

About 1 to 2 mg of the fecal matter is mixed with a drop of 0.85% saline and a cover slip is applied carefully by avoiding air bubbles. Similarly, an iodine mount can be prepared using either Dobell and O'Connor or 1:5 Lugol's iodine solution. The smears are screened under low power objective and suspected objects are confirmed using higher magnification.

A solution of buffered methylene blue (pH 3.6) may be used as vital stain for fresh examination of protozoa. Organisms should be stained for 5 to 10 minutes. The main use of iodine mount is to study the morphology of protozoan cysts as the stain shows nuclear details and glycogen mass but not the chromatoid bars.

Concentration Methods

Concentration procedures are useful in separating the parasites from fecal debris and helpful in growing axenic cultures of the parasites. These techniques are based on the differences in the densities of the parasites and the fecal debris. The concentration techniques mainly fall into two groups; sedimentation in which the parasites are heavier than the solution and are concentrated in the sediment or deposit present at the bottom of the test tube after centrifugation. In floatation techniques, the specific gravity of the solution in which the parasites are placed is heavier than the parasite and hence the parasitic forms float to the surface. Among the various sedimentation and floatation, techniques describe the formalin-ethyl acetate modification of formalin-ether technique and zinc sulfate floatation techniques are widely used. The modification of formalin-ether concentration method of Ritchie by using formalin-ethlyacetate avoids flammability and storage of ether. This technique can be used for specimens to which formalin has been added or specimens fixed in merthiolate-iodine-formalin. If the procedure is properly performed after centrifugation at 1500 rpm four layers should result; ethyl acetate, plug of debris, formalin and the sediment. If tap water is used in the sedimentation technique lysis of *Blastomyces hominis* may occur. If schistosomiasis is suspected the specimen should be preserved in formalin before concentration to prevent hatching.

Faust and his associates first described zinc sulfate centrifugal concentration technique. This method can be used for both unfixed and formalin fixed specimens, although the specific gravity of the zinc sulfate solution differs (Specific gravity 1.20 for fixed specimens and 1.18 for fresh specimens). The disadvantages of this technique are (a) dense schistosome eggs do not concentrate well, (b) opercula often pop and operculated eggs may be missed, and (c) larvae and cysts may collapse. If the modified procedure with formalin-fixed feces is used these disadvantages may be avoided. The advantage of this method is that it leaves rather clean background and had less grit than sedimentation procedure.

Sheather's sugar flotation technique is recommended for concentrating the cysts of *Cryptosporidium* spp because they stand out sharply from the clear background in this solution of high specific gravity. In this technique, 0.5 g of formed stools or centrifuged watery stools can be used. Saline or iodine is not used in the preparation of wet mounts for *Cryptosporidium* spp demonstration.

Baerman's concentration technique has greater sensitivity for the detection of *Strongyloides stercoralis* larvae than do the other conventional techniques. The procedure is useful for the diagnosis, monitoring the therapy and for epidemiological studies. Merthiolate-iodine-formalin fixed stool samples are concentrated using sodium acetate formalin or PVA fixative. Some studies indicated that parasites do not concentrate well from the material fixed in PVA fixative or from material that is fixed in merthiolate-iodine-formalin fixative for extended period.

Hatching Technique for Detection of Viable Schistosome Eggs

About 5 to 10 g of fecal matter is palced in a one-liter flask and water is added while mixing to break up the fecal matter. Add more water to reach a level of 2 to 5 cm from the top of the flask. The entire flask is covered with a foil except the top of the liquid from the light. The flask is allowed to stand at room temperature for several hours. With the help of a hand lens, examine the material at the top of the flask neck for swimming miracidia.

Permanent Stains

Permanent staining is useful for the identification of both trophozoites and cysts of the protozoa. For permanent staining stool sample is fixed either in PVA fixative or in Schaudinn's fixative. Wheatley trichrome stain is widely used. Inadequate removal of mercuric chloride by alcohol-iodine solution (if iodine is very weak) or improper destaining or weak staining by trichrome if it is too diluted with alcohol are some of the troubleshooters of trichrome staining. Trichrome stains,

Cytoplasm of cysts and trophozoites: Blue-green tinged with purple

Nuclear chromatin, chromatoid bars, red cells, bacteria: Stained red or purplish red

Other ingested parasites or yeasts: Green

Parasites eggs and larvae: Red

Acid-fast stain (modified) is generally used for the demonstration of *Cryptosporidium* spp.

Egg Counts

Egg counting methods help in clinical studies to assess the intensity of infection especially due to intestinal nematodes. Methods like Kato thick smear, Stoll's egg counting technique are more scientific but require greater accuracy. The most simple and practical technique is to emulsify 2 mg of fecal matter in a drop of saline on a microscopic slide and count the number of eggs after applying the cover slip. The eggs are counted using a total magnification of X100. The density of the smear is adjusted and standardized using a light meter but it is not required for patient care. The number of eggs per preparation provides a rough index of the severity of the infection.

Aspirated fluid from duodenum or duodenal biopsy are useful for the detection of trophozoites of *Giardia lamblia,* larvae of *Strongyloides stercoralis* and bile stained eggs of helminths or other upper gastrointestinal parasites which may not be detected in feces. String test, in which a weighted gelatin capsule attached to a string, is allowed to swallow by the patient along with small sips of water. The capsule along with the string gradually reaches the duodenum where it is allowed to stay for 4 to 5 hours. Then, the string is removed and the fluid attached to it is squeezed. Wet mount is made out of the extracted fluid for examining the parasites.

Similarly, material obtained by sigmoidoscopy may be useful in diagnosing or monitoring amoebiasis, schistosomiasis and cryptosporidiosis. Swabs should not be used as parasites are killed or trapped by the swab material. Biopsy material should be processed for surgical pathology and PAS stain is particularly useful for the demonstration of amoebae. Biopsy material for the detection of the schistosome eggs is better examined in teased preparations rather than in sections. The cryptosporidia are usually seen at the luminal surface of the epithelial cells of the intestines. These organisms are small and detailed study of the structure requires electron microscopy.

Abscess material is aspirated and wet mounts are examined for the parasites like *Entamoeba histolytica*. The last portion of the aspirate is likely to contain more trophozoites. Since the aspirated pus from the abscess is often thick and difficult to examine it may be treated with streptokinase or streptodornase enzymes to liquefy the specimen (one part of the enzyme to five parts of the aspirated material and the mixture is incubated at 37°C for one hour. The mixture is well mixed and centrifuged at 400 g and the deposit is examined by preparing the wet mount.

Cellophane Tape Method

Cellophane tape is used for the detection of the eggs of *Enterobius vermicularis* and *Taenia* species from the per anal area. The tape must be clear cellophane and should not be cloudy or opaque. If the specimen is difficult to examine, remove the cellophane tape from the microscopic slide carefully; add a drop of toluene, and replace the tape smoothly with an applicator stick. Care is taken to avoid trapping of air. Entire tape including the edges is examined under × 100 magnification (× 10 objective).

Culture of Amoebae and Giardia Species

Cultures for amoebae have improved the detection in some studies. However, the culture methods for pathogenic protozoa are not used routinely. Although the *Giardia* species can be cultured, cultures are not useful for the diagnosis. Several culture media have been described and they are available commercially both for axenic and monoaxenic cultures of amoebae. The culture media are also available commercially. These are complex media and are highly enriched. The prepared culture media are warmed to 37°C before inoculating the stool specimens. *Entamoeba histolytica* microaerophillic and can tolerate an oxygen concentration of 5% but not 10%. The optimum temperature for its growth is 36.5°C. The culture bottles or test tubes are periodically tested under inverted microscope for the growth of the organism.

Larval Maturation

Larval maturation referred as culture can be performed on fecal specimens applied to a wet filter paper. Nematode larvae such as *Strongyloides* or *Ankylostoma* spp mature to filariform larvae in the culture container and migrate from the feces to the water where they are detected microscopically. The procedure can be performed either in a Petri dish or in a large mouthed test tube. The fecal specimen is smeared on to a filter paper strip that is dipped into 3 mL of water. The portion of the filter paper that is smeared with the specimen of feces need not be immersed into the water. The water is examined periodically for larvae by preparing the wet mounts or the tube or plates can be examined under inverted microscope.

Detection of Blood and Tissue Parasites

Parasites that circulate in the blood are generally identified in Leishman or Giemsa stained smears of peripheral blood. Those parasites that are not circulated in the blood may be detected in the skin snips, lesion scrapings body fluids or in the biopsy material. The diagnosis can also be done by demonstrating specific antibodies in the serum or in the body fluids against the antigens of the infecting parasite.

The timing of the collection of blood specimen depends upon the parasite disease suspected. Certain filarial diseases are better detected if the blood specimen is collected between 10 PM to midnight, whereas for other infections specimens are best obtained during the day. In malaria, the number and the stages of the parasite vary in the peripheral blood and vary with different parts of the cycle.

Blood films are best made from the blood specimen that is not treated with any anti-coagulant. A drop obtained from finger prick or ear lobe is usually sufficient. Anticoagulants may interfere with the morphology and staining of the parasite. Care should be taken to observe that the alcohol used to disinfect the finger or ear lobe is allowed to dry otherwise there may be fixation of the erythrocytes and they may interfere with the preparation and staining of the thick and thin film. Thick and thin smears can be prepared from blood with anticoagulant but the staining characters are not satisfactory. If it is unavoidable to use anticoagulant EDTA blood is better than citrated or heparinized blood specimen.

Both thick and thin films are useful. Thick films are more sensitive because the same amount of blood can be examined in 5 minutes, as compared to thin film that may require a 30-minute examination. Thin films are useful to study the effects of the parasite on erythrocytes and provide better morphology of the parasite. Both thick and thin films can be made on the same slide.

The best time to obtain blood for a peripheral smear is a few hours following the chill. Thin smears are sufficient when parasitemia is very heavy and the thick smears are to be made when scanty parasitemia is expected. Buffy coat smears preserve the morphology and gametocytes are more concentrated. Blood smears can be kept without staining for two hours and after staining, they can be stored for two years after mounting.

The smears should be dried quickly to prevent distortion. Any one of the Romanowski's stain like Giemsa, Leishman, May-Grunwald, Jensen, Wright or May-Grunwald Giemsa can be used for staining.

Tissue

Biopsy or necropsy tissue may be examined by histopathology sections or by impression smears. Foe impression smears, the tissue should be blotted to remove as much blood or fluid as possible and then gently pressed against a clean, grease free glass slide to make a series of impressions. The tissue should be dry enough to stick to the slide leave large and irregular films on the slide. Impressions must be close together preferably with slight overlapping for easy scanning. If amoebiasis is suspected impression, smears must be fixed in Schaudinn's fixative and allowed to air dry. For most other parasites, slides are allowed to air dry before fixing them in methanol. Giemsa is the usual recommended stain but other stains such as methanamine silver or iron-hematoxylin may also be used.

Fluids

Tissue aspirates, cyst fluid, bronchial washings, cerebrospinal fluid or other body fluids can be examined after centrifugation and the sediment can be examined by wet mount or by staining with suitable stain depending upon the parasite suspected.

Skin Snips

Skin snips are at times useful for the detection of microfilariae of *Onchocerca* species. Skin snips are taken with a needle and knife. The needlepoint is stuck into the skin and the skin is raised. With a sharp knife or razor blade, the skin is excised just below the needle. The excised skin snip is placed in a small volume of saline in a tube or in a micro titer well. The skin snip is teased well and allowed to stand for 30 minutes or more. The tissue microfilariae migrate from the tissue into the saline that can be examined by wet mount.

Concentration Procedures for Blood Specimens

Most of the concentration procedures described are mainly useful for the diagnosis of the filarial infections. The widely used methods are membrane filters, saponin lysis and Knott's concentration method. Membrane filter technique uses filters of 3 or 5 µm pore size and the technique does not require lysis of erythrocytes. Parasites on membrane filters are often not suitable for morphological studies as compared to stained films. Saponin is used to lyse the red blood cells. The procedure requires collection of 10 mL of blood from a suitable vein and is placed in a tube with an anticoagulant such as EDTA or citrate. The specimen is centrifuged at 150 g to remove plasma. The packed red cells are mixed with 50 mL of 0.5 percent saponin solution in 0.85 percent saline. The mixture is shaken well at intervals for 15 minutes. The lysed solution is then centrifuged and smears are prepared from the sediment. The smears are either examined by wet mount after adding 2 drops of one percent acetic acid and mixed well (microfilaria are killed and straightened). For staining, the smears are allowed to air dry and the dried smears are dipped in buffered methylene blue phosphate solution. The slides are then rinsed in distilled water and after drying them in air, stained with 1:20 Giemsa stain.

Culture Techniques

Culture methods are available for a number of blood and tissue parasites. These methods are primarily used in reference laboratories for research purposes. The cultures of *Leishmania* spp or *Trypanasoma* spp are helpful in the diagnosis as the procedures are relatively simple to use in routine laboratories also. The biopsy material is ground with small volume of saline and the suspension is decontaminated with suitable antibiotic mixture and then inoculated into Novy-MacNeal-Nicolle (NNN) medium. The amastigotes are converted into flagellated forms in this medium.

Urine specimens are examined for the eggs of *Schistosoma heamatobium,* trophozoites of *Trichomonas vaginalis*. Rarely, larvae of *Strongyloides stercoralis* may be found in the urine sample. Occasionally amoebic trophozoites or hydatid sand may be seen in the sputum specimen. Specially induced sputum may be useful for the detection of *Pneumocystis carinii* infection.

Serodiagnosis

Many papers have been published on serological tests for parasitic diseases that have evolved through years from simple gel diffusion to most advanced immunoblots. Major improvements have been made in test parameters because of development of more sensitive techniques and availability of more purified and specific antigens. However, specificity is always a problem in the serodiagnosis of helminthic infections. Recent use of purified glycoprotein antigen of *Taenia solium* has greatly improved the serodiagnosis of cysticercosis. However, many parasitic infections can be diagnosed by simple microscopic examination of feces, blood smears and tissue sections, infections that are deep seated or infections like cysticercosis or hydatidosis may require invasive procedures. These procedures are associated with some risk to the patient. Detection of antibodies can be useful in indicating whether an individual with no previous exposure to a specific infection may have acquired infection while traveling to an endemic area (Table 23.17). Nevertheless, detection of antibodies to parasitic antigens among the individuals residing in an endemic area reflects only past infection unrelated to the status of the patient. Antibody concentration may decline slowly after the patient is cured, but generally lasts from one year to may years and so are not reliable indicators for successful cure. The detection of parasitic specific IgM antibodies can be of value in determining the time of initial infection (e.g. Toxoplasmosis) but these assays are insensitive and lack ability to interpret the results. Added to the problem, at present there are no reference standards for many of the immunological assays to evaluate the specificity and sensitivity of commercially available reagents. There is no proficiency-testing program for any serological tests for parasitic infections at present. Nevertheless, much work has been accomplished in recent times on the development of antigen detecting systems, resulting in commercially available reagents for *Giardia, Cryptosporidium* and *Pneumocystis carinii* and *Trichomonas* spp. Molecular biology shows promise and nucleic acid probes may allow detection of parasitic nucleic acid from the specimens obtained from the patient. Molecular methods are useful for taxonomy and epidemiology. Using recombinant DNA technology, it is possible to obtain

Table 23.17: Antigen and antibody tests for parasitic diseases

Disease	Antibody tests done at CDC	Tests done by Labs	Commercially available Antigen kits
Amebiasis	IHA	Yes	
Babesiosis	IIF	–	
Chaga's disease	IIF, CF	Yes	
Cryptosporidiosis	–	Yes	IIF
Cysticercosis	IB	Yes	
Fascioliasis	–	Yes	
Filariasis	–	Yes	
Echinococcosis	IHA, IB	Yes	
Giardiasis	–	Yes	
Leishmaniasis	IIF, CF	Yes	
Malaria	IIF	Yes	ELISA, IIF
Paragonimiasis	IB	Yes	
Pneumocystosis	–	–	
Schistosomiasis	ELISA, IB	Yes	IIF
Strongyloldosls	ELISA	Yes	
Toxocariasis	ELISA	Yes	
Toxoplasmosis	IIF, ELISA-IgM	Yes	
Trichenillosis	BF	Yes	
Trichmoniasis	–	–	ELISA, DIF

IHA = Indirect hemagglutination, IIF = Indirect immunofluorescence, IB = Immunoblot
ELISA = Enzyme-linked immunosorbent assay, DIF = Direct immunofluorescence

purified antigens that show minimum cross-reactivity with the antibody to the other parasitic antigens. The usefulness of serodiagnosis with respect to the individual parasitic diseases will be mentioned in the systemic parasitology.

Chapter 24

Clinical Mycology

FUNCTIONAL TAXONOMY FOR CLINICAL MYCOLOGIST

Although the classification proposed by Dixon and Fromtling is phylogenetically acceptable and has meaning for academic mycologists but it is of less relevance to clinical mycologists in the day-to-day task of making accurate genus and species identification. The following description of taxonomy is simple and clinically useful.

Zygomycetes

In Greek *'zygon'* means fusion or joining in the manner of a yoke. The old classification Phycomycetes (*Phykon* means seaweed in Greek) has been correctly replaced with Zygomycetes. The sexuality of this group of fungi is characterized by the formation of similar gametes and is called isogamous. The process is known as conjugation and the product of conjugation is zygospore. During the union the ends of two mycelia are swollen, come into contact with each other and the terminal part of the hyphae are segmented by a transverse wall. The similar terminal cells fuse together with the disappearance of the walls between the two conjugating cells. The protoplast masses of both the cells unite to form a zygospore. A zygospore has double wall which is thick and rough. Under favorable conditions the zygospore germinates producing promycelium which bears a sporangium which is similar to one found in the asexual spores. Zygomycetes have no septate hyphae (Coenocytic) and sexual reproduction may be isogamous or heterogamous. The class Zygomycetes contains thè order Mucorales (*Mucere* in Latin means moldy or musty). Mucorales include those Zygomycetes which can reproduce both sexually and asexually. The asexual spores are formed in a sac-like sporangium and sexual spores are zygospores. The term mucor is used to refer the fungal infection caused by the species of the order Mucorales, not just infection caused by *Mucor*.

Ascomycotina (Ascomycetes)

The vegetative body of Ascomycetes may be single celled or both yeast like budding cells and hyphae may be present. The hyphae are septate. Asexual spores or conidia are produced exogenously either from conidiophores or directly from hyphae (blastospores). The sexual reproduction involves sac-like structures, an ascus that contains spores called ascospores which are produced by karyogamy and meiosis. The sexual reproduction is by specialized endogenous spores known as ascospores borne on sac-like structures called asci. The ascospores are derived from the fusion of similar or dissimilar sexual cells. The sexual process may not be hidden during the development (e.g. true yeasts). But in some species the sexual spores are protected by a special structure called perithecium. Within the class of Ascomycotina, the order Eurotiales, the asci are produced within cleistothecium which is a closed structure composed of compact specialized hyphae. Many of the medically important imperfect fungi for which sexual reproduction has been described belong to this order. The members of the family Gymnoascaceae produce special cleistothecia with unorganized peridial hyphae. The genus Arthroderma refers to the sexual forms of dermatophytic fungi like *Trichophyton* and *Microsporum*. The term Ajellomyces refers to the sexual forms of Blastomyces and Histoplasma species. The family Eurotiaceae comprises of species like *Pseudoallecheria boydii* and many of the telomorphs of *Aspergillus* and *Penicillium* species. The cleistothecia of these fungi are more compact and tissue like.

Basidiomycotina (Basidiomycetes)

The vegetative forms of fungi show septate filamentous hyphae. Sexual reproduction is by production of spores in club-shaped organ called basidia and the sexual spores are called basidiospores. The Basidiomycetes are large complex group of fungi some of which show high degree of differentiation. This group includes many plant and insect pathogens, the smuts and rusts, puffballs, bracket fungi, mushrooms and *Filobasidiella neoformans* which is represented in its halophase by the important pathogenic yeast: *Cryptococcus neoformans.*

Deuteromycotina (Fungi Imperfecti)

Fungi of this group comprise of the fungi for which the sexual reproductive cycle has not been discovered. Hence the life cycle is imperfectly known. Dodge describes these fungi as "the fungi imperfecti"and is conceived as a dumping ground until the gaps of our knowledge with respect to their sexual reproduction have fulfilled". These fungi are identified by their asexual spores or conidia which are relatively specific for a given group. The spores may be hyaline or dark, unicellular or multicellular. The spore wall may be smooth or rough, thin or thick. Under the subdivision, the class Blastomycetes contains the imperfect (asexual) yeasts, some of which produce pseudohyphae or true hyphae. The genera include *Cryptococcus, Candida, Malassezia, Rhodotorula, Torulopsis* and *Trichosporon*. The other class Hyphomycetes produces septate mycelia and reproduces by asexual spores that are borne on highly specialized tissue stroma. Most of the pathogenic fungi belong to this class (e.g. *Alternaria, Aspergillus, Epidermophyton, Geotrichum, Histoplasma, Microsporum, Penicillium* and *Trichophyton*). Cell walls of hyphae or conidia or both of dematiaceous fungi contain melanins by which they are darkly pigmented. Saccarado in 1884 classified fungi imperfecti into several orders like Melanchoniales, Sphaeropsidales, Hypomycetales, and Pseudomycetales and mycelia sterilia. Among these orders the fungi belonging to Hypomycetales are of interest to medical mycologists. Hypomycetales are further classified as Moniliaceae, Dematiaceae, Stubaceae and Tuberculariaceae. Only fungi belonging to Moniliaceae and Dematiaceae cause infections in humans and animals. Further classification of Saccarado is based on the characteristics of spores such as shape, color, septation and many subgroups have been described by him. But for a medical mycologist, it is convenient to classify the fungi imperfecti group according to Vuillemin (1919) which was later modified in 1925.

Classification

Tallosporales: Reproducing by Thallospores

a. Blastosporinae, for example, *Candida, Cryptococcus*
b. Arthrosporinae: Reproducing by arthrospores, for example, *Geotrichum candidum, Madurella, Indiella*
c. Mycodermaceae: Septate hyphae with elongated budding forms.

Hemisporales: Reproducing by Hemispores

For example, *Hemispora stellata.*

Conidiophorales: Reproducing by Conidia

a. Aleuriosporineae: Reproducing by aleuriospores, e.g. dermatophytes
b. Sporotrichineae: Reproducing by true conidia but not borne on conidiophores, e.g., *Sporotrichum schenckii*
c. Sporophorineae: Reproducing by true conidia borne on conidiophores. Most of the species of fungi imperfecti belong to this group
d. Phialidineae: Reproducing by true conidia borne on phialides (flask-shaped sterigma), e.g., *Aspergillus.*

Nomenclature

Fungi belong to plant kingdom. Presently they are grouped into a separate kingdom Mycetae (earlier known as Plantae). The kingdom Mycetae is subdivided into classes, orders, suborders, families, tribes, genera and species. The fungi are named as per the binomial nomenclature comprising of generic part which is always Latin substantive and always written with a capital letter. The second part is the specific name of the fungus which is usually an adjective and not written with a capital letter. The species is also named after the name of the discoverer, e.g. *Trichophyton schoenleinni.* In this some prefer to put the discoverer's name with an initial capital letter. While citing the name of a species, the name of the author who described it originally is often appended to the name of the species. When the name is amended and a second name is introduced the name of the original discoverer is put in the parenthesis, e.g. *Microsporum mentagrophytes.* C Robin, 1853, is expressed after amendment as *Trichophyton mentagrophytes* (C Robin) Blanchard 1896.

Medically Important Fungi

Zygomycetes

Rhizopus species
Absidia species
Syncephalastrum species
Circinella species
Cunnighamella species

Aspergillus

A. flavus
A. fumigatus
A. niger
A. terneus

Halinohyphomyces

Penicillium species
Scopulariopsis species
Paeciliomyces species
Fusarium species
Trichoderma species
Acremonium species
Gliocladium species
Chrysosporium species
Scedosporium species
Beauvaria species

Chromomycosis

Claudosporium carionii
Phialophora verrucosum
Fonsecaea pedrosi
Wangiella species
Exophiala species

Phaeohyphomycosis

Alternaria species
Stemphilium species
Epicoccum species
Curvularia species
Bipolaris species
Uloclaudium species
Phoma species
Chaetophorea species
Xylohypha (*Cladophialophora gartiana*)

Dimorphic Fungi

Blastomyces dermatitidis
Histoplasma capsulatum
Coccidiodes immitis
Sporothrix schenckii
Paracoccidiodes brasiliensis

Yeasts

Candida albicans
Candida species
Cryptococcus neoformans
Cryptococcus species
Torulopsis glabrata
Trichosporon species
Geotrichum species
Malassezia furfur

Dermatophytes

Trichophyton rubrum
Trichophyton mentagrophytes
Trichophyton tonsurans
Trichophyton species
Microsporum canis
Microsporum gypseum
Microsporum species
Epidermophyton floccosum

SUPERFICIAL MYCOSIS

Superficial mycosis is mainly confined to the outermost keratinized layer of the skin or grows in the secretion on the surface of mucous membrane. The pathological process does not extend deep like those in cutaneous mycosis. The common clinical conditions causing superficial mycosis are erythrasma, trichomycosis axillaris, piedra, tinea nigra, superficial streptomycosis, tinea versicolor, seborrhec dermatitis and dermatophytosis. Among these clinical conditions dermatophytosis is very common.

DERMATOPHYTOSIS (CUTANEOUS MYCOSIS)

Cutaneous mycosis or dermatophytosis is a clinical condition caused by a group of closely related keratinophilic fungi imperfecti. The infection is common in man and animals and it is commonly known as tineasis. The term tinea dating back to Middle Age refers to circular holes in garments produced by clothes-moth. The appearance is similar to ring like lesions produced by dermatophytic fungi. The term tinea is now used to describe various clinical syndromes caused by dermatophytes. Dermatophytes infect superficial skin, hair and nails without causing any subcutaneous or systemic infection. Tinea infections are also common in dogs, cats, horses and other animals with which man is closely associated. Hence, zoophilic infections in humans are also quite common. The dermatophytes show mycelial filaments in skin, hair or nails and when old they show arthrospores. All of them grow well on Sabouraud's dextrose agar with filamentous colonies and show characteristic appearance. Ringworm or tinea lesions are known to Indians from the time immemorial. The clinical symptoms of the disease have been found in the ayurvedic literature. However, no description of the etiological agent has been mentioned in these works.

General Characters of Dermatophytes

These are keratinophilic imperfect fungi affecting the superficial horny layers of skin, hair and nails. During the infection mycelial forms can be seen in the scrapings during early stage of infection and in old cases arthrospores may be seen. All the species of various genera of dermatophytes grow well on Sabouraud's medium at room temperature (ambient) and show short mycelia with characteristic asexual spores which may be macroconidia or microconidia.

The present classification was described by Ajello in 1968. According to him, there are four genera and each genus has several species except *Epidermophyton* which was only single species.

Genus Trichophyton (15 Species)

T. rubrum
T. mentagrophytes
T. violaceum
T. tonsurans
T. ferrugeneum
T. purpureum
T. megninii, etc.

Genus Microsporum (7 Species)

M. gypseum
M. canis
M. nanum
M. audounii, etc.

Genus Epidermophyton (1 Species)

E. fluccosum

Genus Keratomyces (1 Species)

K. ajelloi

Genus *Trichophyton* is classified into 5 groups:

1. Rubrum group
2. Crateriform group
3. Gypseum group

4. Rosaceum group
5. Flaviform group

Based on hair bait technique dermatophytes fall into two broad groups:

a. **Ecotothrix** forming arthrospores and fungal mycelia are seen around the hair follicle. For example, *M. gymnaseum, T. rosaceum.*
b. **Endothrix** forming arthrospores and fungal mycelia are seen within the hair and they perforate the hair. For example, *T. tonsurans*

Dermatophytes are also grouped based on their predominant predilection to humans, animals or soil.

Anthrophilic

These dermatophytes cause infection in humans only. For example, *Epidermophyton fluccosum, Microsporum audounii, Trichophyton* species.

Zoophilic

These dermatophytes predominantly affect the animals and infection from them is transmitted to humans by close contact. For example, *M. canis, T. gallinae, T. mentagrophytes.*

Geophilic

These fungi responsible for cutaneous mycosis are present mainly in soil and infection in humans occurs due to contact with contaminated soil. For example, *Keratinomyces ajelloi, M. gypseum.*

Clinical Manifestations

Clinically Tinea or ringworm infection due to dermatophytic fungi can occur in several forms, which are briefly summarized in this section.

Tinea capitis or ringworm of the scalp can occur as gray-patch, or communicable ectothrix infection due to *M. audounii* in children. Inflammatory ectothrix with *T. mentagrophytes* of animal origin, black-dot ringworm, an ectothrix infection and fungating exophytic masses (kerions) produced by *T. tonsurans* or favus infection due to *T. schoenleni.* The clinical condition is most frequently encountered and it is due to direct contact or through a variety of fomites. Adults may act as asymptomatic carriers and they contribute to the persistence of infection in a given geographical area. The species may vary from area to area. Contact with domestic pets is the common predisposing factor and familial occurrence of similar infections can occur in 50 to 60 percent of cases.

Tinea corporis or ringworm of the body shows typical annular lesions on the skin of the smooth parts of the body. The lesions show spreading, hemorrhage border. The common species isolated from *T. corporis* are *T. rubrum, T. mentagrophytes* and *T. tonsurans.* The infection spreads from person-to-person by direct contact. *T. rubrum* can survive on the surface of skin for years or even lifetime. The mannan antigens of *T. rubrum* inhibit cell-mediated immunity. The other species like *T. canis, T. gypseum* are isolated occasionally. *T. rubrum* can survive outside the body as spores in the desquamated epithelial cells and promote person-to-person transmission. *Tinea barbe* or the ringworm infection of the beard area is common among the farm workers. The clinical condition is due to *T. mentagrophytes* and the lesions tend to be more inflammatory because of the zoophilic nature of the fungus. *Tinea cruris* or ringworm of the groin appear as circinate and serpigenous. The lesions are inflammatory and vesicular. The margins are enlarged and the infection is very common among athletes. The fungal responsible for infection is *Epidermophyton floccosum*. The infection may occur as epidemic among athletes, soldiers, ship crew due to sharing of towels, linen and clothing.

Tinea pedis or athlete's foot is a very common dermatophytic infection among the humans. The infection is characterized by itching scaling and seeping on soles or intertrigenous scales areas of toes. The infection is common during warm humid climate. The causative fungal species are *T. mentagrophytes, T. rubrum* and *E. floccosum*. The increased amount of keratin in soles and palms makes these sites more vulnerable to infection due to *T. mentagrophytes*. The desquamated skin cells containing the spores of *T. rubrum* are transmitted from person-to-person by fomites.

The ringworm infection of the nails or *Tinea unguium* is the dermatophytic infection of nails. It should be differentiated from onychomycosis caused by a variety of non-dermatophytic fungi such as *Aspergillus, Candida, Geotrichum* species and several other species of dematiaceous hyphomycetes. The infection of nails due to dermatophytes begins either at the lateral or distal edge of the nail plate producing paronychial inflammation. With the progression of infection the nail becomes thick, brittle and in the subunguial region there is accumulation of keratinized debris. *T. unguium* is caused by *T. rubrum, T. mentagrophytes* and *E. fluccosum*. Studies have shown that the peak incidence of *Tinea capitis* was at its peak among the school going children and the incidence of *Tinea pedis* was common among the adolescents. Diabetes mellitus apparently does not predispose to dermatophytosis.

General Characteristics of Dermatophytes

According to the classification dermatophytes fall under the following 4 genera and each genus has distinct morphological features when cultured in the laboratory.

Trichophyton Group

The fungi of this group grow well on Sabouraud's dextrose agar with 0.5 percent Chloramphenicol (to suppress the growth of bacteria) and actidione (to suppress fungal contaminants) and the thick slants are implanted with epithelial scrapings taken from the margin of the lesion, or hair that are plucked from the site of lesion, or nail cuttings obtained under aseptic conditions. The slants are incubated at room temperature or in a BOD incubator. The growth is granular or powdery or glabrous or velvety in appearance. Microscopic examination of a small portion of the colony shows short mycelia. Different species show different types of pigmentation which helps in the identification of species. The color varies from light pink to red, purple, violet, brown or yellow. Microscopically one can see short septate hyphae. Microconidia are either along the sides (en thyrse) or in clusters (en grappe) along the conidiophores. Matured colonies produce long pencil shaped, thin walled macroconidia, racquet mycelium, nodular bodies and coiled hyphae. Microconidia are more prominent. Individual species show variations.

Microsporum Group

All the species of *Microsporum* group grow well on Sabouraud's medium at room temperature. The growth is rather slow and the colonies show powdery appearance, furrowed type or folded type. Pigmentation is less and the colonies may show brownish pigmentation. Microscopically the fungus growth shows less number of microconidia that are arranged singly along the hyphae. They are sessile and smaller in size. Racquet shaped mycelia are seen. Macroconidia are spindle shaped multi-celled and thick walled.

Epidermophyton Group

There is only one species namely *Epidermophyton fluccosum.* The fungus grows well on Sabouraud's medium at room temperature. The growth on the medium is glabrous and folded. The culture is usually yellow or olive green. Microconidia are absent.

Keratinomyces Group

This group also has only one species namely *Keratinomyces ajelloi.* The fungus grows well on Sabouraud's medium at room temperature. Colonies are powdery and show different colors. The macroconidia are large, smooth walled and cylindriform. The hyphae are multi-septate. Microconidia are rare.

Other techniques like Riddle's agar block culture or hair bait technique are also useful for differentiating of the species. Skin testing with trichophytin may show both immediate and delayed type of hypersensitivity. A negative test excludes the possibility of infection due to dermatophytes but a positive test has no clinical value. Commercially available trichophytin preparations are not useful. Serodiagnosis may show elevated IgE, immune complexes and normal IgG titers.

Infected hair may be removed. Earlier topical application like Whitefield's ointment, five percent ammoniated mercury, one percent thymol, 0.5 percent phenyl mercuric nitrate, chryserobin, estrogenic hormone therapy and irradiation were tried. With the discovery of azoles and imidazoles currently the dermatophytic infections are treated with topical application of miconazole nitrate, clotrimoxazole, econazole, ciclopriax or tolnaftate. Griseofulvin when administered orally is very effective but treatment requires prolonged duration. Griseofulvin is poorly absorbed but gets concentrated in the stratum corneum where it acts on hyphae and inhibits their growth. Griseofulvin is given in a dose of 250 to 500 mg/day for adults. The drug is prepared as ultramicrosized form. It is effective against the scalp and nail infections and the drug is given for 2 to 6 weeks for cases of *Tinea capitis* and *Tinea corporis.* For infection of nails the drug may have to be continued upto one year or even for longer period. Recent studies showed that ketoconazole is highly effective in some patients.

SUBCUTANEOUS MYCOSES

Subcutaneous mycosis is due to fungal infection. The fungi that are responsible for this clinical condition are widely distributed in nature, especially in soil and vegetation. These fungi enter the skin or subcutaneous tissue following a trauma. The natural history of the infection depends upon the pathogenic potential of the infecting fungus and the host response. Some fungi can cause distinctive mycosis such as sporotrichosis, rhinosporidiosis, lobomycosis, and rhinoentemopthoromycosis or subcutaneous phycomycosis. On the other hand, subcutaneous mycosis may be due to several fungi that produce single clinical entity known as mycetoma. Fungi causing subcutaneous mycosis are generally confined to skin and subcutaneous tissue. But occasionally they may invade other organ.

Mycetoma

A mycetoma is a localized, chronic granulomatous lesion involving skin and subcutaneous tissues and eventually in some cases the bones. Normally mycetoma are confined to hands and feet but occasionally other parts of the body such as back, shoulders and buttocks may be involved. The lesions contain granulomas, abscesses that suppurate and drain through sinus tracts. The pus contains granules (grains) which are popularly known as sulfur granules. The granules are the microcolonies of fungus that is responsible for mycetoma. The size, color, shape, consistency and texture of these fungal colonies vary with the species and they are often useful in identifying the specific etiological agent. Both *Actinomycetes* and a variety of soil fungi are known to cause mycetoma. Mycetomas hence are broadly classified into Actinomycetoma and Eumycetoma. The organisms responsible for both types of mycetoma are discussed as follows.

Causative Agents of Mycetoma

About 22 species of fungi are commonly isolated from cases of Eumycetoma. Of these species 5 belong to the group Ascomycota and the rest 17 species belong to Deuteromycota.

Ascomycota

Emericella nidulans
Leptosphaeria senegalensis
Leptosphaeria tompkinsii
Neotestestudina rosatii
Pseudoallecheria boydii

Deuteromycota

Acremonium falciforme
Acremonium recifei
Curvularia geniculata
Corynespora cassicola
Curvularia lunata
Exophiala jeanselmei
Fusarium moniliformis
Fusarium solani
Madurella grisea
Madurella mycetomatis, etc.,

The first case of Eumycetoma was reported by Carter in 1830 who established the relationship between the clinical condition and the fungal isolate from a patient in Madurai, Tamil Nadu, India and he named it as 'Madura foot' or 'Madura mycosis'. Later on similar cases were reported from other parts of India and from South America, Mexico, USA and Europe.

All the fungal species responsible for mycetoma produce a uniform clinical and pathological picture and these etiological agents broadly grouped under (a) aerobic Actinomycetoma (due to *Nocardia* and *Streptomyces* species) and (b) Eumycetoma caused by a variety of species of true fungi. Rarely other species belonging to the genera *Aspergillus* and *Penicillium* have been reported as the causative agents of Eumycetoma.

Following trauma, the affected area shows a nodular swelling which is deep seated and fixed. The nodule progresses slowly with indurated area extending in all directions, abscess formation. The abscess ruptures with sinus formation. As the lesion advances, multiple abscesses with sinuses, deformity swelling of long duration and discharge from the sinuses can be seen. The infection involves muscles, fascia and bones due to chronic inflammatory process. The purulent discharge from the sinuses contains granules that vary in size, shape, texture and color depending upon the causative agent. Apart from local tenderness and pain, there is no significant systemic reaction. Involvement of bones may show both lytic as well as proliferative reactions. The clinical diagnosis at this stage is easy and it needs to be confirmed by radiological as well as laboratory diagnosis only to identify the etiological agent.

Mycetoma generally remains localized at the site of infection. The infection is slow but progressive and spreads to the adjacent tissues involving muscle, fascia and bones. Secondary infections with pyogenic organisms aggravate the clinical symptoms and patient may develop septicemia leading to death. The prognosis is very good if diagnosed and treated early.

It is difficult to manage mycetoma. Amphotericin B is recommended for Madurella infection. Alternatively ketoconazole may be used. Topical nystatin and oral potassium iodide are used if the infection is due to *P. boydii*. Flucytosine is effective for *E. jeanselmei* infection. Surgery may be indicated in chronic cases because the drops do not reach the infected tissue in enough concentration due to extensive fibrosis. Invasive infection with *P. boydii* has been successfully treated with amphotericin B. However, some laboratory as well as clinical studies suggests that miconazole is the best choice for treatment.

SYSTEMIC MYCOSIS

Four major dimorphic fungi namely *Coccidiodes immitis, Blastomyces dermatitidis, Histoplasma capsulatum* and *Paracoccidiodes brasiliensis* are responsible for systemic fungal infection. Among these four types of fungi *H. capsulatum* and *C. immitis* are found normally in dry soil or soil mixed with guano (the accumulated excretions of sea birds) whereas the rest two are presumed to exist in nature but the knowledge about their habitats is still not clearly understood. The geographical distribution of these fungi and their prevalence is

Table 24.1: Epidemiological features of primary systemic mycoses

Property	*Histoplasmosis*	*Coccidioidomycosis*	*Paracoccidioidomycosis*	*Blastomycosis*
Saprophytic form	+	+	+	+
Hyaline septate hyphae	+	+	+	+
Tissue form	Yeasts	Spherules	Yeasts	Yeasts
High infection rate in endemic areas	+	+	+	?
> 90% infection is by inhalation	+	+	+	?
Majority of infections are asymptomatic	+	+	+	?
> 90% of infections are self-limited	+	+	+	+
> 90% of infections can occur in				
Immunocompetent patients	+	+	+	
Incidence of infection among the males	80–90%	75–90%	95%	50–90%

delimited. All the four species of fungi are transmitted by inhalation of their spores and produce pulmonary infection. Human to human transmission occurs only in extremely rare instances. Table 24.1 summarizes salient epidemiological features of these systemic fungal infections.

As opportunistic infections, the incidence of these fungal infections with AIDS has sharply increased in recent years.

HISTOPLASMOSIS

The causative agent of histoplasmosis was first seen by Samuel Taylor Darling in 1905 in a patient in the Panama and Canal Zone. The name *Histoplasma capsulatum* was suggested because the yeast-like cells seen in the macrophages were thought to be a protozoan and it was encapsulated. But the organism was later found to be neither a protozoan nor encapsulated. The fungal nature of the infective organism was confirmed by Hausmann and Shenken in 1914 and further reconfirmed by DeMonbreum in 1934. The organism was first cultured from the blood of an infected child. The sexual stage or telomorph of *H. capsulatum* was demonstrated by Kwon-Chung and named *Emmasiella capsulata*. The new term *Ajellomyces capsulatus* was later proposed by McGinnis and Katz.

Histoplasma capsulatum is a dimorphic fungus. The yeast phase is seen in tissue of the infected person while the mycelial phase is seen when cultured in the laboratory. Recent molecular studies revealed that *H. capsulatum* is closely related to *Blastomyces dermatitidis*. The telomorph of *H. capsulatum* is *A. capsulatus*. The mating types are designated as negative (–) and positive (+) and both are equally prevalent in the soil. But 90% of infections are due to negative (–) type.

Acute Pulmonary Histoplasmosis

In humans the route of transmission is always inhalation of the microconidia. The lesions in the lung may run a benign self-limiting. The patients may show symptoms ranging from a mild flu-like illness that clears spontaneously or they may develop moderate to severe infection. The healthy persons develop symptoms proportional to the inoculum size inhaled. In previously sensitized persons, reinfection results in a shorter and milder infection with minimal histological changes. The incubation period varies from one to several weeks. A moderate infection may manifest as cough, dyspnea, chest pain, hoarseness of voice. Severe infection of the lungs may show fever weight loss and night sweats.

The infection may take a chronic course in same patients with cavitations, fibrosis and calcification resembling pulmonary tuberculosis. The infection may mimic bronchiectasis, lymphoblastoma. Pulmonary lesions due to *H. capsulatum* resolve slowly with fibrosis and calcification.

Chronic Pulmonary Histoplasmosis

Chronic pulmonary Histoplasmosis is commonly seen in adult males with some form of underlying pulmonary disease such as chronic obstructive lung disease (COPD), emphysema and abnormal pulmonary spaces (anatomical defects). Chronic infection may manifest as transient pneumonitis and large bullous spaces may become cavitatory type due to infection by *H. capsulatum.* The chronic type of infection may be indistinguishable from chronic pulmonary tuberculosis. The chronic infection may develop immediately after inhalation or after several years of quiescence. The pathological and immunological evidence supports that the late onset is due to reactivation of an old lesion rather than exogenous reinfection. The infection is usually apical. The patients may show low grade fever, productive cough, progressive weight loss and weakness. Prognosis depends on the control of underlying diseases apart from treatment of histoplasmosis (Table 24.2).

Disseminated Histoplasmosis

Histoplasmosis is essentially a systemic infection with yeast form of the fungus invading the reticuloendothelial system. In the disseminated stage of the disease no viscera in the body is spared. Lesions occur in skeletal system, gastrointestinal tract, mesenteric lymph nodes and central nervous systems. Lessons can also be seen in the mucosa of the nose,

Table 24.2: Clinical types of histoplasmosis

	Acute	*Chronic*
Pulmonary	Asymptomatic	Pneumonic or
	Mild	Cavitatory
	Moderate	(Anatomic defect)
	Severe	
Disseminated	Benign	Progressive mucocutaneous
	Progressive	

mouth, pharynx, larynx and in the skin. In the acute disseminated type, the patient may show spiky temperature with hepatosplenomegaly. This may, however, run a benign course with good prognosis. But this often goes into a progressive type with fatal outcome if not diagnosed and treated promptly. Chronic disseminated type presents with ulcerative lesions in the mouth, larynx, tongue and gums. Dissemination may also involve lymph nodes, spleen, liver and bone marrow. It can be completely benign and in apparent except for the presence of calcified lesions. The patients may have anemia, weight loss, hepatosplenomegaly leukopenia and granulomatous lesions with macrophages packed with yeast cell can be observed in all the organs and quite often the adrenals.

Acute progressive histoplasmosis is fatal often fulminant and rapidly fatal. This form of histoplasmosis is an opportunistic disease associated with defective or compromised cell-mediated immunity as seen in patients with progressive HIV infection (AIDS), those receiving immunosuppressive therapy. In endemic areas, children with histiocytosis develop fulminant histoplasmosis (Table 24.2).

Mucocutaneous Histoplasmosis

This is a disseminated form of histoplasmosis characterized by ulcers of the lips, buccal and palatine mucosa, tongue, larynx, pharynx and penis. Ulcers show raised irregular wall with clear floor. The granulation tissue consists of macrophages loaded with yeast form of *H. capsulatum*. The local lymph nodes are often involved. Skin lesions help to establish otherwise obscure nature of the disease.

Other Forms of Histoplasmosis

Very rarely chronic disseminated form of histoplasmosis occurs following primary inoculation of skin or mucocutaneous tissue. The lungs are not involved in this type of infection. The fungus is introduced after the contamination of a traumatic wound. Such infections are anatomically localized as seen in some eye infection or they may chronically progress involving the draining lymphatics of the affected area. Presumed ocular histoplasmosis syndrome (POHS) comprises of choroidal, macular and subretinal lesions and peripapillary atrophy. All cases of POHS show a positive reaction to 'histoplasmin' skin test. The cause for POHS is not clear. Patients with histoplasmosis may have ocular lesions last patients with POHS.

Histoplasmin Skin Test

The antigen histoplasmin is produced by growing mycelia of *H. capsulatum* in broth containing aspargine. The filtrate from the culture is dialyzed and standardized and 0.1 mL of 1:100 or 1:1000 dilution of the standardized antigen is injected intradermally. A positive reaction is indicated by the appearance of induration of $\geq$5 mm diameter within 48 hours. A positive test indicates exposure to the infection. Without the previous history of a negative reaction to the skin test, a positive skin test is of no diagnostic value. Histoplasmin is a crude polyvalent mixture of antigens. Some of the antigens are specific while others show cross-reactivity with other dimorphic fungi. So, skin testing is conducted using a

Table 24.3: Characteristics of systemic dimorphic fungi

Anamorph (Telomorph)	*Ecology*	*Mycelial form*	*Tissue form*
H. capsulatum	Alkaline soil, Bird and bat guano Ohio, Missouri and Mississippi river valley	Septate hyphae	Microcondia
(*A. capsulatus*)	Bird and bat: Guam, Ohio, Missouri, and Mississippi river valley	Hyphae septate globose microconidia tuberculate and non-tuberculate macoconidia	oval yeast of 2–4 μm size
H. capsulatum var duboisii (*A. capsulatus*)	Central Africa	Identical to H.*capsulatum*	Thick-walled yeasts narrow based budding
B. dermatitidis (*A. dermatitidis*)	River banks? Ohio, Mississippi river valley	Hyphae, oval, pyriform, globose, terminal or lateral conidia	Thick-walled yeasts wide based single budding (8–15 μm)
C. immitis	Soil, semiarid region of South Western USA, Central America, and South America	Hyphae and arthroconidia	Spherules (20–60 μm) containing endospores (2–4 μm)
P. brasiliensis	Soil? Central and South America	Hyphae, rare, oval to globose, terminal, or lateral conidia intercalary chlamydospores	Thick-walled, multiple budding yeasts (15–30 μm)

battery of antigens namely coccidioidin, paracoccidiodin, histoplasmin, blastomycin and spherulin.

The protocol used for laboratory diagnosis of other systemic fungal infections (Systemic mycoses) is similar to that described for histoplasmosis (Table 24.3).

OPPORTUNISTIC FUNGI

The modern medical technology has definitely improved the life span of many patients with debilitating diseases or antimicrobial defenses. However, patients receiving corticosteroids, cytotoxic drugs, radiation therapy, broad spectrum antibiotics for the management of cancer, organ transplantation, or undergoing invasive surgical procedures, or having immunological or metabolic disorders such as AIDS or diabetes mellitus or other chronic infections are predisposed to opportunistic infections. Patients with all types of leukemia, Hodgkin's disease, neutropenia due to anticancer therapy, endocrinal abnormalities are more prone to develop opportunistic infections especially due to fungi which are normally nonpathogenic and are frequently found as normal flora of the human body. In general any treatment or condition that reduce the number of functions of phagocytes or impair the cell-mediated immune response, increase the susceptibility to opportunistic fungal infections. The immunocompromized patients are at greater risk for systemic infections due to fungi like *Candida* species, *Cryptococcus* species, *Aspergillus* species and *Zygomycetes* species. These fungi are ubiquitous and almost impossible to avoid exposure to these fungi. In recent years, the incidence of infection due to opportunistic fungi is alarmingly on the increasing side.

CANDIDIASIS

Earlier it was considered that the immense amount of literature that exists about the infections due to *Candida albicans,* a yeast-like fungus is inversely proportional to the seriousness of the disease. Currently it is recognized that this harmless commensal can turn into a deadly foe causing disseminated fatal candidiasis. *Candida* infections are worldwide and superficial or intermediate infections like onychosis, paronychia, epidermophytoses, intertrigo, oral candidiasis, perleche, perianal and vulvovaginal infections as well as infections of the eye and ear are very common. Systemic candidiasis is frequently associated with traumatic conditions or deep seated diseases and endocrinal disorders like diabetes mellitus, hypothyroidism, Addison's disease, malnutrition, steroid therapy, use of broad spectrum antibiotics for prolonged period, agranulocytosis, leukemia and other malignant diseases. Wilson aptly described that "Candida is a better physician and can point out abnormalities in persons much earlier in the course of development of such abnormalities than with our chemical tests in the laboratory".

Historically Legenback in 1893 demonstrated a yeast-like fungus in the lesion thrush which was named as *Oidium albicans* by Robin in 1923. Zopf in 1890 named the yeast as *Monilia albicans.* Berkhout suggested the name Candida to the genus that induced fungi which reproduced by budding and developed pseudo mycelia. The genus *Candida* comprises of several species of which, *C. guillermondii, C. krusei, C. stellitoidea* and *C. viswanathi* are involved in human infections. Majority of human infections are due to, *C. parapsilosis, C. guillermondii* and other species are emerging as opportunistic pathogens. *C. lipolytica* and *C. krusei* have been associated with fungimia and *C. lucitaneae* has been recently recognized as emerging pathogen and it is resistant to amphotericin B.

Chronic macerations of skin, mucous membranes and nails result in infection by endogenous *Candida* species. Physiological changes in the host and immunocompromization contributes to the development of cutaneous or mucocutaneous candidiasis. Mucous membrane candidiasis is often known as thrush. Oral thrush is commonly seen among infants, AIDS patients and among the adults who are treated with broad spectrum antibiotics for prolonged periods or with cytotoxic drugs. The lesions are singular, patchy or confluent. A whitish pseudo-membrane comprising of yeasts and pseudohyphae is seen on the tongue, soft palate and on oral mucosa. Vaginal thrush occurs more frequently among the pregnant women, diabetics and in those women who receive antibiotics and oral contraceptives. Patches of grayish white pseudomembrane are seen on the vaginal mucosa along with yellowish white discharge. Infection may spread to adjacent skin and per anal region. In infants per anal candidiasis is known as diaper rash and it may also be seen in the groin and genital areas. In addition to *C. albicans* other species of the genus can also cause vaginitis, chronic nail infection and paronychia. The skin around the nail is swollen and inflamed resulting in painful condition.

Numerous systemic manifestations can occur following the introduction of *Candida* species into the bloodstream. Candidimia can occur due to indwelling catheters, surgical procedures, trauma to the skin or gastrointestinal mucosa, per sorption or aspiration. The severity of systemic infection is governed by the size of the inoculum, virulence of the infecting species and compromised host defense mechanisms. Occult infections in the form of candiduria, endopthalmitis and macronodular lesions have been reported. Systemic infections tend to localize preferably in the kidneys, lungs and endocardium. Spleen, liver, urinary bladder, brain and other organs are also may be involved. Infection of the kidneys is so frequent because of the filter effect of the glomerular capillaries. Early lesions are found in the cortex of the kidney as small white or yellowish micro abscess or granuloma.

Congenital systemic candidiasis is a very rare infection in newborn children and the infection is usually ascending type from vagina and penetration of intact membranes with infection of the amniotic fluid and subsequent aspiration of the infected fluid by the newborn child. The infection spreads rapidly and the mortality rate is very high.

Chronic mucocutaneous candidiasis is the infection of any or all types of epithelial cell surfaces of the body and it has unique set of predisposing factors and clinical manifestations. The clinical symptoms are limited to skin, oral mucosa, upper respiratory tract, gastrointestinal and genitourinary epithelium. Invasion of deeper tissue is rare. The fungus penetrates the plasma membrane of the epithelial cell that results in the distortion of the cell to a significant level. The organism exists as an intracellular parasite. Chronic mucocutaneous candidiasis (CMC) often begins in the early part of the life and persists for lifetime. The degree of involvement varies with the individuals. Some children develop total skin lesions that recede minimally with treatment. Others may respond to treatment temporarily but permanent cure is rare. The classical lesions are warty, verrucous with horn-like projections growing out from the skin. The lesions become chronic and as the age advances extensive epithelial hyperplasia is seen.

Most patients with chronic mucocutaneous candidiasis have impaired cell-mediated immune response but the precise defect is not known. Patients may not show any consistent deficiency. If the onset occurs between 10 to 30 years of age prognosis is good because the defects in the cell-mediated immunity may get corrected due to treatment. If the onset of chronic mucocutaneous candidiasis is after 40 years of age, it is usually associated with thymoma.

Some patients develop sterile vesicular lesions of the skin due to 'Id' or allergic reaction from the hematogeneous spread of *C. albicans* from the primary focus. This hypersensitivity reaction is known as Candid, Monilid or Levurid. The allergic reaction subsides after healing of the primary focus. Fungus cannot be found in these *Candida* lesions. These allergic lesions are commonly seen in hands and fingers but may be found anywhere in the body.

Topical application of ketoconazole, nystatin or miconazole is useful for cutaneous candidiasis. The drugs of choice for systemic candidiasis are amphotericin B, flucytosine but development of drug resistant has been documented with many strains of *C. albicans.* Chronic mucocutaneous candidiasis has been treated with topical preparations of amphotericin B, flucytosine and miconazole. Ketoconazole has produced dramatic resolution in many patients but the response varies with individual-to- individual and the resolution of lesions is associated with improved immunocompetence. Nevertheless, both the responses are often temporary.

For patients who are at risk of developing systemic candidiasis, a prophylactic treatment with oral ketoconazole or nystatin has been tried in several studies. A low dose or short course of amphotericin B also tried along with antibacterial agents. Controlled trials indicated a low incidence of candidiasis in prophylactically treated patients. Candidiasis should be treated energetically whether it is primary or secondary. *Candida* endocarditis, meningitis and pulmonary candidiasis carry serious prognosis.

CRYPTOCOCCOSIS

The synonyms for this fungal infection are torulosis, European blastomycosis or Busse-Bushke's disease. The genus *Cryptococcus* has many species of which *Cryptococcus neoformans* is the commonest pathogen that causes disease in humans. Other species are occasionally isolated from immunocompromised patients especially those having advanced HIV infection.

Senker in 1864 described yeast-like organism which could be probably this fungal species. The first authentic isolation of this yeast-like fungus was made by Busse in 1894. In 1895 Bushke gave complete description of the organism. Benham in 1954 further studied the organism by conducting the experiments on the original culture described by Bushke and confirmed its name as *Cryptococcus neoformans.*

One of the important antigens of *C. neoformans* is the capsular polysaccharide. By using cross-absorption technique four different antigenic determinants of capsular material namely A, B, C and D have been detected. According to Kwon-Chung the isolates of the sero groups A and D are different from the sero groups of B and C. Serotype A isolates are distributed worldwide and are the most frequent cause of cryptococcosis. Capsular polysaccharide is soluble in water and can be detected from both culture filtrates and body fluids (especially the cerebrospinal fluid).

The initial infection after inhalation of the yeast form of *C. neoformans* can occur in any portion of the lungs and mimics a mild influenza like-syndrome. The infection may resolve spontaneously or it may be asymptomatic. Pulmonary cryptococcosis is rarely fulminant and pulmonary hilar lymphadenopathy; calcification and caseation are rarely seen. Symptomatic patients may have cough, expectoration and weight loss or fever. The tissue response is usually minimal or it may be granulomatous type. Chest X-ray shows variable picture depending upon the type and severity of the infection. In general the lower lobes of the lungs show rounded shadow without any enlargement of hilar shadow. Uncommon presentations like miliary shadows, consolidation may be seen in occasional cases. Calcifications are rare. Localized cryptococcoma in the lung presents as circumscribed subpleural or mediastinal tumor like lesion composed of well-defined gelatinous masses. The size and number of such lesions are variable. Diffuse pulmonary lesions may be hemorrhagic, edematous and patchy that may be either unilateral or bilateral. Cavitations, miliary nodules or mediastinal lymphadenopathy may be seen in some cases. The X-ray appearance may resemble a variety of chronic pulmonary diseases like malignancy, tuberculosis or pulmonary abscess.

Approximately 9 out of 10 cases of pulmonary cryptococcosis may end up in dissemination to central nervous system. Cryptococcal meningitis is more common among the advanced cases of HIV infection. It can also manifest secondary to long-term steroid therapy or other forms of immunosuppression. In majority of the cases the chief symptoms are headache, especially severe and intolerable, nausea, vomiting with or without altered sensorium. Fever and neck rigidity may be totally absent. Patient may present with dementia, cerebellar ataxia, spastic paraperesis and hydrocephalus. Meningovascular lesions may lead to stroke. Except optic nerve involvement other cranial nerve palsies are rare. Lower cranial nerve palsies are more frequently associated with cryptococcal infection than tuberculosis of the nervous system. The infection is chronic and steadily progressive over a period of several weeks. In some patients, the course of the infection is remarkably indolent. Cryptococcomas are rarely seen along with cryptococcal meningitis.

Apart from the dissemination to the central nervous system, in about 20% of cases the infection may spread to lymph nodes, spleen, liver and adrenals simulating Hodgkin's disease or other lymphoproliferative disorders. In 10% of cases, one may see multiple osteolytic lesions in bones. Pustular and ulcerated disseminating lesions of the skin and mucosa which discharge mucinous gray or brownish-red material may be seen in some patients.. This may contain yeast cells of the fungus if examine carefully. Dissemination can occur in any part of the body.

Detection of Cryptococcal Antigen

Detection of cryptococcal antigen for the diagnosis of progressive infection is probably the best antigen detection assay described for infectious diseases so far. Two antigens namely the polysaccharide antigen and protein antigen can be detected using any of the techniques like latex agglutination, co-agglutination or ELISA. For all methods commercial reagents are available. Latex agglutination test may give false-positive results due to interference of rheumatoid factor, hydroxyl ethyl starch, Trichophyton *beigelli* infection, etc. False-negative reactions may be seen if the concentration of the antigen is low or due to prozone effect when the concentration of the antigen is high. In spite of some disadvantages latex agglutination test for the detection of the antigen is easy to perform, can be used both for serum and spinal fluid. The technology is very familiar and does not require any special equipment. Some amount of subjective variation in reading the agglutination reaction, need for the pre-treatment of the specimen and need for meticulous control of the false-positive results are the noted disadvantages of latex agglutination test.

ELISA based assay is more specific and sensitive and quantifiable. The specimen does not require any pre-treatment. But the technique requires expertise and special equipment like ELISA reader and the test is relatively costly.

Cryptococcosis is treated with amphotericin B and flucytosine as per the combination therapy protocol. Patients with advanced HIV infection do not respond to routine combination therapy and they require treatment for long period of time to suppress the infection. Fluconazole has excellent penetration into the central nervous system and treatment with fluconazole prevents recurrences of cryptococcosis.

ASPERGILLOSIS

Aspergillosis is a clinical entity comprising of a number of clinical manifestations caused by fungal species of the genus *Aspergillus*. The word *Aspergillus* is so named due to the resemblance of its spore heads to *Aspergillum* which is a kind of mop used to distribute holy water (Latin: *Aspergere* means to sprinkle). The spectrum of aspergillosis is very wide and caused by a number of species of the genus. The genus *Aspergillus* comprises of a group of rapidly growing hyaline molds. Raper and Fennel described around 700 species in their classical monograph. Rinaldi cited only 19 species. Only four species namely *A. fumigatus*, *A. flavus*, *A. niger*, and *A. terneus* are the most important and most frequently encountered species from clinical species out of 19 species described by Rinaldi.

Individuals with structural abnormalities within the lungs and those with impaired resistance to infection due to metastatic cancer, leukemia, lymphomatous diseases, and steroid usage are more prone to develop infection due to *Aspergillus* species. Hyphae are susceptible to neutrophil killing mechanism but activated macrophages are capable of killing the hyphae and conidia. The products of *Aspergillus* species have been identified that inhibit the activation of the alternative pathway of complement. Allergic forms of aspergillosis involve specific immunopathology without any fungal invasion.

Allergic form of aspergillosis occurs in some atopic patients due to inhalation of antigens of *Aspergillus* species. The individual suffers from an immediate asthmatic reaction that is mediated by reaginic antibody or specific IgE. A positive skin test and history confirm the diagnosis. Bronhoconstriction or consolidation of the lung can occur even without the growth of the fungus in the lung tissue.

Allergic bronchopulmonary aspergillosis is a well-known clinical entity and it is the major allergic form of aspergillosis. The major diagnostic criteria are enlisted at the end of this chapter. Sputum may be positive for culture of *Aspergillus* species. Serum anti-aspergillus precipitins, elevated serum IgE immunoglobulin, and history of recurrent pneumonia are the known symptoms that confirm diagnosis. The soluble *Aspergillus* species antigens react with serum IgG to form immune complexes which can activate complement pathway. This in turn results in induction of neutrophilic infiltrates and a general inflammatory response. The disease is more protracted and may induce chronic changes in the lung tissue.

Non-atopic individuals, when exposed to *Aspergillus* species, develop extrinsic allergic alveolitis which is another form of hypersensitivity reaction to *Aspergillus* antigens. The patients show an Arthus reaction (Type III hypersensitivity) on skin testing and this may precede an immediate type of reaction in some individuals. Inhalation of *Aspergillus* antigens may cause fever, leukocytosis, dyspnea, dry cough, myalgia and rales in the lungs after several hours.

Aspergilloma or fungus ball is a large mass of intertwined and conglomerated hyphae seen in cases of chronic bronchiectasis or tuberculous cavities in lungs. Radiologically one can see a globular shadow in a radiolucent cavity. Aspergilloma is considered as colonization and it may cause very little local reaction and may persist over years without causing much inconvenience to the patient. Repeated sputum cultures may yield same type of fungal species and it can be correlated with radiological findings.

Oculocerebral aspergillosis occurs due to the entry of the fungus through conjunctival mucosa or from paranasal sinuses through lacrimal duct. Contiguous spread to the orbit is also possible. The infection is slowly progressive and may take months or years with formation of granulation tissue in the surrounding tissue and fatty tissue. As a result there may be protrusion of the eye, swelling of the soft tissue, abscess formation; haziness of the paranasal sinuses and the orbit. The lesion may become complicated due to osteomyelitis with necrosis, sequestration, thromboangitis and penetration leading to fatal end. Many cases are not recognized in the early stage due to slow progress of the disease and therefore the appropriate treatment is delayed for long-time until it is too late. Infection of the central nervous system if occurs due to hematogeneous spread the course is more rapid and ocular lesions may be secondary.

Gastrointestinal type of aspergillosis is rare. Apart from the metastatic lesions due to dissemination there may be primary localized necrotizing, purulent and ulcerated lesions in the intestinal mucosa. Peptic ulcer or other forms of ulcers of digestive tract as well as diarrhea are the predisposing factors for intestinal aspergillosis.

The course of invasive aspergillosis, whether localized in the lungs or disseminated depends largely upon the underlying diseases like acute leukemia, granulocytopenia, lymphoma rarely other malignancies or immunosuppression associated with organ or bone marrow transplantation. Patients with long-standing HIV infection may develop invasive pulmonary aspergillosis or obstructing bronchial aspergillosis. The hyphae have special propensity to invade the lumen and the walls of the blood vessels causing hemorrhage, thrombosis and infarction. Disseminated type of aspergillosis may affect the vital organs like kidney, brain, liver, heart and eye.

Primary cutaneous aspergillosis can occur due to *A. flavus, A. fumigatus* or *A. niger.* Secondary cutaneous aspergillosis as a part of dissemination is mainly due to *A. fumigatus.* Primary cutaneous infection is more frequently seen in immunocompromised individuals. Clinically primary cutaneous aspergillosis presents as papules or plaques leading to necrotic ulcers. Primary cutaneous aspergillosis due to *A. fumigatus* rarely occurs in an apparently healthy individual without any systemic involvement. Very little inflammatory reaction is seen in some individuals. The number of hyphae present in the lesion is usually less and there may be well-developed granulomatous lesions.

Another well known and common clinical manifestation of aspergillosis is otomycosis. It is also known as Hong Kong ear or Singapore ear or Panama ear. It is a superficial sub-acute or chronic infection of external auditory meatus and is worldwide in distribution. It is more prevalent in tropics and subtropics. The clinical entity was first described by Andral and Gavarret in 1843. Presently it is one of the commonest diseases seen among the patients attending the ENT outpatient department. In India the clinical entity is all the more important because the patients put oil in the affected ear to relieve the pain and this further creates a favourable condition for the growth of the fungal spores. Depending on the geographical area the incidence of otomycosis varies from 5 to 25 percent of all cases of ottitis externa. Several factors like indiscriminate use of antibiotics or steroids, exposure to warm, humid climate, poor personal hygiene, poor health conditions, chronic infections of the ear, pouring oil or water into the ear predispose the individual to the disease. Natural defenses like fungistatic effect of cerumen, acidic pH of the external auditory canal are if intact, can prevent the infection. Though many fungal species including yeasts and dermatophytes have been reported in the literature, by and large the infection is generally limited to saprophytic molds like *Aspergillus* species, *Penicillium* species and *Pseudo allescheria boydii.* The fungus grows and affixes to the topmost layer of the skin of the external ear. During the course of infection the superficial epithelial cells are cast off and fill the auditory canal with a mass of epithelial debris and fungus. The infection may be either primary or secondary. The exact role played by these fungi in otomycosis is not very clear. The fungus itself may act as a primary pathogen or the fungus simply multiplies under favorable conditions without causing any symptoms or the fungus may be a secondary invader following acute or chronic viral or bacterial infections. The commonest symptoms are itching, obstruction to the external auditory canal leading to partial deafness, tinnitus, dull pain, moderate seropurulent discharge and rarely vertigo.

Allergic form of aspergillosis can be treated with corticosteroids along with antifungal drugs. Disodium cromoglycate is also useful in treating the allergic forms of aspergillosis and it reduces the intensity of the symptoms but it may not prevent the recurrences. Patients with asymptomatic aspergilloma need not be treated. Others may require surgery. Both amphotericin B and flucytosine can be used to treat symptomatic aspergilloma. These drugs can be given as pulmonary lavage to improve the penetration of the drug into the cavity. Local and superficial aspergillosis can be treated with nystatin.

Invasive aspergillosis requires aggressive treatment with amphotericin B as early as possible. However, the overall response is not more than 50%. Aspergillosis of central nervous system has a mortality of more than 90% and so is the case with infected bone marrow transplants. Combination of amphotericin B and flucytosine is effective in some patients with pulmonary aspergillosis. Itraconazole may be specifically effective against aspergillosis as per some of the recent studies and clinical trials.

Prophylactic treatment with low doses of amphotericin B and itraconazole may be useful for patients under high risk of developing aspergillus infection. Itraconazole may be given to prevent relapse in those who are previously treated with amphotericin B.

ZYGOMYCOSIS

Zygomycosis is an umbrella term for a wide range of diseases caused by fungi that belong to the class Zygimycetes. Earlier this entity was named as phycomycosis which is now obsolete. Human pathogens in this class are further subgrouped into two orders; Mucorales and Entomophthorales. Zygomycetes species are the etiological agents of a broad range of mycoses in both normal and immunocompromised individuals, although the infection most common in immunocompromised individuals, especially among the patients with diabetes mellitus.

Zygomacetous infections have been reported from virtually all anatomical sites but Lanodauer and Newcomer in 1962 described four distinct categories; rhino-cerebral, pulmonary, gastrointestinal and cutaneous. Other miscellaneous forms are rarely reported.

The rhino-cerebral type of Zygomycosis is the most common forms seen in clinical settings. This type of zygomycosis occurs after inhalation and deposition of spores on the nasal turbinates. The infection extends to the adjacent paranasal sinuses. It may extend to the ethmoids and retro-orbital tissues and eventually reach the brain through orbital apex. The patient may complain of pain in the face out of proportion to the physical signs in the initial stages. Within a short period, classical black turbinates and palatal ulcers are seen due to infarction of the affected tissues. Black necrotic septum of the nose, blood tinged nasal discharge, fever, facial swelling are the other signs that are frequently observed. These may be rapidly followed by restriction of ocular movements, proptosis, and ptosis and periorbital cellulitis. The third, fourth and sixth cranial nerves may be affected along with papillary dilatation and loss of vision due to central retinal artery occlusion. This is not usually seen in cavernous sinus thrombosis due to bacterial infection. Later on as the disease rapidly progresses, the fifth and seventh cranial nerves may be involved. The infection may rapidly spread to brain resulting in infarction due to direct vascular invasion by the fungus. The infecting agent reaches the brain either by ophthalmic vein or superior orbital fissure and cribriform plate of ethmoid bone. Death occurs in 70% of cases. Patients may have hemiplegia, stupor and coma.

The clinical presentation of respiratory zygomycosis is highly variable. The sporangiospores of the Zygomycetes fungi enter the respiratory tract through the inhalation of aerosols. The acute form of respiratory zygomycosis is severe and characterized by fever, pleuritic chest pain, and leukocytosis. Radiological findings comprise of extensive infiltrates, consolidation or miliary pattern of infiltrates or granulomas, ill-defined infiltrates and wedge-shaped peripheral lesions. Cavitations may occur in some cases and fungus ball has been reported. Subacute pulmonary zygomycosis which is increasingly frequent finding is largely limited to the airways with no or minimal parenchymal involvement. Radiologically one can see ill-defined infiltrates, bronchial pluggings or small peripheral densities. The fungus invades adjacent tissue through blood vessels producing thrombosis, infarction and necrosis. Because of rapid invasion and extensive destruction of the tissue, acute form of pulmonary zygomycosis is associated with high mortality rate.

Gastrointestinal zygomycosis can occur due to species of Mucorales or Entomophthorales. *Absidia corymbifera* is the most frequently isolated species from gastrointestinal zygomycosis followed by *Basidiobolus* and *Conidiobolus* species. Intestinal zygomycosis is a rare infection in humans and usually acquired by the ingestion of fungus or spread from the abdomen or contamination of the ileostomy site. In children intestinal zygomycosis may occur due to mal-nutrition, amoebic colitis, typhoid fever, pellagra and kwashiorkor. The clinical presentation varies with the extent and site of involvement. The clinical presentation may be nonspecific with symptoms of abdominal pain, melena, hematemesis and bloody diarrhea. The fungus as usual invades the blood vessels and produces thrombosis, infarction and necrosis in the gastrointestinal tract and the adjacent tissue.

Cutaneous zygomycosis may present in various forms and it is quite variable in signs and symptoms. Primary zygomycosis can occur due to inoculation of the fungus into the cutaneous or subcutaneous tissue. This can occur in road traffic accidents or by machinery or by using elastoplastic bandages. It can also occur as a result of hematogeneous spread or by direct invasion of the fungus from the organs to cutaneous and subcutaneous tissues. Cutaneous zygomycosis appears initially as an erythematous nodule or plaque which rapidly progresses resulting in an indurated cellulitis often with central black eschar or a central necrotic ulcer. Gangrenous changes may occur along with hemorrhagic bullae. Vascular invasion occurs during the spread of infection to the adjacent tissue. Histological findings include hyperkeratosis, neutrophilic infiltration, and accumulation of proteinaceous fluid and cellular debris. The lesions show a mixture of suppurative and necrotizing inflammatory reaction. Broad non-septate hyphae are seen in the newly invaded blood vessels and tissues. Several species have been isolated from cutaneous zygomycosis and their number is increasing because increasing number of immunocompromised individuals due to severe underlying dieases like advanced HIV infection burns and anticancer therapy.

The mortality of invasive zygomycosis has decreased considerably in recent years but it still remains approximately at 50%. The infection can be treated with amphotericin B and surgical debridement. Recently treatment with hyperbaric oxygen as an adjunct is promising since it inhibits the growth of the fungus. Prognosis depends upon the control of underlying disease and it is best in diabetic patients. Survivors usually have permanent morbidity in the form of facial paralysis, loss of vision, disfigurement and other associated problems.

Chapter 25

Identification of Infectious Agents

LIGHT MICROSCOPY

Most of the laboratory investigations pertaining to pathology and microbiology depend upon microscopic examination of the cells, smears and histological sections that are appropriately stained with dyes of different types or treated with conjugated antibodies to localize the antigens or microorganisms within the cell or tissues. Because most of the cells are too small to be seen by naked eye, the study of cells has depended heavily on the use of microscope. Robert Hook in 1665 first coined the word 'cell' following his observations of a piece of a cork using a microscope that was able to magnify the object by 300 times their actual size. Antoni van Leeuwenhoek in 1670s was able to observe a variety of cells including sperms, red cells, and bacteria which he named them as 'animalcules'. The studies of Matthias Schleiden and Theodor Schwann established the cell theory by 1838. By then it was established that all organisms are composed of cells and they are not formed *de novo* but arise from division of pre-exisisting cells and cells are the fundamental units of all living organisms based on the observations made with the light microscope.

The light microscope is the basic tool for microbiologists, pathologists and cell biologists with ever changing technical improvements allowing the visualization of ever increasing details of cell structure. Contemporary light microscopes are able to magnify the objects to about 1000 times. Most cells are between 1 and 100 μm in diameter, they can be observed by light microscopy, as can some of the subcellular organelles such as nuclei, chloroplasts and mitochondria. However, light microscope has limited power to reveal the finer details of the cell structure, for which the **'resolution'**, the ability to distinguish objects separated by small distance is even more important than magnification. Images can be magnified to the desired extent but such magnification does not increase the level of details that can be observed. The limit of resolution of a light microscope is about 0.2 μm; two objects separated by less than this distance appear as single image and cannot be distinguished from one another. The theoretical limitation of light microscope is determined by (a) wavelength of light (λ) and (b) numerical aperture (*NA*) of the lens (the light gathering power of the microscope lens). According to the following equation:

$$\textbf{Resolution} = 0.61\lambda / NA$$

The wavelength of visible light is between 0.4–0.7 μm, so the value of l is fixed at approximately 0.5 μm for light microscope. The numerical aperture can be envisioned as the size of the cone of light that enters the microscope lens after passing through the specimen and it is expressed as:

NA = η sin α, where η is the refractive index of the medium through which the light travels between the objective and the lens. The value of η for air is 1.0 but objects are not visible because the refractive index of the objectives is also the same. The refractive index can be increased to a maximum of 1.4 by using substances like liquid paraffin or cedar wood oil which have the same refractive index as that of the objective lens. The angle α corresponds to half of the width of the cone of light collected by the lens. The maximum value of l is 90°, at which sin α = 1, so the highest possible value for numerical aperture is 1.4. With these values the theoretical limit of resolution of the light microscope is:

Resolution = 0.61 × 0.5/1.4 = 0.22 μm

Several different types of light microscopy are routinely used in clinical and research laboratories to study the various aspects of the cell structure as well as the tissue organization pattern, the local inflammatory responses and neoplasia in the cells. The simplest and most commonly used one is bright-field microscopy, in which the light passes through the cell and the ability to distinguish different parts of the cell depends upon the contrast resulting from the absorption of light by cell components. In many cases the cells are stained with dyes that interact with proteins or nucleic acids in order to enhance the contrast between the different parts of the cell. Prior to staining the specimens are treated with fixatives or gently heated to fix the cells to the glass slide to preserve their structures. Such staining procedures which are generally used kill the cells and therefore are not suitable for examination of living cells. Without staining the bright-field microscopy cannot distinguish many parts of the cell, which is a major limitation of the bright-field microscopy.

To overcome the disadvantage of light microscopy, optical variations of light microscope can be used to enhance the contrast between the light waves passing through the regions of the cell with different densities. The two most common methods for visualizing the living cells are **phase-contrast microscopy** and **differential interference-contrast microscopy.** Both kinds of microscopy use optical systems that convert variations in the density or thickness between different parts of cell to differences in contrast that can be seen in the final image. The transparent structures like nucleus absorb the light poorly and hence show little contrast. However, the light is slowed down as it passes through these transparent but dense structures and the phase of the light is altered compared to light that has passed through the surrounding structures like cytoplasm. These differences in phase are converted into differences in contrast in phase-contrast microscopy or in differential interference -contrast microscopy which in turn produces improved images of live, unstained cells. The performance of light microscope can be further increased by using video cameras and computers for image analysis and processing. Such systems can substantially increase the contrast of the images of light microscope, allowing the visualization of subcellular organelles like microtubules which are cytoskeletal protein filaments of 0.025 μm in diameter. But this enhancement does not exceed the theoretical resolution of the light microscope. As a result though the tubules can be seen they appear blurred and they cannot be differentiated from adjacent structures. Light microscopy is useful in molecular analysis and by labeling specific molecules they can be seen within the cells. Specific genes or RNA transcripts can be detected by hybridization with nucleic acid probes of complementary sequence and proteins can be detected by appropriate labeled antibodies.

FLUORESCENCE MICROSCOPY

Fluorescence microscopy is widely used in clinical as well as research laboratories. It is very sensitive method for studying the intracellular distribution of molecules. Fluorescence is the emission of light by a substance that has absorbed light or other electromagnetic radiation of a different wavelength. It is a form of luminescence. In most cases emitted light has a longer wavelength and therefore lower energy than the absorbed radiation. Fluorescent dyes are used to label molecules of interest within either fixed or living cells. The fluorescent dye molecule absorbs light usually from ultraviolet region which is invisible and emits the light in the visible spectrum. This fluorescence is detected by illuminating the specimen with a wavelength of light that excites the fluorescent dye and then by using appropriate filters the wavelength of light emitted by the dye is detected. Fluorescence microscopy is used to study a variety of molecules within the cells. One frequent application is to label antibodies directed against a specific protein with fluorescent dye to locate the intracellular distribution of the protein can be determined. Semiconducting nanocrystals known as quantum dots are increasingly being used in place of fluorescent dyes for many applications in fluorescence microscopy because quantum dots fluoresce brighter and are more stable than traditional fluorescent dyes.

In recent years a major advance in fluorescence microscopy has been the use of green fluorescent protein (GFP) derived from pacific jelly fish *Aequorea victoria* to visualize the proteins in the living cells. GFP can be fused to any protein of interest using the standard methods of recombinant DNA, and the GFP tagged protein can then be expressed in cells and detected by fluorescence microscopy. This technique does not require any fixation or staining of the cells. Because of its versatility GFP is widely used in cell biology to localize the different proteins within living cells. Several related fluorescent proteins with different colors derived from marine organisms are now available, further expanding the utility of this technique.

A number of methods such as fluorescence recovery after photo bleaching have been developed to study the movement and interactions of GFP-labeled proteins within the cells. In this method a region of interest in a cell expressing a GFP-labeled protein is bleached by exposing to high intensity of light such as laser and the recovery of fluorescence from the bleached portion over time due to the movement of unbleached GFP-labeled molecules into the bleached region, allowing the rate at which the protein moves within the cell to be determined.

Fluorescence resonance energy transfer (FRET) is useful in analysis of the interactions of two proteins with one another within the cell. The two proteins of interest are coupled to different fluorescent dyes such as variants of GFP that are selected to absorb and emitted distinct wavelengths of light, so that the light emitted by one GFP variant excites the second. The interactions between the two proteins can then be detected by illuminating the cell with a wavelength of light that excites the first GFP variant and then analyzing the wavelength of the emitted light. If the proteins coupled to these GFP variants interact within the cell then the two fluorescent molecules are brought close together and the light emitted by first GFP-variant will excite the second, resulting in emission of light at the wavelength that is characteristic of the second variant GFP.

The images obtained by conventional fluorescent microscopy are blurred due to out-of-focus fluorescence. This can be corrected by computational approach where in the computer analyzes the images and generates sharp images or alternatively use of confocal microscopy allows images of increased contrast. A small point of light, usually supplied from a laser is focused on to the specimen at a particular depth. The emitted fluorescence is then allowed to pass through an aperture so that only light emitted from the plane of focus is able to reach the detector. By obtaining a series of images at different depths, it is possible to reconstruct a three-dimensional image of the sample.

Multi-photon excitation microscopy is an alternative to confocal microscopy that can be applied to living cells and this allows construction of three-dimensional images of the living cells. In principle the specimen is illuminated with a wavelength of light so that the fluorescent dye needs simultaneous absorption of two or more photons which is possible only when the input laser beam is focused at one point. This highly localized excitation automatically provides three-dimensional resolution without any need of passing through an aperture. This technique also minimizes the damage to the specimen and allows three-dimensional images of living cells.

ELECTRON MICROSCOPY

In principle both bright-field and electron microscopes are similar. The illumination source in the electron microscope is a tungsten filament that is heated in vacuum to generate electrons. Rather than having glass lenses to focus light, the electron microscope has set of magnetic coils near the tungsten filament to capture and focus the electron beam onto the specimen. The beam passes through the specimen and the dense areas of the specimen absorb and retard the electron beam whereas the less dense material allows the beam to pass unmodified. After passing through the specimen the electron beam is refocused through a second series of magnetic coils similar to the function of objective lenses in bright-field microscope. The refocused beam is magnified by a third series of magnetic coils and directed to a screen where image can be viewed and transferred to film. The screen is coated with a phosphorus compound that fluoresces upon the contact with the electron beam. There are two types of electron microscopes: transmission type and scanning type. Only transmission electron microscopy is currently used in clinical virology and in cell biology.

Negative Contrast Electron Microscopy

Electron microscope is the only instrument with which one can see the ultrastructure of the cells directly. The electron microscope was developed in 1930s and it was used in biology by Albert Claude and George Palade in 1940s and 1950s. The typical morphology is easy to recognize under electron microscope because it can achieve greater resolution due to short wavelengths of the electrons and theoretically it is possible to get a resolution of 0.002 nm. However, in electron microscope the numerical aperture is a limiting factor and one can achieve a numerical aperture of 0.01 and as a result under optimal conditions the resolving power of electron microscope is 0.2 nm and this is further reduced with biological specimens due to lack of inherent contrast. Nevertheless, the resolution is 100 times more than that of the light microscope. One of the major limitations of electron microscopy is the cost, requirement of trained staff and its apparent insensitivity. Electrons pass through the biological material without much deviation, and the contrast is necessary to make the structures visible. Such contrast is provided by soluble salts of electron-dense heavy metals like uranium, tungsten and molybdenum. Because of their smaller structure, uranium salts are devoid of visible structure and they can easily enter the interstices of the cell and provide high resolution. However, their pH is in very narrow range and hence acts as poor contrast substances compared to tungsten salts. The potassium or sodium phosphotungstate with a pH range of 5.0 to 8.0 is very commonly used in clinical virology as a negative stain, although the chemical has some detrimental effect on the living cells.

The preparation of specimens for negative contrast electron microscopy is relatively simple. Suitably processed virus containing specimen or virus suspension is mixed with the contrast and the mixture is placed on a microscopic grid. All but a small amount is then drawn off with filter paper and the residual virus-stain mixture is allowed to dry. The dried grid is then inserted in the microscope and virus particles are examined at a high magnification of 50,000 X. Several modifications of electron microscopy such as negative staining, thin section electron microscopy, metal shadowing, and immune electron microscopy are being used as research tools for studying the ultra structure of the viruses and bacterial cells.

The clinical presentation of many infectious diseases are alike and it is always not possible to establish the identity of the infectious agent to be it a bacteria, virus, fungus or parasite based on the clinical features. It is therefore necessary to identify the infectious agent to establish the etiology, for prompt treatment and to implement immediate preventive measures to prevent the outbreaks. For example, if the diarrhea is due to cholera, immediately the health authorities should be alerted so that necessary measures will be taken to see the quality of the drinking water, leakages in the sewage system, etc. This will enable us to prevent the spread of the disease.

There are many techniques for diagnosis and identification of the infectious agents ranging from simple examination of the specimen under microscope to more sophisticated techniques like identification of the genes. However, all the available techniques are not feasible to carry out and require the help of reference laboratories.

WET FILM EXAMINATIONS

Aspirated fluids such as pus, peritoneal fluid, pericardial fluid as well as blood, urine, sputum, etc. can be examined directly under the microscope. Similarly, a small portion of feces can be emulsified in a drop of saline placed with a glass slide and covered with a cover slip. This preparation can be examined under the microscope. The technique is simple and enable us to identify various infectious agents such as *E. histolytica, Giardia lamblia, Trichomonas, vaginalis, cysts* of various parasites, larvae of parasites, microfilarias, fungal elements, pus cells with bacteria. Simple examination of wet film gives us a lot of useful information and many diseases can be diagnosed easily and rapidly. Various types of microscopes such as light microscope, darkground microscope, phase contrast microscope can be used for this purpose. Using electron microscope which can magnify the images of the infecting agent upto 1 lakh times even viruses can be seen directly in the specimens, and based on their morphology; diagnosis can be arrived at by using special microscope like fluorescent microscope. Many infectious diseases can be diagnosed rapidly.

STAINING OF THE INFECTIOUS AGENTS

Infectious agents such as fungi, bacteria, viruses, and cysts of the parasites cannot be seen even under microscope (except that when they are suspended in liquid medium) because their refractive index is same as that of air. Hence, to observe them with the help of the microscope, it is necessary to stain them with some coloring agents known as dyes. Robert Koch introduced the technique of staining the bacteria with special dyes belonging to the group—pararosaniline dyes. By staining the infectious agents, we can easily identify them under the microscope. There are many techniques of staining among which the following are used commonly.

Gram Stain

Sir Christian Gram noticed that when bacteria are stained with one of the para rosaniline dyes like crystal violet, gentian violet, certain bacteria retain the color of these dyes even after decolorization with absolute alcohol or acetone whereas others lose the color and become colorless. When a counter stain like safranin or dilute carbol fuschin is used these decolorized bacteria take up the counter stain and appear as pink in color. Those bacteria which retain the primary dye even after decolorization are called gram-positive and those which are decolorized and take up the counter stain are known as gram-negative (Figs 25.1 and 25.2). This classification is very useful in bacteriology.

Procedure

Take a clean, scratch free glass slide and pass it over a Bunsen flame 4 or 5 times with the help of forceps and allow it to cool.

Take the specimen such as pus, sputum or any aspirated fluid with the help of a bacteriological loop (made of nichrome wire) and spread it on the glass slide in a circular or oval shape so as to form a thin smear of 2 × 2 cm size.

Allow the smear to dry by airing gently. The smear should not be too thick or too thin. A properly made smear will enable us to read the printed matter through it.

After air drying pass the smear over the Bunsen flame quickly 3 or 4 times so that the smear gets fixed to the slide. The smear should not be overheated otherwise it gets charred.

Now mark the slide on the opposite side for identification purpose.

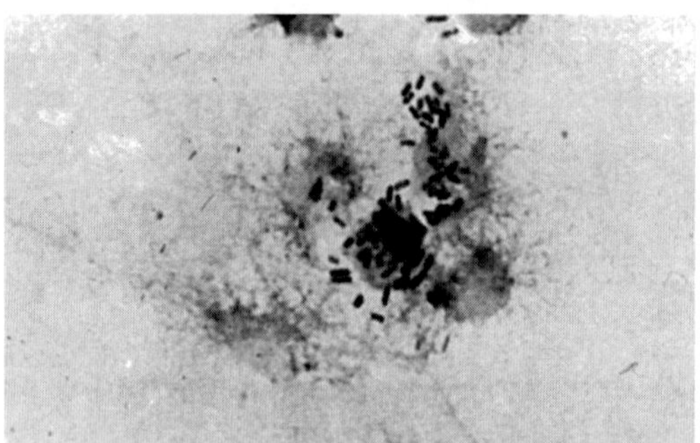

Fig. 25.1: Pus cells with gram-negative bacilli. Gram stain of urine smear (×100) (*For color version, see Plate 12*)

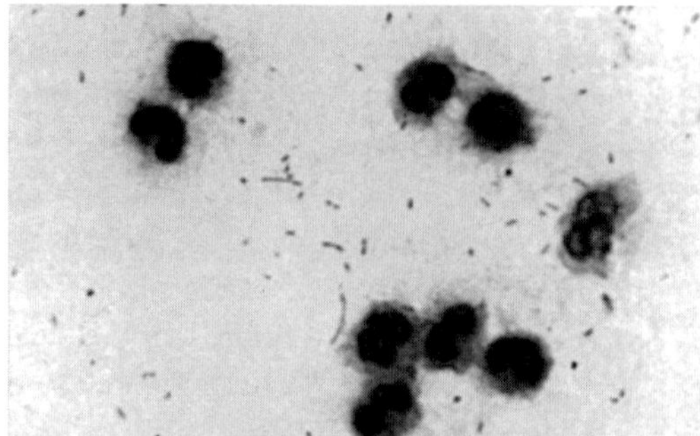

Fig. 25.2: Pus cells with gram-negative bacilli (×100) (*For color version, see Plate 12*)

Place the slide on the staining rack and cover the smear with crystal violet solution (1%) for 1 minute.

Wash the slide with running water and cover the smear with Grams iodine solution which helps in fixing up the dye to the cell wall of the bacteria and allow it to act for 1 minute.

Again wash the slide with running water. Handle the slide in a slant position and pour absolute alcohol drop by drop. The smear gets decolorized and one can see purple color coming out of the smear; continue pouring the absolute alcohol till a faint color of the stain is seen.

Immediately wash the slide with running water and cover the smear with one percent safranin or dilute carbol fuchsin for 30 seconds.

Wash the slide with running water. Dry the slide by blotting and observe under the light microscope by measuring the slide with liquid paraffin or cedar wood oil. Use oil immersion lens (100x) for observing bacteria.

- Gram-positive bacteria appear as purple colored
- Gram-negative bacteria appear as pink colored
- *Examples*:
  - Gram-positive cocci: Staphylococci, streptococci, pneumococci
  - Gram-positive bacilli: *Corynebacterium diphtheriae, Clostridium tetani, Clostridium perfringens, Bacillus anthrax*
  - Gram-negative cocci: *Neisseria gonorrhoeae, Neisseria meningitides*
  - Gram-negative bacilli: *Escherichia coli, Vibriocholerae, Pseudomonas aeruginosa, Klebsiella pneumoniae, Salmonella typhi, and Shiegelle* species.

Ziehl–Neelsen Stain

Some of the infectious agents like tubercle bacilli resist decolorization with acid. Such bacteria retain the dye even after decolorization with acid whereas others are decolorized with acid and take up the counter stain. Those bacteria which are resistant to acid decolorization are known as acid–fast bacilli (AFB) and they appear pink (the color of the dye used) (Fig. 25.3) and the rest take up the counter stain and appear blue in color (Figs 25.4 and 25.5).

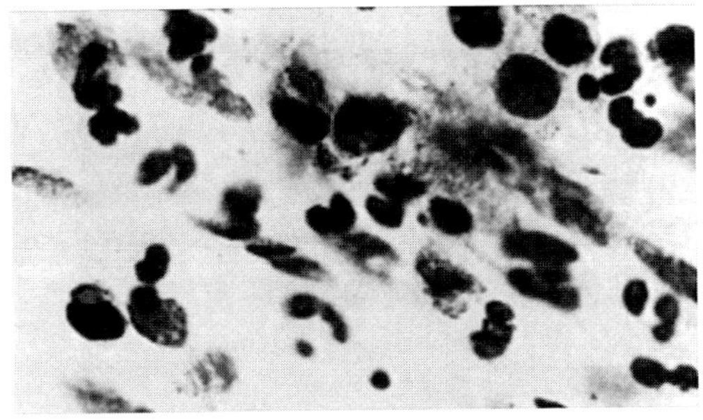

Fig. 25.3: Intracellular acid–fast bacilli. Note bundle of pink-colored slender rods. Z–N stain (×100) (*For color version, see Plate 13*)

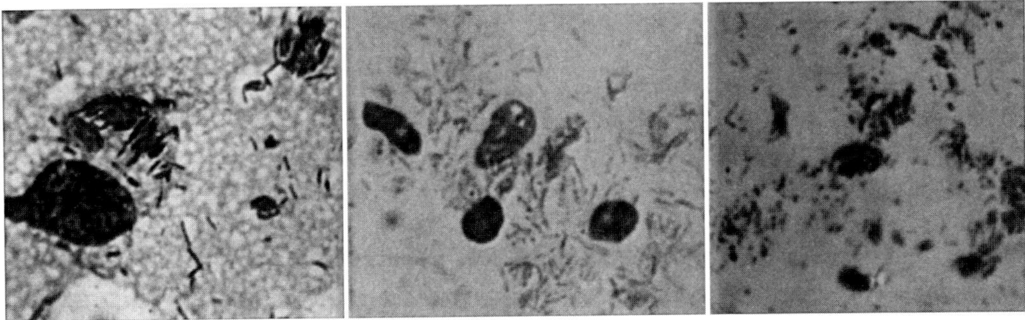

Fig. 25.4: Pink-stained acid-fast bacilli (Z–N stain). Note the different morphological forms (*For color version, see Plate 13*)

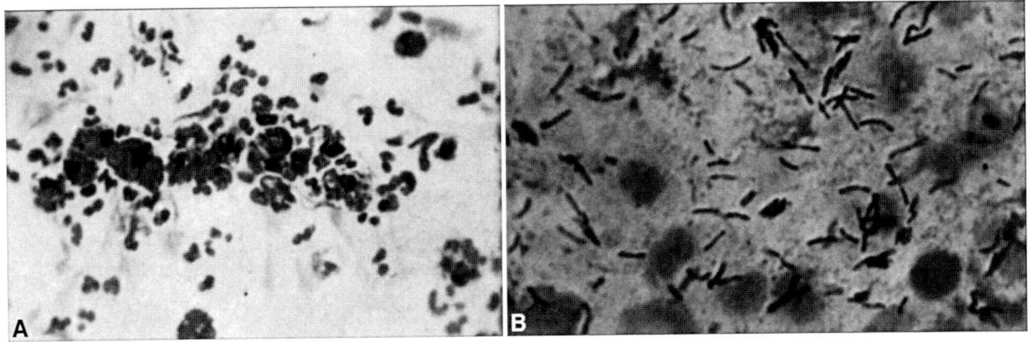

Fig. 25.5: (A) Ziehl–Neelsen stained smear of a nasal scraping from a patient with lepromatous leprosy showing red staining AAFB—*Mycobacterium leprae*—in globi. **(B)** Sputum from a patient with tuberculosis stained by the Ziehl–Neelsen method to show red acid and AAFB—*Mycobacterium tuberculosis* (*For color version, see Plate 13*)

Procedure

Prepare the smear from the specimen as described for Gram's stain. Cover the smear with strong carlol fuchsin solution (1 g of basiofuchsin dissolved in 100 mL of 5% phenol) and gently heat the slide from below using a spirit lamp. Heating should be done intermittently without charring the slide. Only fumes should come from the slide and the solution on the slide should not be boiled. Staining with intermittent heat is continued for 5 minutes.

Pour out the stain and wash with running tap water gently.

Hold the slide in slanting position and pour 25% sulfuric acid drop by drop till a faint pink color comes out of the slide (alternatively slide can be decolorized with a mixture of 97 mL absolute alcohol + 3 mL hydrochloric acid).

Wash the slide with water and counter stain the slide with one percent Löeffler's methylene blue for 1 minute.

Wash the slide and dry with blotting or on a hot plate. Put a drop of liquid paraffin on the smear and observe under the oil immersion lens.

At least 100 fields must be searched before the slide is reported as negative for acid-fast bacilli.

Acid–fast bacilli appear as bright pink slender rods.

The others take up blue stain. Leprabacilli are less acid-fast and hence only 5% sulfuric acid should be used for decolorizing the smears taken for the demonstration of leprabacilli.

Nocardia bacilli resist one percent acid decolorization. Hence, smears suspected of this infectious agent should be decolorized with one percent sulfuric acid (Modified Ziehl-Neelsen stain of Kinyoun).

Albert's Stain

Albert's stain is useful for the demonstration of characteristic diphtheria bacilli from the swabs taken from the tonsillar area or posterior pharyngeal wall or larynx of suspected cases of diphtheria (Table 25.1).

The smear is prepared and fixed by heat as per the description mentioned earlier.

Cover the smear with solution A for 3 to 5 minutes and wash with water. Cover the slide with solution B for 1 minute, wash with water. Blot and dry.

Put a drop of liquid paraffin over the smear and observe under oil immersion microscope.

The diphtheria bacilli are seen as thin rods arranged in L, V or cuneiform shape or pallisade arrangement with bluish purple granules and greenish cytoplasm.

Blood smears can be obtained by Leishman or Giemsa stain for the demonstration of malarial parasite, *Leishmania denovani*, *Microfilariae*, etc. (Fig. 25.6).

Special staining techniques are available for the staining of spirochetes, trophozoites of *E. histolytica* or *G. lamblia*, cell wall of the bacteria, capsule, and flagella of the microorganisms.

Table 25.1: Procedure for Albert's stain

	Solution A	*Solution B*
• Toluidine blue	1.5 g	Iodine 2 g
• Malachite green	2 g	Potassium iodide 3 g
• Glacial acetic acid	10 mL	Distilled water 300 mL
• 95% alcohol	20 mL	Dissolve the ingredients in water and store in an amber colored bottle
• Distilled water	1000 mL Dissolve the ingredients in water and allow to mature for one day. Then filter before use	

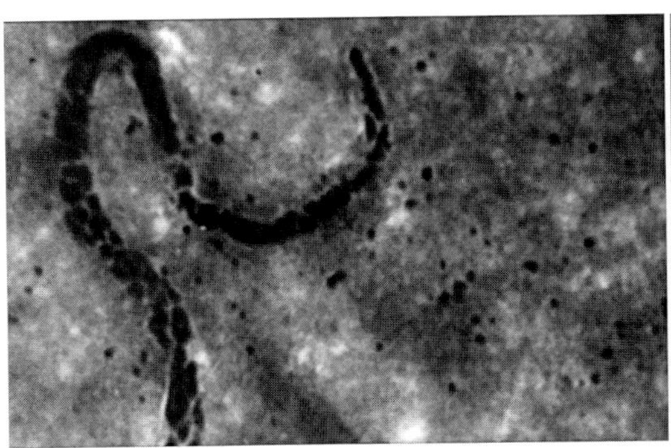

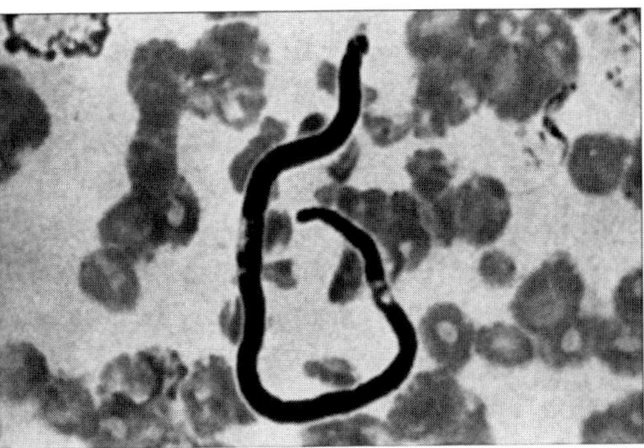

Fig. 25.6: Microfilaria in blood smear (*For color version, see Plate 14*)

Fungi can be stained by lactophenol cotton blue stain. For details of staining of different infectious agents reference books should be consulted.

CULTIVATION OF INFECTIOUS AGENTS

In order to identify the correct infectious agent, it is necessary to culture these organisms in the laboratory under appropriate conditions. Growing the organisms from the specimens obtained from the infected patients is known as culturing the microorganisms. Just like human beings, microorganisms also require carbohydrates, proteins, fats, vitamins, minerals and water for their growth and multiplication. By combining these essential nutrients, a number of recipes have been designed known as culture media. (Fig. 25.7) These can be in liquid form or semisolid or solid form. To liquid culture media agar agar, which is a polysaccharide obtained from seaweeds, is added in a concentration of 1.5 to 2.0 percent to get solid media. Agar agar has got unique properties that it melts at 100°C and solidifies at 45°C. It is not utilized by microorganism and hence it is nutritionally inert.

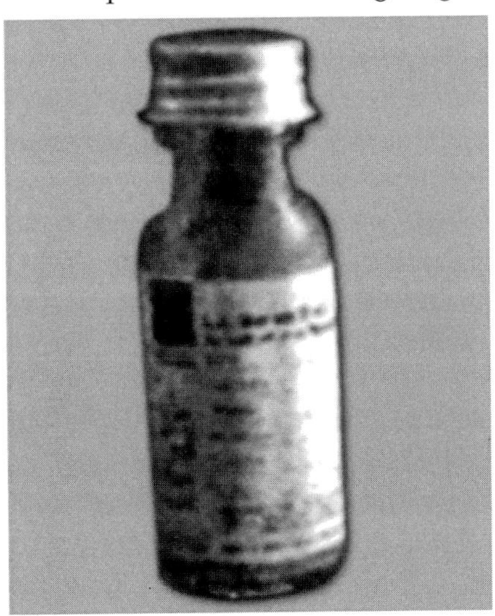

Fig. 25.7: LJ medium bottle used for the cultivation of *M. tuberculosis* (*For color version, see Plate 14*)

Culture media used in the laboratory are usually prepared from meat infusion (by boiling meat and obtaining the extract) or peptone (golden yellow powder obtained from the meat by acid hydrolysis), milk protein, yeast extract, extracts from brain, liver, and heart, or synthetic media which is made by combining all essential amino acids, vitamins, minerals and water in the required proportions. The media thus prepared for cultivating the microorganisms are classified as:

1. Simple media: e.g. nutrient broth, peptone water, and nutrient agar.

2. Enriched media: To the simple media animal protein in the form of human or sheep blood, serum or acitic fluid or egg yolk are added.
3. Differential media: These are usually employed in the identification of enteric bacilli such as *Escherichia coli, Klebsiella pneumoniae, Salmonella* and *Shiegella*. These media contain peptone sodium chloride and sugars like lactose and an indicator such as neutral red.

   The organism which ferment lactose produces acid and in the acid medium the indicator changes its color and as a result the colonies of bacteria appear colored and those bacteria which do not produce acid from the sugars appear colorless, e.g. MaConkey medium: *Escherichia coli* produces pink colonies on this medium, *Salmonella* produces colorless colonies on this medium.
4. Selective media: Special chemical substances are added to the simple or enriched media so that the chemical suppresses or inhibits the growth of other bacteria that is required. For example,
   - Potassium tellurite blood sugar—It promotes the growth of diphetheria bacilli
   - Crystal violet blood agar—It promotes the growth of streptococci.
5. Enrichment media: Liquid selective media are called enrichment media. They help in increasing the isolation of bacteria causing disease and inhibit the normal harmless bacteria known as commensals. For example,
   - Selinite-F broth—It increases the yield of *Salmonella* and *Shigella*
   - Alkaline peptane water—It improves the yield of vibrios.
6. Transport media: Many microorganisms are very sensitive to heat, sunlight and they die when the specimens are sent to laboratory without taking proper precautions to protect them till they are inoculated onto the nutrient media.

For example, buffered glycerol saline in which stool specimen is mixed and sent to the laboratory.

Venkatraman and Ramakrishnan medium in which stool sample is mixed and sent to the laboratory for the isolation of cholera bacilli, Stuarts transport medium and Amies transport medium are used to transport specimens to the laboratory; minimal essential medium, Hank's balanced salt solution or Dulbecco's medium for the transportation of specimens for the isolation of virus.

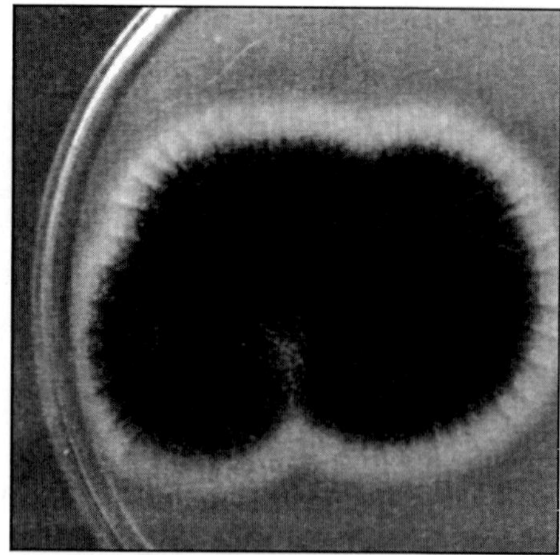

Fig. 25.8: *Aspergillus niger* growth on Sabouraud's agar medium

For the isolation of fungi special media like Sabouraud's dextrose agar (Fig. 25.8) thioglycolate broth, and chlamydospore agar are used for better yield. Many fungi can grow on blood agar and nutrient agar. All fungal cultures should be cultured in duplicate. One culture should be incubated at 37°C and the other one at room temperature between 24 to 28°C.

Since viruses grow within the living cells for the isolation of viruses, fertilized eggs of hen or infant mice or suckling guinea pigs are used. Because large number of animals are required for the isolation of viruses, the animals are replaced by tissue culture. Organs like kidney, lung or placenta are taken aseptically and they are cut into small pieces. These pieces are treated with trypsin which separates the tissue into individual cells. These cells are placed in sterile test tubes containing nutrients which support the growth of the living cells. The living cells take up the nutrients and divide and get attached to the glass surface to form a sheet of living cells.

These sheets of living cells are known as 'cell lines' which can be easily maintained in the laboratory by supplying required nutrients. These cell lines when inoculated with specimen like blood, wine, fluids obtained from the patients suspected of having viral infection, the viruses get attached to the living cells in the test tube and multiply. By studying the morphological changes in the infected cells one can diagnose viral infections and by disrupting the cells from the virus particles by special techniques. Examples for cell lines are monkey kidney cells, human embryonic lung tissue, HELA cells (cells derived from cancerous tissue), etc.

Parasites like *Entamoeba histolytica, Giardia, Trichomonas,* malaria and the larvae of several worms can also be cultured on specially designed nutrient media (e.g. Diamond's medium). Bacteria, viruses, fungi can be identified by their macroscopic appearance on the nutrient media or cell lines, by their physical and chemical properties, their ability to produce disease in laboratory animals, clumping of or agglutination of human or animal red blood cells or their lysis.

Apart from nutritional requirement microorganisms require optimum temperature (37°C), oxygen, carbon dioxide, hydrogen ion concentration (pH) for their growth.

DETECTION OF ANTIBODIES IN THE BLOOD

Sometimes it is not possible to culture the infectious agent in the laboratory. Under such conditions, the presence of infectious agent can be identified by detecting specific substance known as antibodies in the blood of the patient. Whenever a person gets infected due to bacteria or virus or fungi or parasite, the immune system of the body promptly reacts and produces these specific antibodies against the individual infectious agent which help the body in clearing the infection. These antibodies combine with infectious agent or its cell component neutralizes the effect of the infectious agent and helps the body to recover from the effect of the infection. These antibodies can be detected in the blood of the patient by various laboratory techniques like precipitation, agglutination, complement-fixation, neutralization and immobilization. These antibodies can also be detected by the most sensitive and specific methods like radioimmunoassay (RIA) or enzyme-linked immunosorbant assay (ELISA). For all these tests one should send 5 mL of clotted blood in a plain sterile vial or test tube.

ANIMAL CELL CULTURES

Since viruses replicate only in living cells, it is necessary to provide cells in one or the other form if the viruses are to be cultured or isolated from specimens received in the laboratory.

Earlier, for propagation of viruses, tissue or organ culture and animal inoculations were practiced, but currently most widely used method is cultivation of viruses in cell cultures. Cultured cells are categorized on the basis of source, karyotype and multiplication potential. More than 3000 cell lines are now available which are maintained by European collection of animal cell cultures, the American type culture collection (ATCC), Statens Seruminstitut, Copenhagen, Institut Pasteur, Paris and WHO.

Types of Cell Cultures

Cell cultures may be primary or continuous. **Primary cell cultures** are started from tissues taken from laboratory animals or from human material obtained during the surgery. Some tissues like foreskin are not pathological. Tissues taken from young or embryonic animals give better results. The tissue obtained under sterile conditions is minced and the cells are liberated using agents like trypsin or versene and after filtration they are finally suspended in growth medium. Once the primary cells have been subcultured sufficiently, they are seeded into glass or plastic tubes or flasks to get a sheet of cells called cell line. Cell lines can be classified as diploid (having the same chromosome number as the somatic cells of the species from which they are derived) or heteroploid (with an altered chromosome number). Primary cell lines cannot be propagated indefinitely because they tend to suffer a reduction in growth rate and a loss of ability to propagate the viral infection after 20 to 50 passages. On the other hand, the **continuous or aneuploid cell lines** derived from cancer cells or transformed cells can be maintained indefinitely by periodical subculturing. The most commonly used cell cultures are monolayer cultures, with a single layer of cells attached to the surface of the culture vessel. Some cell types are anchorage independent and they can be grown with agitation, in suspension in a liquid medium. To grow cells in suspension the levels of calcium and magnesium in the medium are reduced to inhibit attachment, and higher levels of nutrients and buffers are required to support the high cell densities that are attained in the suspensions unlike that of monolayer cells. Most established cell lines can be grown in suspension form with some exceptions that are encountered occasionally. Embryos and tumors are commonly used as starting material because they contain rapidly growing cells. Embryo fibroblasts are one of the most widely studied types of animal cells. Embryonic stem cells are established in culture from early embryos and they maintain their ability to differentiate into the entire cell types present in adult organisms.

Shell vial cultures contain a cell monolayer grown on one side of the coverslip in a Leighton tube type. The inoculated tube is centrifuged at a low speed, which apparently distorts the cell surface and renders more susceptible to virus attachment. After 48 to 72 hours irrespective of any visible cytopathic effect (CPE) the coverslip is washed gently and can be subjected to immunofluorescence assay or nucleic acid hybridization. This technique is very suitable for rapid identification of adenoviruses, cytomegaloviruses and respiratory syncitial viruses.

Insect cell lines are continuous cell lines derived from SF9 ovary (fall army worm, *Spodoptera frugipedra*) and from mosquitoes. These cell lines are cultured in special media and are very susceptible to infection with baculoviruses. The mosquito cell lines are used to culture many mosquito-borne viruses.

Microcultures are now very popular that are grown in a 96-well microculture plates with flat bottoms. They are ideal for neutralization tests, ELISA, monoclonal antibody testing and many other screening assays. Macrocultures in standard tubes are still preferred for primary virus isolation because of the convenience in setting up stationary or roller cultures in ordinary incubators, reading the monolayers for CPE and for obtaining sufficient volume of virus culture for sub passagings as well as for genetic analyzes and storage.

Specialized culture systems have been devised to meet special needs such as co-cultivation. Immortalized microvascular endothelial cell cultures derived from foreskin are sensitive to a number of viruses under special conditions. Extra cellular matrix systems are being used to support the three-dimensional growth of cells. Finally large volume culture systems such as culture vats, cells on the surface of the Sephadex beads or other microcarriers and cells on spirals of sterilin or plastic film are extensively used in the industry to prepare vaccines, interferons and monoclonal antibodies.

Several cell culture systems are useful in propagation of the viruses, detection of bacterial exotoxins and in studying the adhesion assays. Once a cell culture has been inoculated with patient specimen, viruses can be detected by the development of visible CPE in cells infected with viruses. The appearance of the CPE and its timing will often give a clue to the identity of the infecting virus. The other methods for detecting and characterizing viruses in cell culture include:

Hemadsorption

Because of incorporation of viral hemagglutinins into the cell membrane, infected cells may be detected by adsorption of the erythrocytes from various animal species.

Immunofluorescence

Viral antigens may be detected in infected cells by using specific antibodies conjugated with a fluorescent dye. Viral antigens may be detected well before the appearance of CPE.

Nucleic Acid Probes

Viral nucleic acids may be detected by specific probes that are labeled with either enzyme or an isotope.

Reverse Transcriptase Assay

Retroviruses growing in lymphocyte cultures may be detected by means of their unique RNA dependent DNA polymerase activity.

ENZYME-LINKED IMMUNOSORBENT ASSAY (ELISA)

One major advance in biotechnology and biomedical sciences is in the field of immunology. This has made possible the development of a wide variety of methods that can be applied for diagnosis of diseases like tuberculosis, leprosy, filariasis, malaria and amoebiasis, etc. and for early diagnosis of pregnancy. One such technique is enzyme-linked immunosorbant assay (ELISA) or enzyme immunoassay (EIA), was introduced almost 4 decades ago has pervaded almost every branch of biology and medicine. Its simplicity, speed, specificity and sensitivity as well as practicality have led to its use in developed and developing countries alike. The impact of the technique is so great that it has created multibillion dollar industry.

Realizing the importance of this powerful yet cost-effective technique for epidemiological studies involving mass screening, Voller et al. explored the use of disposable polystyrene plates with 96 wells as a carrying surface for the antigen. Advantages of using such plates were obvious. They were easy to handle, inexpensive and small quantities of reagents and samples were enough to carry out the assays. The results could be glanced with naked eye within minutes. The micro plate technology led to parallel development of accessories such as fixed and variable multi-channel micropipettes capable of dispensing required volume within minutes to the entire plate, the micro plate washers both semi-automatic and automatic, vertical beam photoelectric colorie meters (ELISA readers) for end point as well as kinetic analysis. Soon several publications devoted to the trouble shooting in ELISA and a variety of solutions were offered to these problems. The problems of variable binding from plate to plate and batch to batch, polystyrene beads were proposed as an alternative mode for presenting the immunosorbent. The bead technology particularly became popular in Japan and with a major producer of diagnostics, viz. Abbott. Over the years the improvements in the binding characteristics of the ELISA plates and availability of small strips of 8, 12 and 16 and even single well rather than an entire plate of 96 wells making small sample runs more practical, has put the micro plate ELISA on a firm footing.

However, some of the deficiencies of these new modifications also became evident. Sandwich techniques for estimation of serum components used polyclonal antibodies that required long incubation periods and tedious washing steps. Two site sandwich assay techniques using different antibodies for coating and labeling which would be directed toward two different sites on antigen simplified the assay system and reduced the incubation time from 16 to 2 hours without compromising with specificity. The introduction of monoclonal antibodies further changed the scenario completely by increasing the sensitivity and specificity.

In 1982, a new immunosorbent was introduced to the field of ELISA in the form of nitrocellulose membrane which showed a very good binding capacity to soluble antigens, antibodies and bacterial cells. A suitable enzyme and a substrate which would form colored insoluble product ensured a marked contrast between the white background and dark color at the site of reaction. The reagent to be adsorbed onto the nitrocellulose was applied as dot and the visibility of the dot depended on density of concentration of the reagent and not the amount. This assay came to be known as Dot-ELISA. In 1985, a new format of Dot-ELISA was introduced in to the market ushering the era of STAT ELISA tests—rapid yet retaining the sensitivity and specificity. The application of multilayer film technology so far applied in clinical chemistry was extended to ELISA in 1980s and it was mostly designed for the drug assays. A major advance in the field of ELISA technology was seen in enzyme amplification technique which resulted in the development of assays with unsurpassable sensitivity. The enzyme amplification technique used reagents like avidin-biotin, enzyme cycling and enhanced chemiluminescence. The avidin-biotin system originally described from immunohistochemical staining for tissue by Bayer and Wilcheck was extended to ELISA because of very high affinity of avidin to biotin that resulted in avidin-biotin ELISA with several times more sensitive than conventional ELISA and RIA. Using enzyme cycling as proposed by Stanley et al. an alkaline phosphatase based ELISA was developed for estimation of TSH to detect very low levels of TSH with high accuracy. In this procedure NADP was used as the substrate and the NAD generated was cycled through alcohol dehydrogenase and diaphorase and the end product was measured photometrically.

A number of modifications of ELISA are available and they are used as per the requirement.

Indirect ELISA is useful in detecting the antibody against a specific antigen. The micro plates are coated with antigen and the test sample (e.g. serum, CSF or other body fluids) is added to the micro well of the plate. Any antibody specific to the antigen will be bound to the available sites. After incubation and washing the bound antibody is detected by incubation with enzyme-labeled specific anti-immunoglobulin followed by the addition of enzyme substrate. The enzyme acts as an amplifier, even if only few enzyme-linked antibodies remain bound, the enzyme molecules will provide many signal molecules. The enzyme can go on producing color indefinitely but if more primary antibody is present in the test sample, more enzyme-conjugated antibody will bind and the color develops faster.

Double antibody sandwich ELISA is useful for antigen detection in the test sample. In the assay system the antigen to be detected is sandwiched between two similar or different antibodies of which one is labeled with the enzyme. The use of secondary antibody conjugate avoids the expensive process of creating enzyme-linked antibodies for every antigen one might want to detect. By using enzyme-linked antibody that binds the Fc region of other antibody a variety of antigens or antibodies can be detected.

Competitive ELISA is useful for identification and quantitation of either antigen or antibody. In antigen determination by this method, antigen present in the test sample competes for sites on the antibody with labeled antigen added to the medium. The color change is inversely proportional to the amount of antigen present in the sample.

Inhibition ELISA works on the same principle as that of competitive ELISA but in this system the two antigens (antigen in the test sample and enzyme-labeled antigen) are added one after the other. This method is useful especially when test serum contains both antigen and antibody of interest in the immune reaction. Inhibition ELISA is also useful in determining the identity of the specific antigen or antibody.

Anti-C3 ELISA is used to detect disease specific circulating immune complexes or specific antigen present in the circulating immune complexes. Test specimens are incubated in micro titer plate wells that are previously coated with rabbit or goat anti-human-C3 antibody. The antigen in question in bound immune complexes is detected by further incubating the wells with enzyme-labeled specific antibody.

In designing the micro-plate ELISA procedures the following parameters must be considered for obtaining specificity and sensitivity of the assay.

The choice of the micro-plate is important. Micro plates suitable for ELISA are available from several manufacturers. Rigid polystyrene plates are most commonly used and are available in untreated, irradiated and tissue culture-treated forms. Each form has different surface characteristics that may be more appropriate for binding an individual antigen (protein). Polyvinyl chloride plates are also used for ELISA. Before designing an ELISA, several different types of plates should be evaluated to determine which is most suitable for a given assay.

DOT AND SLOT BLOT ASSAYS

Dot blot and slot blot techniques are modifications of standard ELISA. Both are rapid techniques to screen a single serum specimen against a number of ligands or a number of sera against one or more ligands. The whole ligand or a fraction of it is directly applied to or filtered through nitrocellulose or a comparable membrane. The ligand upto 2 µg in a 2 µl test dose is pipetted carefully onto nitrocellulose or other suitable membrane sheet for a dot or applied with a pen for a slot blot. Alternatively, the ligand in the 200 µl sample is filtered in to selected membrane sheet. The geometric configuration is the major difference between the assays. The slot blot configuration is preferred for quantitation by densitometry.

After the application of the ligand the membrane is allowed to dry and blocked with a skimmed milk solution and an immunoassay similar to that of ELISA is carried out.

CASSETTE ELISA

Cassette ELISAs are also known as lateral flow through tests or flow through tests or lateral flow through immunochromatographic assays. These are simple devices intended to detect the presence or absence of a target analyte in the sample. Most often these tests are used for medical diagnostics, either for home tests, point of care testing or laboratory use. These are attractive alternatives for micro plate procedure when small numbers of specimens are tested. These assays can be performed more quickly than micro plate assay and typically the entire procedure can be carried out in less than 10 minutes. Cassette EIAs or lateral flow immunochromatography assays use elevated concentrations of reactants to drive the assay to completion. The results in these devices can be read visually.

In principle the antigen or antibody is immobilized at a specific location on the selected membrane such as nitrocellulose and fixed in a disposable cassette. Serum sample to be tested is allowed to flow along the solid substrate through capillary action or allowed to filter in to absorbent material below the membrane in the cassette base. The unbound antibody or antigen is washed or the sample applied to the test it encounters a colored reagent which mixes with the sample and transits the substrate encountering the lines or zones which have been pre-treated with an antibody or an antigen. Alternatively after an additional washing a substrate mixture that will generate insoluble enzyme product is added. Positive result is indicated by a colored product at the spot where the antigen or antibody was immobilized. An attractive feature of these assays is that internal positive and negative controls can be incorporated at additional sites on the membrane. Simple visual interpretation of the device yields test result and validation procedure.

ELECTROBLOTTING

Electroblotting is a technique widely used in biotechnology to transfer proteins or nucleic acids onto membrane made of polyvinylidene fluoride (PVDF) or nitrocellulose after gel electrophoresis and this technique is widely used in molecular biology, biochemistry and immunogenetics. The proteins or nucleic acids thus separated are further analyzed using specific antibodies, ligands, lectins or stains as probes. The technique was patented by William J Littlehales in 1989. This technique relies on current and transfer buffer solution to drive the proteins or nucleic acids onto a membrane on which they are immobilized. Following electrophoresis a standard tank or semi-dry blotting transfer system is used. A stack is prepared in the following order from cathode to anode: sponge, three sheets of filter paper soaked in transfer buffer, gel containing separated proteins or nucleic acids, PVDF or nitrocellulose membrane and three sheets of filter paper soaked in the transfer buffer. The membrane on to which the proteins or nucleic acids are to be transferred must be located between the gel and the cathode as the sample and the current will be moving in that direction. The prepared stack is placed in the transfer system and current of suitable magnitude is applied for a suitable period of time depending upon the material used. Proteins may react with antibodies giving rise to the term immunoblotting or they may react with ligands or lectins which are known as affinity blotting. Several modifications of electro blotting such as Southern blotting, Western blotting, Northern blotting, Eastern blotting and Southwestern blotting and all of them apply same principles.

IMMUNOELECTROPHORESIS

A number of biochemical methods used for separation and characterization of proteins based on electrophoresis and reactions with antibodies are grouped under a general name immunoelectrophoresis. All variants of immunoelectrophoresis utilize immunoglobulins or antibodies that react with proteins to be separated and characterized. Several variants of immunoelectrophoresis were introduced during the second half of the 20th century and they were extensively applied in biochemistry and protein chemistry.

Immunoelectrophoresis is performed in one percent agarose gel slabs of about 1 mm thickness buffered at high pH (about 8.6). The electrophoresis in agarose under native conditions preserves the native structure and activities of the proteins under investigation. Immunoelectrophoresis can also be used for characterization of enzyme activities and ligand binding in addition to their separation by electrophoresis. The introduction of immunoelectrophoretic analysis boosted the protein chemistry and allowed separation of a number of serum proteins and also revealed the existence of several immunoglobulin classes with electrophoretic heterogeneity.

The principle of electrophoresis is the formation of precipitate lines at the equivalence point of the antigen and its corresponding antibody. In this technique it is important that the ratio between the quantities of antigen and antibody is in correct proportion. When the antibody is in excess, statistically at most one antigen binds to each antibody and when the antigen is in excess at most one antibody binds to each antigen. Yet at a specific antigen and antibody ratio (equivalence point) huge macromolecules are formed. They consist of antigen-antibody-antigen-antibody sequence and are immobilized in the gel matrix as immunoprecipitate. The white precipitate lines are visible and they can even be stained with any of the protein stains. Immunoelectrophoresis is specific and highly sensitive because distinct zones are formed. Immunoelectrophoresis is generally performed under three principles.

Counterimmunoelectrophoresis

This principle was first described by Bussard in 1959. In an agarose gel exhibiting high endosmosis, the pH of the buffer is set at 8.6 because at this pH the immunoglobulins or the antibodies are practically immobile since they do not carry any charge. The sample and the antibody are placed in the respective wells and allowed to move toward each other. The charged antigen migrates electrophoretically and the antibodies are carried by electro-osmotic flow. When both react at the zone of equivalence white precipitin lines are formed which can be viewed directly or stained by any protein stain. Counter immunoelectrophoresis can be either discontinuous or continuous type. In discontinuous type a gradient of ionic strength is produced as the agarose gel is made in 0.015 M buffer and the electrophoretic tank contains 0.75 M buffer. Since the gel has a low ionic strength the speed of the charged particles is increased. Thus discontinuous counter immunoelectrophoresis (DCIE) differs from continuous immunoelectrophoresis (CIE) only in the speed of movement of the reactants. But the sensitivity and specificity are the same. In continuous electrophoresis, buffer can be stored and re-used for at least 20 times whereas in discontinuous electrophoresis it should not be re-used for more than three times. The advantage of DCIE is rapidity and that of CIE is economy of the buffer.

Zone Electrophoresis

According to Graber and Williams, first a zone electrophoresis is performed in the agarose gel followed by a diffusion of an antigen fraction toward the antibody which is pipetted out into the trough cut in the side parallel to the electrophoretic run.

Rocket Electrophoresis

Rocket electrophoresis as described by Laurell in 1966 and the related methods analyze and quantify the antigens. The antibody in definite concentration is incorporated in the agarose gel matrix and the antigen in question is allowed to migrate toward the antibody. Because of the high pH of the buffer selected the antibody is immobilized because it does not possess any charge. As the antigen migrates one antibody will bind to one antigen until the ratio of concentrations corresponds to the equivalence point of the immune complex. As a result rocket-shaped precipitin lines are formed, the enclosed area is proportional to the concentration of the antigen ion in the sample. A series of modifications have been developed including two-dimensional ones. Presently immunoelectrophoretic techniques are not widely used for two reasons. First, the procedures are rather work intensive and need some manual expertise and secondly these techniques need large quantities of polyclonal antibodies. Presently gel electrophoresis followed by electro blotting is most preferred choice for protein characterization because of its high sensitivity and ease of operation as well as low requirement for specific antibodies. Further proteins are separated on the basis of their molecular weight which is not possible with immunoelectrophoresis. However, immunoelectrophoresis is still useful when non-reducing conditions are needed.

POLYMERASE CHAIN REACTION (PCR)

Polymerase chain reaction (PCR) technology hailed as one of the most important scientific developments of our generation. During its 20 year history, this Nobel Prize winning technology has become essential research and diagnostic tool for improving human health and quality of life. The use of PCR technology has greatly increased scientists' ability to study the genetic material. By imitating nature's ability to replicate DNA, PCR can amplify minute quantities of genetic material from millions to over billions of times within a few hours, allowing for the rapid, reliable detection of genetic markers for infectious diseases, especially diseases caused by viruses and other fastidious organisms which are difficult to culture routinely or takes long-time for the culture, cancer and genetic diseases. Using PCR based tests; physicians now have the greater insight into progression and management of life-threatening infections such as HIV and hepatitis viruses (HBV and HCV, etc.) as well as to identify genetic variations that may predispose people to diseases like cardiovascular disorders or cancer.

Birth of PCR

While driving along Highway 128 north of San Francisco on one Friday night of April 1983, Kary B Mullis, a DNA chemist of Cetus Corporation conceived the idea of PCR. Struggling to formulate a simple method for determining the identity of a specific nucleotide along the stretch of DNA, he suddenly envisioned being able to isolate and amplify a specific nucleotide by starting and stopping polymerase action. This flash of inspiration marked the birth of the polymerase chain reaction concept–a simple, yet elegant process that enables the production of virtually unlimited copies of a specific DNA sequence in a test tube. Kary B Mullis received Nobel Prize in 1993 for this breakthrough discovery.

With coordinate efforts of a team of scientists from Cetus Corporation, Mullis' idea of PCR was developed into an experimental system. In 1985, Cetus filed for first PCR patent application and published first article on PCR in *Science*. In 1986, PCR technology was successfully used in forensic testing for DNA typing of the HLA-DQA genetic sequence variant locus. Enthusiastically embracing this promising technology, scientists were on the verge of realizing the diagnostic potential of PCR.

Basic Principle of the PCR

Polymerase chain reaction is used to amplify specific fragment of DNA strand known as DNA target. Most PCR methods typically amplify DNA fragments upto 10 kb although some techniques allow the amplification of the fragment upto 40 kb.

A basic PCR set up requires several components and reagents which include:

DNA template that contains DNA region to be amplified.

Two primers that are complementary to the 3′ends of each of the sense or anti-sense strands of DNA target.

Taq polymerase or another DNA polymerase with a temperature optimum at 70°C at which it is stable.

Deoxyribonucleic acid phosphates (dNTPs) required as the building blocks from which the DNA polymerase synthesizes a new DNA strand.

Buffer solution that produces a suitable chemical environment for optimum stability and activity of DNA polymerase.

Divalent cations like Mg^{2+} or Mn^{2+}.

Monovalent cations like potassium ions.

The reaction volume of PCR is generally varies from 10 to 200 µl in a small reaction tubes in a thermal cycler. The thermal cycler heats and cools the reaction tube to achieve temperatures required for each step of reaction. Many models of thermal cyclers are available and they use Peltier effect which permits both heating and cooling of the block holding the PCR tubes simply by reversing the electric current. The thin-walled reaction tubes permit the thermal conductivity and allow rapid thermal equilibrium. Most thermal cyclers have heating lids to prevent condensation at the top of the reaction tubes.

Real Time PCR

During the biological processes, the changes induced in the cell by various artificial or natural agents can be studied by many ways such as examining the changes in the transcripts that may indicate changes in the corresponding protein synthesized or presence or abscence of a bacterial or viral or other pathogens, increase in the levels of transportation of a transgene or inhibition of expression of an endogenous gene. In all these cases, quantitative real-time PCR technology is of great value in getting the required information.

Earlier nucleic acid quantification was carried out by the addition of radiolabeled UTP or deoxythymidine triphosphate (dTTP) to cell cultures or to one of the many *in vitro* experimental preparations and measuring their incorporation by trichloroacetic acid precipitation. However, such radiolabeled quantification was not satisfactory for identifying or quantifying specific gene transcripts. Southern or Northern blotting techniques allowed the identification of a particular gene specifically but these methods were not useful for quantification. Subsequently improvements in RNA transcript quantification came with the RNAse protection experiments. The protected products were separated by using denatured PAGE and expose to film. The phosphoimager greatly improved the quantification of separated nucleic acids due to expanded dynamic range and improved software analysis. The introduction of polymerase chain (PCR) reaction in biotechnology by Kary B Mullis in 1983, resulted in quantification of transcripts from a given sample became possible with the advent of competitive RT-PCR. Utilizing the RNA promoter, truncated *in vitro* transcribed RNA could be made and quantified. Known amounts of the RNA product were spiked in to the RT reaction and converted into cDNA along with the target sequence in the unknown sample. Subsequently, both the truncated standard and the unknown target sequences were amplified using PCR. The amplified DNA was separated using denatured PAGE. In some cases radioactive deoxynucleotide base was added for labeling the amplified DNA and quantified using a film or phosphoimager. In other methods, the gels were stained with ethidium bromide or SYBR Green. Quantification of unknown band was carried out by comparing the signal from the spiked and quantified DNA standard. This method was most accurate, although it still had detection problem. In 1996, Applied Biosystems Inc (ABI) made real-time PCR commercially available with the introduction of the 7700 instrument. Since then real-time PCR became the most sensitive method for detection and quantification of nucleic acids. The technique put an end to all major problems encountered in earlier techniques. However, there are two problems for real-time PCR that still remain unaddressed. They are a) method of quantification, i.e. kind of standard, assay quality and calculation methods, b) how to properly normalize different samples to correct for differences in the nucleic acid input from sample to sample.

The common question that may bother a beginner in molecular biology is 'What exactly is the meaning of real-time quantitation PCR'? In order to be truly real-time one should be able to watch the growth of amplification curves during PCR on a computer monitor. But in real practice this is not the case. The original real-time software program does not allow the visualization of amplification curves as they progress throughout the run. Some systems use software that perform the data analysis using final data sets from whole plate and some systems use the software that allows the follow-up of the progress of amplification curve in each well in real-time. Even then the instruments are not exclusively real-time type. The real-time PCR is a continuous collection of fluorescent signals from one or more polymerase chain reactions over arrange of cycles which are converted into numerical values for each sample.

FLOW CYTOMETRY

Flow cytometry is a technique of quantitation of single cell analysis. The flow cytometry uses the principle of light scattering, light excitation and emission of fluorochrome molecules to generate multi-parameter data from particles and cells in the size ranging from 0.2 to 150 μm. The cells are suspended in a stream of fluid and passed through electronic system which allows the simultaneous analysis of physical, chemical or both characteristics of upto thousand of cells per second. Flow cytometry is routinely used in the diagnosis of health disorders particularly blood cancers. Nevertheless, it has several other applications in both research and clinical practice. A variation of this technique enables physical sorting of cells or particles based on their properties so as to purify the population of interest.

Wallace H Coulter in 1953 patented the first impedance–based flow cytometry device developed using coulter principle. Mack Fulwyler invented the forerunner of today's flow cytometers particularly the cell sorter in 1965. Wolfgang Göhde from the University of Műnster developed the fluorescence-based flow cytometers in 1968 and obtained patent for the same. Subsequent developments in the fields of computer sciences, laser technology, monoclonal antibody production, cytochemistry, fluorochrome chemistry led to the development of flow cytometers that can be commercialized. The first commercial flow cytometers was large, complex and difficult to operate and maintain. They were primarily used in research laboratories. However, the enormous value of flow cytometry in medical and biological sciences was quickly appreciated and the cost and complexity gradually decreased as its analytical capabilities increased. The present state-of-art flow cytometers are capable of analyzing upto 13 parameters (forward scatter, side scatter and 11 colors of immunofluorescence) per cell at the rate upto 100,000 cells per second. Automation and robotics are increasingly being applied to flow cytometry to reduce the cost of analysis and improve the efficiency. During early stage of development absorption method was preferred by the researchers to fluorescence method. By the middle of 1970s several manufacturers started producing flow cytometers commercially and the first FACS (Fluorescence activated cell sorting) instrument was introduced by Becton and Dickinson in 1974. The original name for flow cytometry technology was 'Pulse cytophotometry' (German: *impulszytophotometrie*) based on first patented application of fluorescence-based flow cytometry. Eight years after the introduction of the first fluorescence-based flow cytometry, the name flow cytometry became popular and the name was decided at the 5th American Engineering Foundation Conference on Automated Cytology in Pensacola (Florida) in 1976.

Flow cytometers use the principle of hydrodynamic focusing for presenting the cells to the laser or any other exciting light source. The sample is injected into the center of the sheath flow. The flow chamber is conical in shape, and the reduced diameter of the chamber forces the cells into the center of the stream. In this process, the cells pass through the laser or source of light one cell at a time. As the cells or the micro particles of interest intercept the light source, they scatter the light and the tagged fluorochrome is excited to a higher energy state. As the molecule relaxes to a lower state, the energy is released as a photon of light with specific spectral properties unique to the fluorochrome used. One unique feature of flow cytometry is that it measures the fluorescence per cell or particle which is in contrast to spectrometry wherein the percent of absorption and transmission of specific wavelength of light is measured for a bulk volume of the sample.

Scattered or emitted light from the cells or particles are converted to electrical pulses by optical detectors. Collimated (parallel light wave forms) light quanta is picked up by confocal lenses focused at the intersection point of the cell and the light source. The light is sent to different detectors by using optical filters. Photomultiplier tube is commonly used in flow cytometers as the detector and this photomultiplier tube converts light into electrical pulses. The electrical pulses originating from light detected by photomultiplier tube are then processed by a series of linear and log amplifiers. Logarithmic amplification is most often used to measure the fluorescence in the cells. This type of amplification expands the scale for weaker signals and compresses the scale for strong or specific fluorescent signals. The different signals or pulses thus amplified are further processed by an analog to digital converter which then allow for the events to be plotted on graphical scale.

Chapter 26

Prevention of Communicable Diseases (Infectious Diseases)

INTRODUCTION

"Prevention is better than cure" is a well-known proverb. Many infectious diseases can be controlled and even they can be eradicated if we follow the principles of prevention. These principles are very simple but need dedication and awareness in implementing them in the routine practice. In this chapter, the principles of prevention of communicable diseases (infectious diseases) are discussed.

IMMUNIZATION

Immunization is possible to prevent many infectious diseases by artificially exposing the person to the killed or live attenuated bacteria or viruses, who is not exposed to these infectious agents before. When the person is given either whole bacteria or viruses or its components, the individual resistance power gets boosted up and subsequently he/she will be prevented from developing the diseases even if he/she comes in contact with the infectious agent. The immunizations was first introduced by Edward Jenner to prevent the smallpox. This was soon widely practiced and to prevent the smallpox and it was eradicated from the world. Similarly, immunizations were carried out for other diseases. Today we have wide range of microbial products which are used for the prevention of a number of diseases. The immunization programs are mainly targeted to prevent the diseases in children. The schedule of immunization is discussed in Table 26.1.

Apart from the above immunizing agents which are given routinely under the extended program of immunization (EPI) (except hepatitis B which is not covered but parents are advised to vaccinate their children at their own expense). Nursing staff should get immunized against hepatitis B and other contagious diseases, there are other immunizing agents for prevention of disease like rabies, Japanese encephalitis (brain fever). Influenza, typhoid fever, cholera, anthrax, etc. These are selectively given to those who have the risk developing these diseases.

Table 26.1: Schedule of immunization

• Birth	• BCG to prevent childhood tuberculosis • Oral polio vaccine Ist dose • Hepatitis B vaccine Ist dose
• 6 weeks	• Diphtheria-polio-tetanus (DPT or triple antigen) Ist dose • Oral polio vaccine 2nd dose • Hepatitis B vaccine 2nd dose
• 10 weeks	• DPT 2nd dose • Oral polio vaccine 3rd dose
• 14 weeks	• DPT 3rd dose • Oral polio vaccine 4th dose
• 6–9 months	• Oral polio vaccine 5th dose • Hepatitis B vaccine 3rd dose
• 9 months	• Measles vaccine
• 15–18 months	• Measles-mumps-rubella vaccine (MMR) • DPT first booster dose • Oral polio vaccine 6th dose
• 5 years	• DPT-second booster dose • Oral polio vaccine 7th dose
• 10 years	• Tetanus toxoid (for tetanus) 3rd booster dose • Hepatitis B vaccine booster dose
• 15–16 years	• Tetanus toxoid 4th booster dose

NUTRITION

A well-balanced nutritious diet helps in preventing many infectious diseases. Malnutrition is one of the important factors that decides the outcome of many diseases like diarrheas, tuberculosis, etc. Balanced diet should consist of (a) daily requirement of protein (1 g/kg body weight). This amounts to 15 to 20 percent of the energy intake. Next comes the fat requirement, which should be limited to 20 to 30 percent of the daily intake. Along with this main nutritional requirements, the diet should also contain required amounts of micronutrients such as vitamins, trace elements like zinc, manganese, phosphorus, calcium-selenium, etc. The energy derived from various foods is measured in terms of kilocalories/gram or kilojoules/gram. The daily requirement of calories for an individual varies with age, sex and the type of work. The dietary pattern differs widely in different parts of the world and it is largely influenced by climatic conditions of the region, socio-economic status, religion, customs, taboos, tastes and habits of the people. Children and pregnant women should take more calories than the recommended daily intake (Table 26.2).

The daily diet should consist of carbohydrates (rice, wheat, ragi, etc.) protein (dhals, meat, fish, eggs), fats (oils, ghee, butter), vitamins, minerals, which are present abundantly in milk, green leafy vegetables, fruits. Persons who recently recovered from an acute

Table 26.2: Recommended daily intake of energy

Groups	Body weight in kilogram	Energy allowance per day kilocalories
1. Infants		
• 0–6 months	118/kcal/kg/day	
• 7–12 months	108/kcal/kg/day	
2. Children		
• 1–3 years	12.03	1220
• 4–6 years	18.87	1720
• 7–9 years	26.37	2050
3. Adolescents		
• 10–12 years	34.30	2420 (males) 2260 (females)
• 13–15 years	47.03	2660 (males) 2300 (females)
• 16–18 years	56.50	2820 (males) 2200 (females)
4. Adults		
• Males	55.00	2400 light work 2800 moderate work
• Females	45.00	1900 light work 2200 moderate work 3000 heavy work
• Pregnancy lactation	+285 throughout pregnancy +500 first 6 months +400 for 6–12 months	

disease should take more proteins, fresh fruits, vegetable and milk. A well-balanced diet offers good protection from many diseases.

SAFE DRINKING WATER

Water is essential for life, 80 to 90 percent of the body weight is due to water content. Normally persons should take 1 to 1.5 liters/day to replace the loss through perspiration, urine and stools. Water not only required for digestion of food but also is essential to maintain body complexion and skin elasticity. The water we drink everyday should be free from infectious agents, and it should be tasty and refreshing. Water also contains many minerals, which are essential for life. Many of the ill-healths in the developing and underdeveloped countries are due to lack of safe drinking water (Fig. 26.1).

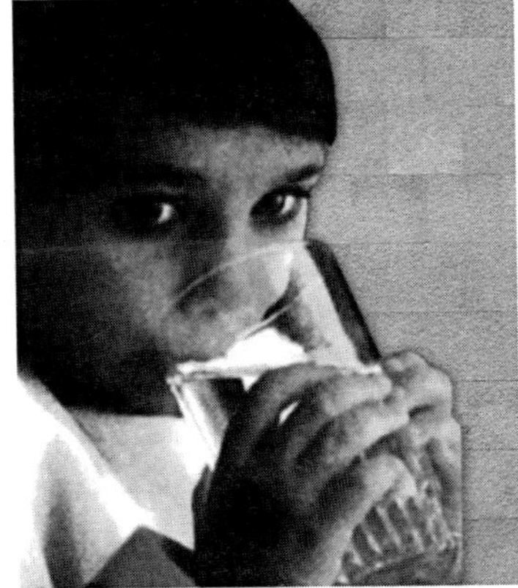

Fig. 26.1: Safe drinking water prevents many infections (*For color version, see Plate 14*)

BIOLOGICAL WASTE MANAGEMENT

Biomedical waste means any waste, which is generated during the diagnosis, treatment or immunization of human beings or in research activities pertaining thereto or production or testing of biological products (e.g. vaccine preparation from microorganisms or from their metabolites such as toxins and biochemical or immunological reaction intended for use in the diagnosis, immunization or treatment).

Biomedical waste generated in a hospital is classified into infectious and noninfectious wastes.

1. *Infectious waste:* Pathological waste including tissues organs, body fluids, syringes, IV tubing, blood bags and other items contaminated with blood, pus and other body fluids. Items like plaster casts can be considered infectious only when they are contaminated with blood and other body fluids. Human anatomical waste or surgical waste includes resected organs, and amputated limbs, pathological specimens. Waste from microbiology laboratory such as cultures, media, serum samples, body fluids, swabs, needles, IV tubing, cannulas, cotton swabs, bandages maps, etc. are all included in the infectious waste.
2. *Non-infectious waste:* This constitutes nearly 85% of the entire hospital waste generated. It is similar to household waste. It can be broadly classified into the following wastes:
   i. Kitchen waste: Left over food, vegetable peels, natural kitchen waste are biodegradable. The other kitchen waste include plastic tea cups, wrapping, plastic paper, etc.
   ii. General office waste: Wrapping paper, office papers, cartoons, packing material, plastic sheets, bouquets, newspapers, etc. constitute the general office waste.

Classification of Biomedical Waste (Table 26.3)

- Category 1 : Human anatomical waste
- Category 2 : Animal waste (animal killed during animal experiment)
- Category 3 : Microbiology and biotechnology waste
- Category 4 : Sharps such as needles, blades, scalpels, saws, nails, broken glass

Table 26.3: Waste categories and disposals

Color codes	*Types of container*	*Waste category*	*Treatment/disposal*
Yellow	Plastic Nonchlorinated bag	Cat 1, Cat 2 Cat 3 and Cat 6	Incineration or deep burial
Red	Disinfected container plastic bag	Cat 3, Cat 6 and Cat 7	Autoclaving, chemical treatment, microwave oven
White translucent	Puncture proof	Cat 4, Cat 7	Autoclaving, microwave oven, chemical disinfection
Black	Plastic bag	Cat 5, 9 Solid chemical waste Kitchen and office waste	Disposals in secured Landfill Landfill

- Category 5 : Discarded medicines and cytotoxic drugs
- Category 6 : Solid waste
- Category 7 : Solid waste (general or kitchen waste)
- Category 8 : Liquid waste
- Category 9 : Inceneration ash
- Category 10 : Chemical waste

Separation of waste helps in the followings:

A. Reducing the risk of infection to the medical staff.
B. Reducing the cost of treatment of waste.
C. Reducing the risk of spreading the infection in the community.
D. Recycling wherever possible, e.g. formaldehyde from theaters can be reused for autopsy and in pathology.

Disposal of the Waste

1. Bins must be emptied at least twice a day or when the bags are three-fourths full or more often for theaters, if needed. The plastic bags in the bins must be tightly closed and carried on wheelbarrow. The waste handlers should wear apron, masks, gloves and gumboots.
2. Liquid waste such as body fluids should be left into general sewage system after treatment with disinfectant like sodium hypochlorite or two to three percent carbolic acid (phenol).
3. Sharp needles be put in puncture proof container and should be sent for incineration or autoclaving. Needles, sharps should be cut with a needle cutter so that they cannot be reused by illegal means.
4. IV tubing, gloves used should be cut before putting into the yellow container.
5. Incharge should keep records for the waste disposed from her ward (Table 26.4).

Some Do's and Dont's

Do's

1. Segregate waste as per the category.
2. Put the separated waste in correct bin as per Table 26.3.
3. Ensure that the plastic bag has biohazard symbol or label.
4. Remove plastic bags when they are three-fourths full, tie the bag properly.
5. Remove the bags on wheelbarrows.
6. Cut the needles before putting them in puncture proof containers.
7. Wear protective dress while handling the waste, materials.
8. Always snip the IV bottle, cut IV sets, cut the used gloves (if they are not returned for autoclaving).
9. Keep the record of waste disposal up-to-date.

Dont's

1. Put the waste indiscriminately.
2. Put the waste in the wrong container.
3. Fill the bags till the neck.

Table 26.4: Record keeping in hospital waste management

1. Sister incharge/Dept. Incharge											
Mark (✓) or (×) Date	*1*		*2*		*3*		*4*		*5*		*6*
M—Morning, E—Evening	*M*	*E*	*M*	*E*	*M*	*E*	*M*	*E*	*M*	*E*	*M*
1. Waste segregated											
2. Disposables treated/mutilated											
3. Hypochlorite solution made											
4. Needle cutter/burner working											
5. All bins lined with bags											
6. Number of bags for disposal — Yellow — Red — Green — PPC											
7. Everything collected by sweeper											
8. Safety gear worn											
9. All bags tied/labeled											
10. Sister incharge—(M) Sister incharge—(E)											
11. Name of sweeper—(M) Name of sweeper—(E)											
12. Checked by WMO*											
13. Action taken by WMO*											

* Waste management operations (WMO)

4. Handle waste without protective clothing.
5. Drag the bags after removal.
6. Recap the needle.
7. Mix infectious waste with noninfectious waste.

SOME DISINFECTION PROCEDURES

Airways and Endotracheal Tubes

Use single use disposable or autoclave or disinfect with two percent glutaraldehyde.

Ampoules

Wipe neck with 70% alcohol and allow to dry before opening.

Bedpans

- Handle only after wearing gloves and apron
- Empty with a disposable wooden spatula and paper

- Wash with tap water
- Disinfect with phenol two percent for 10 minutes followed by tap rinse (1 hour in gastrointestinal infection).

Urinals

Empty and wash with detergent, then put it in a big drum of water at 80°C for 10 minutes or chemically disinfect in two percent phenol for 15 minutes. Rinse well.

Bedding

- Blanket: Change on discharge/every week and send to laundry
- Bedsheet: Change everyday or whenever soiled
- Bedframe: Clean after discharge with detergent and water.

Mattresses

- Cover with water impermeable cover: Wipe cover with detergent before bed making. Wipe with two percent phenol or five percent Savlon, one percent hydrogen peroxide after wash if contaminated. Fumigate for heavy contamination
- Pillows: Treat them like for mattresses.

Blood Spill

Cover with absorbent material, pour one percent hypochlorite or two percent carbolic acid and leave for 10 minutes, remove with gloves on. Then wash the area with a disinfectant.

Bloodstained Linen

Soak in fresh bleach solution (bleaching powder 14 g/L) for 30 minutes send to laundry.

Bowls

Mop with two percent carbolic acid or five percent lysol or one percent hypochlorite. Rinse with waste and keep inverted. Surgical bowls—autoclave.

Cheatle Forceps

Autoclave or boil. Store forceps in two percent Savlon to be changed daily.

Thermometers

- Auxillary: Store dry after cleaning with 70% alcohol or keep in two percent Savlon and change daily
- Rectal: When not in use keep in two percent Savlon, change daily. Before use wash in soap water, clean with 70% alcohol and dry.

Mops

Use disposable mops wherever possible. Change mop daily in operation theater. For wards and other areas after use wash in detergent thoroughly and dry in the sun. Immerse in two percent phenol overnight if there is heavy contamination.

Buckets

Should be washed, dried and kept inverted.

Catheters

Discard or autoclave.

Cystoscope

Immerse in two percent glutaraldehyde for 9 to 10 hours.

Endoscope

Two percent glutaraldehyde for 10 to 30 minutes in between the procedures.

Handwash

Use plenty of soap and running water (soap used should be Savlon, Dettol or carbolic).

Instruments

Autoclaving.

Chapter 27

Infection Control Guidelines

INTRODUCTION

Hospital-acquired infections or nosocomial infections are those acquired during hospital care, which are not present or incubating at the time of admission. Infections occurring more than 48 hours after admissions are usually considered as hospital acquired infections. Based on clinical and biological criteria approximately 50 potential infection sites have been identified by CDC, Atlanta. Nosocomial infections may be epidemic or endemic. The endemic infections are the most common. Short epidemic outbreaks may occur in some units due to failure of aseptic procedures or due to immunocompromisation. Infection acquired by staff or visitors to the hospital may also be considered as nosocomial infection.

The following simplified criteria provide definition for common infection that could be used for surveys in facilities with limited access to sophisticated diagnostic techniques (Table 27.1).

Other hospital acquired infection, include soft time infection, gastroenteritis, sinusitis, other enteric infections, eye and conjunctival infections, endometritis and other infections of the reproductive organs during the childbirth.

Table 27.1: Classification of nosocomial infections

Type of hospital-acquired infection	*Simplified criteria*
Surgical site infection	Purulent discharge, abscess, cellulitis at the surgical site during the month after the operation
Urinary tract infection	Positive urine culture with at least 10^5 bacteria/mL without any symptoms
Respiratory infection	Respiratory symptoms appearing during hospitalization along with at least two of the following signs Cough Purulent sputum New infiltrates in the chest Radiograph consistent with infection
Vascular catheter infection	Inflammation, lymphangitis or purulent discharge at the insertion site of the catheter
Septicemia	Fever rigors and at least one positive blood culture

The microbial flora responsible for hospital acquired infection includes bacteria, viruses, fungi and parasites. Bacteria are the most common pathogens of nosocomial infection and the bacteria may be commensal flora when the host is compromised or pathogenic bacteria such anaerobic rods (*Clostridium* spp) or members of the family Enterobacteriaceae. Gram-negative bacilli such as *Pseudomonas aeruginosa* and *Pseudomonas* spp are often isolated from water and damp areas. Selected other bacteria are unique risk in hospitals; *Legionella* spp may cause pneumonia due to inhalation of contaminated aerosols (air conditioning, showers and therapeutic aerosols).

Virus such as hepatitis B and hepatitis C may cause infection due to transfusion, dialysis, injections and endoscopy. Respiratory syncytial virus, rota virus and enteroviruses transmitted by inhalation or hand-to-mouth contamination. Other viruses like cytomegalovirus, varicella-zoster, HIV, and influenza may also be transmitted. Some parasites like *Giardia* can easily be transmitted among adults and children. Many fungi cause opportunistic infections in immunocompromised patients. Environmental contamination by airborne pathogens is also a concern in designing hospital construction or expansion of the existing hospital.

The reservoirs of various microorganisms are the permanent or transient flora of the patient, flora from another patient or the hospital staff or the flora from the health care environment such as water, damp area, disinfectants, linen and other supplies. Appropriate housekeeping normally limits the risk of bacteria surviving. Food, dust, droplets generated by coughing, sneezing, speaking may cause nosocomial infection. **The routes of transmission are mainly (a) direct contact form hands, clothing of the staff, linen, (b) ingestion (feco-oral transmission), and (c) indirect contact from fingers, fomites, shared articles and contaminated instruments (Tables 27.2 and 27.3).**

Table 27.2: Differential nosocomial infection risk by patient and intervention

Risk of infection	*Type of patients*	*Type of procedures Noninvasive*
Minimal	Non-immunocompromised; no significant underlying disease	No exposure to biological fluids
Medium	Infected patients or patients with same risk factors	Exposure to biological fluids
High	Severely immunocompromised, multiple injuries, severe burns, organ transplant	High-risk invasive procedures

Table 27.3: Aseptic procedures appropriate for different levels of risk of infection

Risk of infection	*Asepsis*	*Antiseptics*	*Hands*	*Clothes*	*Devices*
Minimal	Clean	None	Simple hand washing or alcohol rub	Street clothes	Clean or disinfected at intermediate or low-level
Medium	Asepsis	Standard antiseptic-product (e.g. sterillium)	Hygienic hand washing alcohol rub	Protection against body fluids	Disinfection at high level sterilization
High	Surgical asepsis	Specific major products	Surgical hand washing or surgi-cal alcohol rub	Surgical wear	Sterilization or high level disinfection

All devices entering sterile body cavities should be sterile.

HAND HYGIENE

The hands play an important role in the patient care. With hands we touch the patient, carry the equipment, furniture, manipulate, rearrange, feel, push, point out and greet. They are the body's main connecting link to the surrounding environment. Most of the nurse-to-patient, physician-to-patient and patient-to-care giver, contacts take place using the hands. Patients are reassured with hand holding a hand on the shoulder or rubbing and simple touching. The healing touch of the hand is well known since centuries. The hands play an important role in transmitting pathogenic microorganisms. In order to avoid transferring these pathogenic organisms, nursing staff or other health care workers should ensure that their hands are as clean as possible before providing direct patient care.

Ignaz Semmel Weis was the first to demonstrate the importance of person-to-person transmission of infections by the hands. He also noticed that handwashing reduced the incidence of infections. Lord Lister used carbolic acid to wash the hands before and after attending the patient, and he proved that infection rate was significantly reduced with handwashing with a germicidal chemical like carbolic acid.

Handwashing is a complex learned behavior and requires continuous education and motivation. Recognizing the importance of handwashing for preventing the spread of nosocomial infections, medical and nursing schools are increasingly teaching the skills and rationale for effective handwashing. As a fundamental lifetime hygiene practice handwashing must be valued, taught, learned and practiced from an early age.

The complex anatomy of the hands provides an ideal environment for the multiplication of microbes. The skin over the hands contains resident flora which can be cultured repeatedly. They are usually harmless except when they are introduced into the body by invasive measures such as injections, IV lines or trauma. The microbial flora that are most commonly resident are gram-positive cocci like *Staphylococcus epidermidis*, micrococci, gram-positive bacilli. Resident flora are not removed easily by simple washing or scrubbing but they are inactivated by topical antimicrobial agents such as antiseptic lotions, creams or antibiotic preparations but significant regrowth occurs within 24 hours. The transient microbial flora is loosely attached to the upper layer of the skin and may be pathogenic. They are relatively short-lived and can be removed easily by soap and water. Among the transient microbial flora *Staphylococcus aureus*, streptococci, gram-negative bacilli like *E. coli*, *Pseudomonas* and viruses are common and they are the most common organisms responsible for infections.

FACTORS THAT INFLUENCE THE EFFECTIVENESS OF HANDWASHING

1. **Active ingredient or product used:** An antimicrobial product such as alcohol or iodine compounds or chlorhexidine gluconate are used in high-risk areas where frequent invasive procedures are performed on patients with compromised immunological status. Among these agents alcohols are cheap and effective and can be used in day care centers, disaster situations (accidents), emergency vehicles, or nursing homes. Iodine compounds have broad-spectrum microbicidal activity but it is decreased in the

presence of organic matter such as blood, pus and other body fluids. Chlorhexidine gluconate has good persistent antimicrobial activity. When these compounds are used for handwashing the instructions given on the label should be read carefully and followed before they are used.

2. **Frequency of washing:** The appropriate frequency for handwashing is dependent on numbers and types of the patients contacts. Plain soap removes soil, debris, transient and a few resident organisms. In situations where frequent handwashing is necessary, e.g., more than twice/hour, squamous cells from the loosened skin are shed and these cells contain viable bacteria. As a result frequent washing with plain soap increases the bacterial counts. Hence, wherever frequent handwashing is indicated antimicrobial soaps should be used instead of ordinary soap.
3. **Amount of soaps/antiseptics used:** When plain soap is used just for removing the dirt, the amount of soap used seem to be of little importance and 1 ml of liquid soap is sufficient. Alcohol containing antiseptic soap solutions are effective only in the presence of moisture. Therefore, sufficient amount of soap solution should be used to keep the hands wet throughout washing. For a 10 seconds wash 3 ml of antimicrobial soap solution is sufficient. For a 5 minutes surgical scrub of hands and arms 25 ml of alcohol is required.
4. **Duration of wash:** It is recommended that a minimum of 10 to 15 seconds is necessary for effective handwashing. For surgical purposes 5 minutes are adequate. If alcohol is used it may be possible to reduce the time to one or two minutes. However, studies are required to prove the efficacy of surgical handwashing for 1 to 2 minutes.
5. **Technique:** Even when hands are washed, areas of greater microbial contamination are missed. Most of the people spend more time and soap in washing palms and dorsal areas of hand which are usually clean. The vast majority of pathogenic organisms live under the nail region (sublingual areas). This is of particular importance especially when gloves are worn frequently or for prolonged time, the bacteria can leach out during glove wearing and contaminate the hands. Additionally, the nails should be trimmed and kept as short as possible. Ring wearing may interfere with thorough hand scrubbing. Many people feel that glove wearing is a substitute for handwashing. But in practice increased use of gloves could actually result in dirtier hands. This could be due to two reasons; first, skin bacteria multiply rapidly in the warm moist environment of the gloves. Second, undetected punctures in the gloves are common and hands are unlikely, even when gloves are used to be free from contamination.

The major problem related to hands hygiene is the failure to wash hands at all. Handwashing is frequently omitted even for invasive procedures. Handwashing like other habitual behavior is very difficult to change. It should be noted by all who directly handle the patient that hand hygiene is essential component in an intentional program of barriers such as gloves, masks, gowns and chemicals for infection prevention (Table 27.4).

Patients are admitted to intensive care units for the purpose of receiving life-saving treatment. Paradoxically the hospital environment exposes them to a potentially life-threatening complication—hospital acquired or nosocomial infection (Nosokome = Hospital). A combination of patients impaired body resistance and the use of sophisticated

Table 27.4: Factors that influence handwashing effectiveness

Factors	*Impacts*
1. Active ingredient or product used	• In approximate order of antimicrobial activity • Alcohols • Iodine compounds chlorhexidine gluconate plain soap
2. Frequency of washing	• Plain soap—no effect. With antimicrobial soap increased frequency increased activity
3. Amount of soap used	• Plain soap—no effect
4. Duration of wash	• Antimicrobial soap 3 to 5 mL is recommended • < 10 seconds and > 1 minute for routine washing has not been studied.
5. Technique	• Areas of with highest microbial counts are often missed.

invasive devices are responsible for contracting nosocomial infections. The other patients and the hospital staff play an important role in transmitting the infections to an already suffering patient.

HOSPITAL-ACQUIRED INFECTION

In spite of availability of a number of treatment modalities, nosocomial infections still rank among the major causes of morbidity and mortality in the intensive care units of the hospitals. Scrupulous attention must be paid to preventive measures ranging from the simple discipline of handwashing to the most advanced treatment modalities. We must recognize that patients are bound to develop infection and be prepared to treat them when they occur with the help of appropriate microbiological investigations.

Changes in the pattern of nosocomial pathogens that have occurred over past years must be taken into account while selecting the most appropriate antibiotic therapy. In the past gram-negative organisms predominated but in the recent years the proportion of infection caused by gram-positive organisms has rapidly increased. Today, the antimicrobial choice has to take an account of this changing scenario as well as the trends in antimicrobial resistance.

The incidence of hospital acquired infection varies from one hospital to another and this may range from 5 to 40 percent. The main types of hospital acquired infection are:

1. **Hospitals acquired pneumonia:** This accounts for 10 to 25 percent of all hospital acquired infections and it is the leading cause of death among all the nosocomial infections. Pneumonia is particularly common in the intensive care units largely because of the high proportion of patients receiving mechanical ventilation. Typical symptoms of pneumonia may be absent in these patients. Diagnosis is based upon invasive techniques such as culturing of protected brush specimen sampling or bronchoalveolar lavage and examination of Gram-stained smears for leukocytes and bacteria.
2. **Bloodstream infections:** This can be primary bloodstream infections which occur without any recognizable focus of infection at any other site at the time of taking the blood

sample for blood culture. Typical examples include bloodstream infections associated with intravenous or intra-arterial catheter lines. Secondary blood culture infections, which develop following a documented infection with the same microorganism at another site. For example, a blood culture showing growth of *Staphylococcus aureus*. Patient may be defined as having bloodstream infections if the blood culture is positive for a bacterium or fungus, more than 48 hours after admission to hospital along with the presence of signs and symptoms of infection such as fever, chills, leukocytosis, raised ESR. An unexpectedly positive culture or one positive culture in a series of negative blood cultures from the same patient can often be considered as contaminant. However, any positive blood culture even in the absence of clinical symptoms must be evaluated carefully.

3. **Urinary tract infections:** These are very common among the patients who undergo invasive procedures such as cystoscopy or who have individually catheters. Risk of urinary tract infections are more in females and in immunocompromised patients such as diabetics, chronic renal failure patients.
4. **Surgical wound infections:** Surgical wound infections are common in hospitals wards and intensive care units are no exception. Overall surgical wound infections account for about 40% of all nosocomial infections in surgical patients. The highest rates of wound infections are found after colon surgery, coronary artery, bypass surgery and gastric surgery.

The most common pathogens of nosocomial infections are *Escherichia coli*, *Staphylococcus aureus*, enterococci, *Pseudomonas aeruginosa* and other like coagulase-negative staphylococci, *Candida albicans*, *Klebsiella pneumoniae*, *Proteus* species and *Enterobacter*.

Prevention of Nosocomial Infections

1. **Basic hygiene:** The nursing staff should observe basic hygiene such handwashing use of face mask, gloves in order to prevent the transmission of infection by contact. Barrier nursing such as keeping the patients with infection in a sideward with careful attention to hygiene reduces the risk of transmission of infection to other patients in intensive care units.
2. **Aseptic precautions:** Before undertaking any procedure on patient, the skin should be disinfected using as infectants like 70% absolute alcohol or chlorhexidine or povidone-iodine. Ventilator tubing should be changed as when necessary (usually once in 48 hours).

Patient should be given proper balanced diet. If he/she is not able to take orally, parenteral nutrition is recommended. Oral feeding should be considered as early as possible as it balances gut flora and avoids colonization with opportunistic pathogens like *Candida albicans*.

Appropriate antibiotics should be administered based on microbiological investigations and antibiotic sensitivity reports.

The environment should be kept clean. The floors, walls should be washed with a detergent or five percent phenol and if necessary should be fumigated.

Wash Your Hands

1. Before taking food or any beverage (soap and water).
2. Before and after attending the patient for checking the temperature, blood pressure pulse, etc. (soap and water).
3. Before and after giving a sponge bath to the patient (soap and water).
4. Before and after bed make (soap and water).
5. Before and after starting and intravenous or central line or inserting a vasofix (70% isopropyl alcohol or sterillium).
6. Before and after giving IV, IM injections, or drawing blood specimens use (70% isopropyl alcohol or sterillium for skin disinfection).
7. Before and after dressing a surgical wound or any oozing wounds. (70% isopropyl alcohol or sterillium).
8. Before and after emergency resuscitation such as cardiac arrest, Shock etc (70% isopropyl alcohol or sterillium).
9. No need for the washing hands if you don't touch the patient or any of the articles surrounding the patient but simply talk to him to find his/her requirements or enquiring about his/her health status or greeting him/hcr.

   Before and after suction of nasogastric aspirations or tracheal aspirations (70% isopropyl alcohol or sterillium).
10. Before and after suction of nasogastric aspirations or tracheal aspirations (70% isopropyl alcohol).
11. After coming into contact with any of the secretions such as saliva, vomiting or blood and other body fluids (first clean thoroughly with soap and water followed by washing with 70% isopropyl alcohol or sterillium).
12. Before and after removal of sutures or staples or indwelling catheters (70% isopropyl alcohol or sterillium).
13. Before and after clinical examination of the patient (soap and water).
14. Before and after attending an injured person in a road traffic accident (70% isopropyl alcohol or sterillium).
15. In case of accidental needle pricks, cuts due to sharps or glass pieces, first wash the affected part with soap and water using running water and then apply either betadine cream or liquid. Determine the status of the patient (That is whether he/she is HIV or HBsAg positive).
16. After disposing of the infected cotton gauge, used IV bottles, cannulas, IV catheters (that are to be cut before putting them into the appropriate waste bin) wash with soap and water.
17. After using the toilet (soap and water).
18. The amount of isopropyl alcohol required for hands washing is 3 ml/wash. If the hands are dirty first wash with soap and water before washing with 70% isopropyl alcohol or sterillium.

PERSONAL HYGIENE

1. All staff shall maintain good personal hygiene. Nails and hair are periodically trimmed and kept clean
2. Clothing: Staff shall wear a personal uniform or street clothes covered with white coat.
3. In special areas like burn units, intensive care unit, uniform trousers and short-sleeved gowns are used. In other units, women can wear short-sleeved dress.
4. The clothing material shall be easily washable and decontaminatable type.
5. The clothing shall be changed if it is exposed to blood or body fluid or if it becomes wet due to sweating or other body fluid exposure.

Shoes

1. In restricted areas or in aseptic units or in units, where number of immunocompromised patients are kept, staff shall wear dedicated shoes which are easy to clean.
2. If necessary that shoes and slippers are sterilized by ethylene oxide gas.

Caps and Masks

1. These are used in aseptic unit, operating rooms or while performing of a selective invasive procedure.
2. Caps shall completely cover the hair. Masks of cotton wool gauze or paper are ineffective.
3. Paper masks with synthetic material for filtration are effective barrier for microorganisms.
4. Masks are used in operating rooms, to care immunocompromised patients and to puncture body cavities.
5. Staff shall wear masks while caring patients with airborne infection or while performing bronchoscopies or similar examinations. A high efficiency masks are recommended.
6. Patients with infection which may be transmitted by the airborne route must wear surgical masks when they are outside their isolation rooms.

Gloves

1. Sterile gloves are used for surgery to care immunocompromised patients, or during invasive procedures involving entry into the body cavities.
2. Nonsterile gloves are used for all patient contact where hands are likely to come into contact with wounds or mucous membranes.
3. Staff wear nonsterile gloves to care for patients with communicable diseases transmitted by contact, to perform bronchoscopies or similar such procedures.
4. Hands are washed after removing the gloves.

Safe Injection Practice: Ampules or Vials are Decontaminate with 70% Alcohol

1. a. Required to prevent transmission of infections between patients with injection.

   b. Unnecessary injections are eliminated.
   c. Sterile disposable needle and syringes are used.
2. After use the needle is cut with needle cutter as the tip of the syringe is also cut. Used needles are placed in the thick puncture proof screw capped white container having 1% sodium hypochlorite solution.
3. Contamination of medications are prevented especially the eye drops, ear drops, lotions and creams
4. The ampoules are via decontaminator with 70% isopropyl alcohol or sterillium or before breaking or operating the injection ampoule or vial.

PREVENTION OF TRANSMISSION OF INFECTIONS FROM THE ENVIRONMENT

Proper methods such as cleaning, disinfection and sterilization procedures are used to minimize the transmission of microorganisms from equipment and the environment.

Cleaning of the Hospital Environment

To keep the hospital environment clean and free from dust and soil routine cleaning is carried out.

Majority of the microorganism is present within the 'visible dirt' and the main purpose of routine cleaning is to eliminate this visible dirt. Depending upon the likelihood of contamination and the level of asepsis required the hospital area falls into one of the following four groups.

Zone A

No patient contact. Requires only normal domestic cleaning (e.g. administration, library)

Zone B

Care of the patients who are not infected and are not immunocompromised. These areas are cleaned by a procedure that does not raise dust. Dry sweeping or vacuum cleaners are not recommended. Cleaning should be done with water and a detergent. Areas that show visible contamination with blood or body fluids are disinfected before cleaning.

Zone C

Area where infected/isolated patients are kept. This area in cleaned with a detergent/ disinfectant with separate cleaning equipment for each room.

Zone D

Area where highly susceptible patients are located or protected areas such as operation theaters, delivery room, intensive care units, premature baby units, casualty departments, transplantation unit, postoperative wards, acute medical care, and dialysis unit. These areas are to be cleaned using a detergent or disinfectant solution and separate clearing equipment.

- All horizontal surfaces of zones B, C, D and all toilet areas are cleaned daily.

- Bacteriological testing of the environment is not recommended except in selected circumstances like
  a. Epidemic investigation for which environmental source is suspected.
  b. Dialysis water monitoring for bacterial counts (< 2000 CFU of coli form bacilli/ mL of dilution water and less than 2000 CFU of coli form bacilli/ml of dialysate).
  c. Quality control when changing the cleaning procedure.

UNIVERSAL PRECAUTIONS IN THE OPERATING ROOMS

Preoperative

An indication of the infectious nature of the patients should be made in the routine operations lists.

Preoperative shaving should be eliminated. If there is excess hair, clippers can be used to trim the hair. Patients should be anesthetized in the operating rooms rather than anesthetic bay.

Unnecessary equipments should be removed from the theater.

Personnel

1. The surgeon incharge of the patient is responsible for seeing that all the members of the team know the nature of infection hazards and the precautions to be taken.
2. The anesthesiologist should be informed before preoperative visit so that he is able to fully assess the patient. The anesthesia team should also follow the same principles of infection control as the surgical team.
3. The team is limited to essential members.
4. Personnel with skin abrasions or oozing dermatitis or wounds of the skin must be excluded from the operating team.

Protective Apparel

All persons must wear:

1. Water proof long-sleeved cuffed wrist gown.
2. Water proof over boots.
3. Masks.
4. Protective goggles or glasses to protect against the splashes wherever appropriate.
5. The members of the scrub team should wear double gloves.

Terminal Cleaning of Operating Room and Instruments

1. Disposable waste should be placed in a yellow contaminated waste plastic bag and sealed linen should be placed in a plastic bag and then inserted into linen bag.
2. Instruments are carefully cleaned under running water using detergents and then they are sent for steam sterilization after proper packing. The sink is cleaned with 1:10 dilution of sodium hypochlorite (5.25% stock solution). Heat sensitive instruments are sterilized by two percent glutaraldehyde for 1 hour.

3. Scalpel blades, needles are discarded in puncture proof plastic container with screw cap that contains 1:10 dilution of sodium hypochlorite (To be filling upto 1/3rd of the container).
4. Spill over of blood and body fluids on the floor should be treated with 1:10 dilution of sodium hypochlorite. After 10 minutes the ward boy or aya should wear gloves and mop the area with newspaper and discard the paper in the yellow bag. Again mop the area with 1:10 dilution of sodium hypochlorite.
5. Operating table instrument should be cleaned with diluted solution of sodium hypochlorite.

Recovery

1. The patient should be nursed in isolated area in case of HIV or HBsAg infection.
2. Staff in this area should wear the protective apparel as mentioned earlier.
3. Disposable suction apparatus may be used otherwise the suction apparatus should be cleaned with diluted sodium hypochlorite and then with a detergent.
4. Nondisposable instruments if not heat sensitive should be autoclaved or treated with two percent glutaraldehyde.

Operating Room Techniques

The principle of "confine and contain" should be followed.

Nontouch technique should be followed in the OT and passing needles, blades, other sharp instruments directly to the hand must be avoided. A neutral zone using a sterile dish in which the sharp objects must be placed to minimize the chances of needle stick injury of knife injuries.

Blood soaked sponges are kept in a sterile bowl and carefully counted in to a plastic bag when five have accumulated.

A wound dressing should be used that will contain exudates within an impervious outer covering.

Accidental Inoculation or Contamination

1. The affected area is thoroughly cleaned with running tap water and washed thoroughly and cleaned with an antiseptic soap.
2. Bleeding is encouraged for a short time by local venous occlusion.
3. Report the accident to the senior staff member and to the infection control committee for further follow-up and treatment.

Equipment

Wherever possible use disposables.

Anesthesia Machine

Filters should be used to protect the head of the machine. Terminal cleaning of the machine is done by using 0.2% sodium hypochlorite. All contaminated anesthesia equipment should be pasteurized after proper cleaning or cleaned with two percent glutaraldehyde. Use disposable wherever possible.

UNIVERSAL PRECAUTIONS FOR HEALTH CARE WORKERS

1. Do not eat, smoke or drink within the working area.
2. Wear gloves only after washing the hands either with soap and water or isopropyl alcohol. Glove wearing is not a substitute for hand washing.
3. Gloves should be worn for touching blood, body fluids, mucous membranes and weeping wounds. They should also be worn while inserting a vasofix.
4. Gloves should be changed after the contact with each patient.
5. Masks and protective eye wear or face shields are to be used during the procedures that are likely to generate droplets of blood or other secretions.
6. Gowns and aprons should be worn during procedures that are likely to generate splashes of blood or other body fluids or while attending patients met with road traffic accidents.
7. Hands should be washed thoroughly if contaminated with blood or body fluids. Hands should be washed immediately after removing the gloves.
8. Care should be taken to prevent injuries by needles, scalpels and other sharp devices during procedures.
9. After using the syringes the needles and the tip of the syringe should be cut with a cutter and the cut needles are placed in a white puncture proof plastic container with screw cap. One-third of the container should be filled with 1:10 dilution of 5.25 percent stock solution of sodium hypochlorite (liquid bleach).
10. Resuscitation equipment should be used once only and discarded or be thoroughly cleaned and disinfected.
11. Health care workers who have educative lesions or weeping eruptions should refrain from all direct contact with patient and from handling the patient until the condition resolves.
12. Pregnant health care workers should be familiar with and strictly adhere to precautions to minimize the risk of exposure.
13. Isolation precautions should be used as necessary if associated conditions such as infectious diarrhea or tuberculosis are diagnosed or suspected.
14. No touch technique should be practiced while dressing the wounds or venipuncture.
15. All health care workers should be vaccinated against hepatitis B, hepatitis A (optional), varicella-zoster (optional) and other preventable diseases like tetanus, diphtheria, Pertussis and poliomyelitis.
16. All needle stick or sharp instrument injuries should be reported in the prescribed proforma. If there is more than 6 months lapse after taking a tetanus toxoid, a booster alone is required otherwise there is no need to take tetanus toxoid infection.

PROTOCOL FOR HIV OR HBSAG POSITIVE PATIENTS IN THE OPERATING ROOM

Patients presenting to the operating room with either confirmed or suspected HIV or HBV infection are afforded the same care as any other patient presenting for an operation. However, the following precautions should be taken.

Preoperative

- An indication of the infectious nature of these patients should be made in the routine operating lists.
- Preoperative shaving of the body parts of the patient should be avoided.
- Unnecessary equipment should be removed from the operation theater.

Personnel

- The surgeon incharge of the patient should be responsible for seeing that all members of the team know about the infection hazards and insist on the precautions to be taken.
- The anesthesiologist should be informed before the preoperative visits so that he can fully assess the patient. The anesthesia team should follow similar precautions.
- Staff with exudative lesions or open wounds should not be allowed into the theater
- The team should be limited to essential members. An extra nurse and **technician/ attender** will be required to be stationed outside the operating room door to fetch any equipment or drugs needed.
- All persons attending the patient should wear full protective clothing such as.
  - Gloves
  - Plastic aprons
  - Gowns
  - Eye protection wear.

Theater

- The posting of the patient should be at the end of the operating list to allow ample time for the theater and scrub room to be decontaminated after surgery.
- The patient should be induced in the theater and should recover fully in the theater.
- The operating table should be covered with a water proof sheet.
- Adequate quantities of suitable disinfectant must be made available.
- Specimen bottles should be labeled with ***'Biohazard'*** and safely transported to the laboratory.
- After surgery the operating room and all equipment must be thoroughly cleaned with hot soap water and 1% sodium hypochlorite.
- (*Note:* Sodium hypochlorite must not be used on stainless steel. Use 2% glutaraldehyde or 1% lysol).

Spillage

- If there is a spillage of body fluids or blood
- The area should be saturated with one percent sodium hypochlorite for 30 minutes.
- It should be mopped by an acknowledgable person using gloves and newspaper and sent for safe disposal in a yellow plastic bag.
- This should be followed by mopping with the regular disinfectant used for floors and other areas.

Instruments

- They should be autoclaved before washing.
- After cooling, they are washed with soap and water and rinsed well several times.
- All the instruments are again re-autoclaved for further use.
- Brushes that are used for cleaning should also be autoclaved.

For Non-autoclavable Equipment

- Immerse in two percent glutaraldehyde for 1 hour.
- After removing the instrument the glutaraldehyde solutions should be discarded.
- Instruments are then thoroughly cleaned with warm water and soap.
- Rinse in two percent glutaraldehyde and leave to soak for 3 hours.

Suction Bottles

- Suction bottles should contain 30 ml of two percent glutaraldehyde or 60 ml of one percent sodium hypochlorite.
- After surgery they should be emptied and autoclaved.

Sharps

The principle of 'Confine and contain" should always be used. A non-touch technique should be adapted in the operating theaters and avoid passing needles, blades or other sharp instruments from hand-to-hand.

- Always use a sterile dish on the table to place all the sharp objects.
- Accidental injuries should be reported to the senior member of the staff immediately.
- The injured part should be thoroughly cleaned with running water and soap. The wound is dressed with antiseptic.
- If there is a need, tetanus toxoid should be given.
- The person should be followed up and should be screened for HBsAg and HIV subsequently if necessary.

Equipment

- Wherever possible disposable should be used
- Anesthetic machines should be cleaned with one percent sodium hypochlorite and detergent.

Terminal Cleansing of Operating Room and Instruments

1. **Disposable waste:** Should be placed in an 'Yellow bag' labeled as ***'Biohazard'*** and handed over for safe disposal as per the regulations of management of biological waste.
2. **Linen:** Should be soaked in 1% sodium hypochlorite for ½ an hour and then sent to laundry for regular washing.
3. **Instruments:** Already mentioned above.

4. **Sharp instruments:** Already mentioned above
5. **Blood and other body fluids:** Already mentioned above.

Recovery

- The patient should be nursed in an isolated area of the recovery room.
- Staff in this area should wear protective apparel.
- Disposable suction apparatus must be used.
- Any non-disposable equipment should be autoclaved or disinfected or pasteurized.
- The room should be cleaned with one percent Sodium hypochlorite after the patient is discharged.

Disinfectants which are Effective Against HIV and HBsAg

Fresh sodium hypochlorite 1%	30 minutes
Glulltaraldehyde 2%	60 minutes
Formaldehyde 5%	60 minutes
Ethyl alcohol 70%	60 minutes
Isopropyl alcohol 50%	60 minutes
Lysol 1%	60 minutes
Hydrogen peroxide 3%	60 minutes

PREVENTION OF COMMON ENDEMIC NOSOCOMIAL INFECTIONS

The four most common nosocomial infections are urinary tract infections, surgical wound infections, pneumonia, and primary bloodstream infection. Each of these is associated with an invasive medical device or invasive procedure. Specific policies and practices to minimize these infections must be established, reviewed and updated regularly, and compliance monitored (Table 27.5).

Urinary Tract Infections (UTI)

Urinary tract infections are the most frequent nosocomial infection; 80% of these infections are associated with an indwelling urethral catheter. Interventions effective in preventing nosocomial urinary infection include:

- Avoiding urethral catheterization unless there is a compelling indication
- Limiting the duration of drainage, if catheterization is necessary
- Maintaining appropriate aseptic practice during urinary catheter insertion and other invasive urological procedures (e.g. cystoscopy, urodynamic testing, cystography)
- Hygienic hand wash or rub prior to insertion and following catheter or drainage bag manipulation
- Sterile gloves for insertion
- Perianal cleaning with an antiseptic solution prior to insertion
- Non-traumatic urethral insertion using an appropriate lubricant
- Limiting the duration of drainage, if catheterization is necessary

Table 27.5: Measure of prevention of infection

Infection	Proven effective	Proven not effective
Urinary tract infections	Limit duration of catheter aspect technique at insertion; maintain closed drainage	Systemic antibiotic prophylaxis; bladder irrigation or instillation of normal saline antiseptic or antibiotic Antiseptic added to drainage bag Antimicrobial-coated catheter Daily antiseptic perianal cleaning
Surgical site infections	Surgical technique Clean operating environment Staff attire Limiting preoperative hospital stay Preoperative shower and local skin preparation of patient Optimal antibiotic prophylaxis Aseptic practice in operating room Surgical wound surveillance	Fumigation Preoperative shaving
Pneumonia	Ventilator-associate Aseptic intubation and suctioning Limit duration. Non-invasive ventilation Others Influenza vaccination for staff isolation policy. Sterile water for oxygen and aerosol therapy. Prevention of *Legionella* and *Aspergillus* during renovations	Digestive decontamination for all patients Changes of ventilator circuit every 48 or 72 hours
Vascular device infections	All catheters Closed system Limit duration Local skin preparation Aseptic technique at insertion Removal in infection suspected Central lines Surgical asepsis for insertion Limitation of frequency of dressing change Antibiotic-coated catheter for short-term	Antimicrobial creams for skin preparation

- Maintaining appropriate aseptic practice during urinary catheter insertion and other invasive urological procedures (e.g. cystoscopy, urodynamic testing, cystography)
- Hygienic hand wash or rub prior to insertion and following catheter or drainage bag manipulation sterile gloves for insertion
- Perianal cleaning with an antiseptic solution prior to insertion
- Nontraumatic urethral insertion using an appropriate lubricant
- Maintaining a closed drainage system.

Other practices which are recommended, but not proven to decrease infection include:

- Maintaining good patient hydration
- Appropriate perianal hygiene for patients with catheters
- Appropriate staff training in catheter insertion and care

- Maintain unobstructed drainage of the bladder to the collection bag with the bag below the level of the bladder.

  Generally, the smallest diameter catheter should be used. Catheter material (latex, silicone) does not influence infection rates.

  For patients with a neurogenic bladder:
- Avoid an indwelling catheter if possible
- If assisted bladder drainage is necessary, clean intermittent urinary catheterization should be used.

Surgical Wound Infections (Surgical Site Infections)

Factors which influence the frequency of surgical wound infection include:

Surgical Technique

- Extent of endogenous contamination of the wound at surgery (e.g. clean, clean-contaminated)
- Duration of operation
- Underlying patient status
- Operating room environment
- Organisms shed by the operating room team

A systematic program for prevention of surgical wound infections includes the practice of optimal surgical technique, a clean operating room environment with restricted staff entry and appropriate.

Staff attire, sterile equipment, adequate preoperative preparation of the patient, appropriate use of preoperative antimicrobial prophylaxis, and a surgical wound surveillance program reduces the incidence of surgical site infections. Surgical wound-infection rates are decreased by standardized surveillance for infection with reporting of rates back to individual surgeons.

Operating Room Environment

Airborne bacteria must be minimized, and surfaces kept clean. A recommended schedule for cleaning and disinfection of the operating theater is:

- Every morning before any intervention: cleaning of all horizontal surfaces
- Between procedures: cleaning and disinfection of horizontal surfaces and all surgical items (e.g. tables, buckets)
- All the end of the working day: complete cleaning of the operating theater using a recommended disinfectant cleaner
- Once a week: Complete cleaning of the operating room area, including all annexes such as dressing rooms, technical rooms, cupboards.

All items used within a sterile field must be sterile. Sterile drapes must be placed on the patient and on any equipment including the sterile field; these drapes must be handled as little as possible. Once a sterile drape is in position, it must not be moved; shifting or moving the sterile drape compromises the sterile field.

For selected high-risk surgery (e.g. orthopedic procedures with implants, transplantation) further specific measures for operating room ventilation may be considered.

Operating Room Staff

Hand Washing

Surgical hand disinfection should be performed by all persons participating in the operative procedure (see hand hygiene).

Operating Room Attire

Operating staff must wear sterile gloves. The reported occurrence of glove punctures ranges from 11.5 to 53 percent of procedures, and double gloving is therefore advisable for procedures with a high risk of puncture such as total joint arthroplasty. Double gloving is also recommended when operating on patients known to be infected with blood borne pathogens such as the human immunodeficiency virus (HIV), hepatitis B, or hepatitis C (10). Gloves should be changed immediately after any accidental puncture.

All persons entering the surgical theater must wear surgical attire restricted to being worn only within the surgical area. The design and composition of the surgical attire should minimize bacterial shedding into the environment.

All head and facial hair, including sideburns, and neckline, must be covered. All personnel entering in the operating suite must remove any jewellery; nail polish or artificial nails must not be worn.

Full coverage of the mouth and nose area with a surgical mask for everyone entering the operating suite is necessary

Sterile surgical gowns must be worn by all persons participating directly in the operation. Waterproof gowns or aprons should be worn for procedures at high risk of blood contamination.

Operating Room Activity

- The number of persons entering the theater during an operation should be minimized.
- Unnecessary movement or conversation should be avoided.

Preintervention Preparation of the Patient

For elective procedures, any existing infections should be identified and treated before surgery. The preoperative stay should be minimized. Any malnourished patient should have nutrition improved before elective surgery.

The patient should normally be bathed or showered on the evening before the intervention, using an antimicrobial soap. If hair removal is required, this should be done by clipping or with a depilatory rather than by shaving.

The operative site must be washed with soap and water, and then an antimicrobial preoperative skin preparation applied from the center to the periphery. The area prepared must be large enough to include the entire incision and adjacent skin sufficient for the surgeon to work without contacting unprepared skin.

The patient must be covered with sterile drapes; no part is uncovered except the operating field and areas needed for the administration and maintenance of anesthesia.

Surgical Wound Surveillance

Prospective surgical wound surveillance should be undertaken for selected procedures.

Infection rates should be stratified by the extent of endogenous bacterial contamination at surgery: clean, clean-contaminated, or dirty.

Surgical wound infection rates may also be stratified by duration of operation and underlying patient status.

Individual surgeons should be provided their own surgical wound infection rates in a confidential manner, with a comparator of overall rates for the facility or region.

Nosocomial Respiratory Infection

Nosocomial respiratory tract infections occur in different patient groups. In some cases, the hospital environment may play a significant role. Recommendations to prevent these infections include:

Ventilator-associated Pneumonia in the Intensive Care Unit

Appropriate disinfection procedures and use of tubing, respirators, and humidifiers to limit contamination.

No routine changes of respirator tubing.

Avoid antacids and H_2 blockers.

Sterile tracheal suctioning.

Nursing in head-up position.

Medical Units

Limit medications which impair consciousness (sedatives, narcotics).

Position the comatose patients to limit the potential for aspiration.

Avoid oral feeds in patients with swallowing abnormalities.

Prevent exposure of neutropenic or transplant patients to fungal spores during construction or renovation.

Surgical Units

All invasive devices used during anesthesia must be sterile.

Anesthetists must use gloves and mask when undertaking invasive tracheal or venous or epidural care. Disposable filters (for individual use) for endotracheal intubation effectively prevent the transmission of microorganisms among patients by ventilators.

Preoperative physiotherapy prevents postoperative pneumonia in patients with chronic respiratory disease.

Neurological Patients with Tracheostomy (with or without Ventilation)

- Sterile suctioning at appropriate frequency.

- Appropriate cleaning and disinfection of respiratory machines and other devices.
- Physiotherapy to assist with drainage of secretions.

Infections Associated with Intravascular Lines

Local (exit site, tunnel) and systemic infections may occur. They are most common in intensive care units. Key practices for all vascular catheters include:
- Avoiding catheterization unless there is a medical indication
- Maintaining a high level of asepsis for catheter insertion and care
- Limiting the use of catheters to as short a duration as possible
- Preparing fluids aseptically and immediately before use
- Training of personnel in catheter insertion and care.

Peripheral Vascular Catheters

- Hands must be washed before all catheter care; using hygienic hand wash or rub
- Wash and disinfect skin at the insertion site with an antiseptic solution
- Intravenous line changes no more frequently than change of catheters, with the exception of line changes after the transfusion of blood or intravenous lipids, and for discontinuous perfusions
- A dressing change is not normally necessary
- If local infection or phlebitis occurs, the catheter should be removed immediately.

Central Vascular Catheters

- Clean the insertion site with an antiseptic solution
- Do not apply solvents or antimicrobial ointment to the insertion site
- Mask, cap, and sterile gloves and gown must be worn for insertion
- The introduction of the catheter and the subsequent catheter dressings require a surgical hand wash or rub
- Follow appropriate aseptic care in accessing the system, including disinfecting external surfaces of hub and ports
- Change of lines should normally not occur more often unless there is an indication
- Change dressing at the time of the change of lines, following surgical asepsis
- Use sterile gauze or transparent dressing to cover the catheter site
- Do not replace over a guide wire if infection is suspected
- An increased number of catheter lumens may increase the risk of infection. A single lumen catheter is preferred wherever possible
- Antimicrobial impregnated catheters may decrease infection in high-risk patients with short-term (<10 days) catheterization
- Use the subclavian site in preference to jugular or femoral sites
- Consider using a peripherally inserted central catheter, if appropriate.

Central Vascular Totally Implanted Catheters

- A preoperative shower and implantation under surgical conditions in an operating room

- Local preparation includes washing and antisepsis with major antiseptic solution as for other surgical procedures
- Mask, hat, sterile gloves and gown must be worn; the introduction of a catheter and the dressing require a surgical hand wash or rub
- Maintain a closed system during the use of the device; a change of lines should normally occur every 5 days for continuous use, and at each intervention for intermittent use; a change of line is necessary after the transfusion of blood, and for discontinuous perfusions.

PREVENTION OF FOOD AND WATER-BORNE INFECTION

Quality and quantity of the food are the essential factors for patient convalescence. Ensuring safe ford is an important service delivery in health care.

Bacterial food poisoning is generally characterized by acute gastroenteritis that occurs after ingestion of contaminated food or water. The infection or intoxication is manifested by abdominal pain and diarrhea with or without vomiting or fever. The symptom may occur within one hour to more than 48 hours after eating the contaminated food. Usually, large numbers of organisms actively multiplying in the food served are required to initiate the symptoms of food poison. Water, milk, solid foods are all the vehicles of transmission. A wide variety of microbial agents are known to cases of food poisoning. Among the most commonly encountered organisms are given in Table 27.6.

Because of the increasing complexity of handling, the frequency of food-borne infection are increasing. Mass–catering and increase in the importation of potentially contaminated food products from the countries are important factors for increasing food-borne illnesses.

Adequate number of organisms in the food, presence of adequate nutrients for the organism to multiply, mistune and warmth for multiplication of the organism or production of toxin between preparation and consumption of food are important risk-factors for food poisoning.

Many inappropriate food handling practices permit contamination, survival and growth of the infecting bacteria. The most common errors that contribute to outbreaks of food poisoning are:

- Preparation of food more than half-a-day in advance of needs
- Storage at room temperature
- Inadequate cooling
- Inadequate reheating

Table 27.6: Microorganisms responsible for food and waterborne infection

Bacteria	*Salmonella* spp, *Staphylococcus, Clostridium perfringens* *Clostridium botulinum, Bacillus cereus* *Escherichia coli, Campylobacter*
Virus	Rotavirus, Calicivirus
Parasites	*Giardia lamblia, Entmoeba histolytica*

- Use of contaminated processed food prepared in premises other than those in which the food was consumed
- Under working
- Cross-contamination from raw to cooked food
- Contamination from food-handling.

Hospital patients may be more susceptible to food-borne infection and suffer more serious consequences than healthy persons. Hence, it is mandatory to maintain high standards of food hygiene. Foods-born outbreaks are promptly investigated and controlled.

Prevention of Food Poisoning

- Clean work area is to be maintained
- Cooked food is protected from cross-contamination with raw food.

Appropriate cooking techniques are to be followed and the recommendations to prevent the growth of organism in the ford should be followed. Scrupulous personal hygiene among food handlers should be maintained especially hand washing. Staff should change work clothes at least once a day and the hair should be kept covered.

Persons suffering from an infection disease in prevented from handling the food and all such infection are to be reported.

Purchased food must be good quality and bacteriologically safe.

Storage facilities must be adequate and correspond to the requirements of the type of the food. The quality of perishable goods should not exceed an amount corresponding to one day consumption.

Dry goods, preserved and canned food should be stored in dry, well-ventilated storage areas and stocks are rotated.

Frozen food storage and preparation should follow the manufactures instruction and be kept at temperature of at least –20°C. Frozen food should not be refreezed.

The catering system environment is washed often and regularly with tap water and detergent or disinfectant samples of the prepared food should be stored for a specified time period to allow retrieval for testing should an outbreak occur. Food handlers are continuously educated and monitored for safe practices.

Water

The physical, chemical and bacteriological standards of water should meet the local regulations. The institution is responsible for the quality of water once it enters the building. For specific uses water taken from the public network must obtain be treated for medical use (physical and chemical treatment).

Drinking water must be safe for consumption. Unless adequate treatment is provided fecal contamination may be sufficient to cause infection through food preparation washing, the can of the patient and even through steam or air inhalation (*Legionella pneumophilia*). Even water that conforms to accepted criteria may carry potentially pathogenic organisms. Micro-organism with nosocomial infection such as wound infection, respiratory tract infection and other sites (semicritical equipment such as endoscopes rinsed with tap water after they are disinfected).

The following organisms are commonly encountered in water-borne infection.

Gram-negative Bacteria

Pseudomonas aeruginosa, Aeromonas hydrophilia, Burkholderia pseudomallei, Stenotrophomonas maltophilia, Serratia marcescens, Falvobacterium eningosepticum, Acenitobacter calcoaaceticus, Legionella pneumophilia, Mycobacterium spp *(Atypical mycobacteria)*

The temperature of the hot water network promotes the development of *Legionella* spp within the protozoan phagosomes, tap water facilities the multiplication of several bacterial species including *Stenotrophomonas maltophilia*. Equipment that uses tap water may be a risk in health care institution; water used for flowers and holy water has also been implicated in nosocomial infection.

Method used for monitoring the quality of water must suit the use. Bacteriological, medical and biochemical methods not necessarily adapted to environmental analyzes and may lead to falsely reassuring results. Important considerations for water ecosystem are biofilm and level of stream for the microorganisms (must receive an exposure to physical and chemical disinfecting agents). This biofilm is a dynamic reservoir for microorganisms.

Bacteriological test may not always give true estimates of contamination because of the presence of agents such as disinfectants.

STERILIZATION AND HIGH-LEVEL DISINFECTION

Sterilization

Sterilization is a process of freeing an article from all living organisms including bacterial and fungal spores and viruses.

All skin and mucous membrane piercing instruments (needles, lancets, scalpels, scissors, etc.), other instruments and equipment coming in contact with organs and tissue during surgical procedures must be sterilized before use.

Sterilization can be achieved by heat (dry and moist) ionizing radiation (gamma radiation, ultraviolet), chemical (formaldehyde, ethylene oxide) and filtration.

However, the only practical and dependable method of sterilization in Health Care Settings is moist heat-steam under pressure utilizing different types (simple, steam jacketed, etc.) of autoclaves. It is important to note that temperature achieved in an autoclave depends on pressure of the steam and not pressure of the steam and air; 15 lbs pressure of steam will correspond to 121°C whereas if 50% air is present, the temperature achieved will be only 112°C whereas if 50% air is present, the temperature achieved will be only 112°C. Table 27.7 illustrates the temperature achieved at same pressure but steam with different amount of air.

The time taken to achieve sterilization depends on the pressure of steam and temperature achieved. Sterilization can be achieved at 15 lbs/sq inch pressure (15 lb/psi) equivalent to one atmospheric pressure and a temperature of 121°C in 15 to 20 minutes (holding time).

Table 27.7: The effect of air on temperature at same pressure (lb/sg in) (psi).

Gauge pressure, i.e. pressure above atmospheric (lb/sq in) (psi)	Temperature in degree centigrade		
	Complete air discharge	Half air discharge	No air discharge
10	115	105	100
15	121	112	100
20	126	118	109
30	135	128	121

An electric or gas oven can be used for sterilization of instruments (blunt instruments, all glass syringes, glassware, etc.) and material (wax, oils, powders, etc.) which are impermeable to steam and can withstand a temperature of 170°C. Household oven can be used for this purpose. The holding time ranges from 60 to 120 minutes depending on the contamination of the material to be sterilized and temperature achieved.

Testing for Sterilizing Efficacy of Autoclave

In hospital settings where sterilization is done centrally (Central Sterile Supply Department, CSSD), it is necessary to monitor if each load has been properly sterilized. There are number of variables in sterilization by autoclave like pressure indicated by autoclave may not be only of steam due to inadequate removal of air resulting in achieving lower temperature at the same pressure, overloading of an autoclave thus inhibiting free passage of steam between the articles, breakdown of electricity during the process of autoclaving particularly during the holding time after the maximum temperature has been achieved. It may be noted that autoclave tapes on packs merely provide an indication that the process has been carried out at or more temperature at which color of the tape changes but not that the contents are sterilized.

It is, therefore, necessary to carry out periodically biological test by putting disk or strips containing at least 10^6 spores of *B. stearothermophillus* (NCTC 10003, or ATCC 7953) in one or more packs in coolest and least accessible part of the autoclave chamber. After autoclaving, check the strip if all the spores have been destroyed or not by culturing in suitable liquid medium (Tryptone soya broth) at 56°C for 5 days.

High Level of Disinfection

High level of disinfection is a process of destroying all microorganisms; however, some spores may survive particularly if initially present in large numbers.

High level of disinfection can be achieved by continuous boiling for 20 to 30 minutes. This is simplest and most reliable method for freeing an article from most of the pathogenic microorganisms including HIV and HBV, in situations where sterilization by autoclaving is not possible.

High level of disinfection can also be achieved by exposure to vapors of ethylene oxide (Ethylene oxide sterilizer) and formaldehyde (Formaldehyde disinfector and low temperature steam formaldehyde sterilizer) or by soaking in chemical disinfectants like activated glutaraldehyde and carbolic acid for prolonged period.

Instruments and equipments like vaginal specula, proctoscope laryngoscope, flexible fiberoptic endoscope, etc. which come in contact with intact mucous membrane but do not penetrate; it should ideally be sterilized, however, if sterilization is not possible they must be exposed to thigh level of disinfection.

Syringes, needles and other skin piercing instruments can also be used after high level of disinfection by boiling when autoclaving is not possible.

Chemical disinfectants must never be used for syringes and needles.

HIV is resistant to ultraviolet and gamma radiation and X-rays. Dry cleaning also does not inactivate or kill HIV.

Thorough cleaning and washing has great role in freeing an object of organic matter and most of the microorganisms. Washing with warm detergent removes most of the pathogenic microorganisms. This must preceded sterilization and disinfection process.

Disinfection

Disinfection is a process of destruction or removal of organisms capable of giving rise to infection. Disinfectants are capable of killing vegetative bacteria, fungi, viruses and rarely spores. Through long usage, the term 'disinfectant' has become closely associated with chemical substances.

The disinfection must never be used when sterilization is possible. Disinfectant may not kill even the susceptible organisms since disinfectants take time to act which varies with the microbial load, presence of organic matter, temperature, pH, etc.

Instruments and equipment that come in contact with intact skin but do not pierce, it should be disinfected between each patient contact.

Disinfection of skin and mucous membrane must be carried out before use of any skin piercing instrument or equipment.

Contaminated instruments equipment and material must be disinfected to make it safe to handle before sterilization (autoclaving) of re-useable material or disposal of material which is not to be reused.

Contaminated floor, surfaces like trolley tops, table tops, trays, clothes linen, beddings, bed, crockery, enamel and stainless steel utensils and other articles like bedpan, urine bottles, bowls, etc. should be disinfected before use. Environment of operation theatre, ward or other rooms may require disinfection rarely.

In the recent years, a variety of disinfectant preparations in hospital use have been found to harbor pathogenic bacteria giving rise to outbreaks of infection. It is, therefore, essential to have a suitable disinfection policy for a hospital.

Most of the disinfectants used for health care purposes in this country, if used in proper concentration, are effective against HIV and HBV. However, chemical disinfectants may not be depended upon for satisfactory disinfection of blood and blood contaminated material, since blood and other organic matter may inactivate the disinfectant used. Further, it may not reach the virus present in the blood clot. Therefore, objects to be disinfected should be thoroughly cleaned by detergent in warm water and dried before disinfecting. It is not only necessary to use proper concentration of disinfectant for different situations but also it is necessary to maintain this concentration as the strength may decrease due to improper preparation and storage. Soaking the wet instruments in disinfectant fluid may result in dilution of the disinfectant which is being used. Thus, it is necessary to remove all contamination from the instruments before immersing them in disinfectant fluid may result in dilution of the disinfectant which is being used. Thus, it is necessary to remove all contamination from the instruments before immersing them in disinfectant fluid. Chemical disinfectants must not be used for needles and syringes (Table 27.8).

Table 27.8: Concentrations/dilutions of the different disinfectants to be used in 'clean contaminated' and 'grossly contaminated' conditions

Disinfectants	*Recommended conc./dilution*	
	Clean contaminated	*Grossly contaminated 'dirty'*
I. Chlorine releasing compounds Available chlorine	0.1%	1.0%
1. Sodium hypochlorite Liquid bleach (Usually 5% available chlorine)	I g/L (1000 ppm) 20 mL/L	10 g/L (10000 ppm) 200 mL/L
2. Calcium hypochlorite (Usually 70% available chlorine)	1.4 g/L	14.0 g/L
3. Sodium dichloroisocyanurate (NaDCC) (Usually 60% available chlorine) (More stable, available as tablets of 1.5 g available chlorine)	1.7 g/L	14.0 g/L
4. Chloramine-T Slow chlorine release (More stable than 1, 2) (25% available chlorine)	20 g/L	20 g/L
II. Iodine compounds		
1. Tincture of iodine (Iodine 0.5% + Alcohol 70%)	2.5%	2.5%
2. Povidone iodine (PVI) (Usually 10% Sol. (1% iodine) Povidone iodine (Betadine)	2.5%	2.5%
III. Aldehydes		
1. Glutaraldehyde (Activated) (Cidex: 2% glutaraldehyde)	2.0%	2.0%
2. Formaldehyde-formaline (40% Solution of formaldehyde)	5% (2% formaldehyde)	10% (4% formaldehyde)
IV. Alcohols		
1. Ethyl alcohol	70%	70%
2. Isopropyl alcohol	70%	70%
3. Methylated spirit (Denatured alcohol)	70%	70%
V. Hydrogen peroxide	6% (Freshly prepared)	Not recommended
Bottles/bowls	Phenols/chlorhexidine	

Contd...

Contd...

Disinfectants	*Recommended conc./dilution*	
	Clean contaminated	*Grossly contaminated 'dirty'*
Surfaces Floor/walls/trolleys/furniture/sinks/wash basins	Wash with detergents, disinfect with chlorine acid/PVI/ hexachlorophenes	
Humidifiers and incubators	Fill daily humidifiers with sterile distilled water containing % silver nitrate. Clean and disinfect with chlorine releasing compounds/ activated glutaraldehyde/alcohol or carbolic acid	
Crockery/cutlery	Wash with warm detergent solution keep in boiling water for 10 minutes or expose to steam. No chemical disinfectant should be used	
Syringes and needles	Chemical disinfectant must not be used for needle and syringes.	
Instruments, Cheatle's forceps	Keep in concentration recommended for grossly contaminated articles of PVI/Chlorhexidine + cetrimides/ chloroxylenols, glutaraldehyde. Change the disinfectant daily.	
Sharp instruments Skin piercing and invasive	Keep in concentration recommended, for grossly contaminated situations, activated glutaraldehyde for at least 10 hours	
Instruments Equipment Catheters Cystocope or endoscope Laparoscope	Chemical disinfection only as last resort, if sterilization by heat is not possible Immerse in activated solution of glutaraldehyde for 4 to 10 hours or more for sterilization Only vegetative bacteria, fungi and viruses are killed by immersing in surface disinfectants for 30 minutes.	

The widespread use of disinfectants in the hospital and undue reliability on the 'disinfected' material warrant a regular monitoring of the disinfectants in hospital use. The manufacturers usually supply information regarding the activity of disinfectant against a variety of organisms as well as other relevant details regarding toxicity, corrosiveness and compatibility. However, disinfectants are only useful when used in proper concentration for appropriate time. It is however, better to carry out an independent test to determine or confirm the in-use dilution, necessary for the particular purpose.

All endoscopes are subjected to high-level disinfection and it involves six steps.

1. Clean mechanically external surfaces, ports and internal channels with water and an enzymatic detergent (follow the manufacturer's instructions while using the enzymatic detergent). Disconnect the camera from the scope.
2. Rinse and drain the channels.
3. Immerse the endoscope in two percent glutaraldehyde placed in a suitable plastic container with lid and perfuse the disinfectant into the suction/biopsy channel air and water channel and expose at least for 20 minutes.

Table 27.9: Disinfection time for various endoscopes

Endoscope	*Disinfection*
Flexible endoscope	20 minutes between patient, beginning and at the end of the list 60 minutes on a known case of pulmonary TB or immunocompromized patient
Cystoscope	10 minutes between the patient beginning and at the end of the list, 60 minutes on suspected case of tuberculosis
Gastrointestinal endoscope	20 minutes between the patient 20 minutes beginning and at the end of the list 60 minutes on a HIV reactive case and immunosuppressed patient
Arthroscope and laparoscope	20 minutes between patients

4. Endoscopes are cleaned or rinsed with sterile water after removing them from the disinfecting container. If this is not feasible, use tap water followed with alcohol rinse.
5. The insertion tube and the inner channels should be dried by means of forced air after disinfection and before storage.
6. Endoscopes should be stored in a way that prevents contamination. Cross-infections are more common when the disinfection is inadequate.
7. Automatic endoscope re-process machines have been linked with outbreaks of infection and colonization. Hence, they are not recommended for use.

Cleaning of the Endoscopes

Cleaning of the endoscopes just before sterilization is extremely effective in eliminating microorganisms with a mean log (99.9%) reduction in microbial contamination.

If cleaning is not possible and organic matter with high microbial load is present, immerse in 2.4 percent alkaline glutaraldehyde for 45 minutes at 25°C may be necessary for 100% tuberculocidal effect.

However, with proper cleaning with enzymatic detergent, 20 minutes exposure at room temperature is 100% effective (Table 27.9).

PROLONGED IMMERSION IN DISINFECTANT IS NOT A SUBSTITUTE TO CLEANING BEFORE STERILIZATION/DISINFECTION

Laparoscope and Arthroscope

Laparoscope, arthroscope and other endoscopes that enter normally sterile tissue should be subjected to sterilization procedure, and if sterilization is not feasible high-level disinfection should be done.

If high-level disinfection is used, a sterile water rinse is required to prevent contamination with tap water microorganisms.

After proper rinsing the endoscope must be dried accordingly to a method that does not recontaminate them.

OCCUPATIONAL HEALTH

Health Maintenance

1. Employment physical screening includes:
   a. Physical screening assessment (including review of immunization status).
   b. Tuberculin skin test (unless known positive reactor).
   c. Chest X-ray, if indicated.
2. Annual physical screening—completed by the Office of Occupational Health:
   a. Physical screening assessment.
   b. Tuberculin skin test (unless known positive reactor). (Required for All "Volunteers" and "Sisters" as well as other regular full-time and part-time employees).
   c. A screening assessment is completed on known TST reactors.
   d. Assessment/documentation immunizations.
      i. Review of adult required immunizations.
      ii. Referral to appropriate health care provider as indicated.

Health Education

1. Information on infection control and health issues is provided to new employees during orientation. The employee is informed of his/her job classification category, the exposure control plan and the hepatitis vaccine program. An introduction to the Infection Control Manual is given.
2. Individual counseling is provided to employees by the Occupational Health and Injury Services as indicated (i.e. exposure to blood/body fluids or health-related issues).

Immunizations

Hepatitis B Vaccine

a. New employees are offered the hepatitis B vaccine in orientation. They are requested to sign a consent/refusal form that is forwarded to the Office of Occupational Health. Employees will report to the Occupational Health to schedule/receive the vaccine.
b. Current employees may request the vaccine and receive it at a scheduled date and time.
c. The vaccine is also offered following a true exposure to blood/body fluids, if the employees have not previously been vaccinated.

Influenza Vaccine

a. The influenza vaccine is offered annually. Employees are notified of the dates and times that the vaccine will be administered.

Tetanus Vaccine

a. Employees are advised to maintain their tetanus immunization status, with boosters every ten years and as indicated by injury.

Measles Vaccine

a. Employees born in or after 1957 are advised to verify measles immunization or evidence of measles immunity.
b. Employees who cannot verify immunity will be referred to their private physician or the public health department for evaluation/immunization.

Chickenpox Vaccine

a. Employees who cannot verify immunity will be referred to their private physician or public health department when appropriate.

Procedure for Completing Hepatitis Immunization

1. All consent/refusal forms for hepatitis B vaccine received in Occupational Health will be entered into the computer database. New employees are instructed, during orientation, to report to the Occupational Health office to the schedule, an appointment to begin the vaccination series. Current employees are notified of the routine dates and times of vaccine administration at the time of their annual physical screen and upon inquiry.
2. New employees documenting that they have received the hepatitis B vaccine will be offered screening for an anti-HBs (antibody screening). If the individual is negative for the antibodies, the vaccine will be offered and administered as request.
3. Employees will receive a series of three hepatitis B vaccines, the initial dose followed by a second dose one month later and a third dose five months after the second dose.
4. Employees are scheduled for antiHBs (antibody screening) two months after third dose of hepatitis B vaccine.
5. If the antibody screening is negative (no antibodies formed) a second series of 3 immunizations will be offered.
6. In the event of a true exposure, employees who have a negative antiHBs may receive the hepatitis B vaccine series again.

Emergency Care

Exposure to Blood/Body Fluids

a. The hospital must designate a process for providing post–exposure prophylaxis or HIV to employees within 2 hours of exposure. This procedure must be published and known to the staff.
b. Assessment for the need for post-exposure prophylaxis for hepatitis is available to all staff through the office of Occupational Health. Staff has to report to Occupational Health for evaluation and referral on the first regular working day following exposure.

Illness from Communicable Disease

a. Employees with known or suspected communicable diseases/conditions shall notify their supervisors and the office of Occupational Health.

b. Employees who have acute infections with communicable diseases must seek treatment by their private physician or the local emergency room/urgent care center.
c. The employees are prohibited from direct client care until the communicable disease/ condition is resolved.
d. A written certification that the employee is no longer a danger to clients or other employees is required prior to return to work.
e. All documentation of medical information regarding the communicable illness must be sent to the office of Occupational Health to be placed in the employee's record.

EMPLOYEES WHO REPORT THAT THEY ARE HIV POSITIVE

Kamineni hospitals will comply with Centre for Disease Control and Prevention (CDC) guidelines relating to invasive procedures and the HIV status of employees. In the event that a health care worker reports to his or her supervisor that he or she is HIV positive, that individual's duties will be reviewed by a team comprised of the employee, his or her supervisor, the clinical director, and any other person indicated and agreed upon by the people listed here. This team will determine if any limitations must be placed on that individual's assigned duties based on the infectious process involved.

Maintenance of Health Records

Medical information is maintained in a confidential record in the human resources department. Information regarding immunizations, blood and body fluid exposures and reports of communicable disease is maintained in the Office of the Occupational Health. Information can only be released with the written consent of the employee as required by law (Table 27.10).

Staff must assess the risk of exposure to blood or body fluids for each situation and determine what PPE is needed. If a staff member is unsure what PPE to use, that staff member must consult his or her supervisor before proceeding.

Methods of Minimizing the Risk of Transmission of Infection

1. Hand washing facilities or the approved waterless antiseptic hand cleanser will be accessible at all times.
   Supervisors will ensure that employees wash their hands and other skin surfaces.
   i. Immediately if contaminated with blood or other body fluids, and
   ii. Immediately or as soon as feasible after removing gloves and other PPE
2. Engineering and work practice controls minimize the opportunities for exposure to blood-borne pathogens.
3. Personal protective equipment will be used in situations in which occupational exposure remains after engineering and work practice controls are instituted. Supervisors will ensure that appropriate PPE is used.

Table 27.10: Tasks posing risk of contact with blood and body fluids and recommended protective measures

Task	*Recommended protective measure*			
	Gloves	*Gown/Apron*	*Eyewear*	*Mask*
PO medication administration	X			
PO medication administration	X			
Oral examination	X			
Genitourinary examination	X			
Rectal examination	X			
Enteral feeding	X			
Assisting client bathing	X			
Assisting client toileting	X			
Assisting client eating	X			
Assisting client	X			
Assisting client brushing teeth	X			
Handling contaminated linen, clothing, equipment, instruments, etc	X	S		
Cleaning contaminated items, floors, work surfaces	X	S	**	**

X = Routinely only for identified potential contact of non-intact skin with blood/body fluids
S = Only if soiling by blood/body fluids is likely
** = Only if splash, splatter or aerosolization of blood, body fluids is likely

4. Safety needles and sharps will be used unless an exception is made by the Facility Infection Control Committee with approval by the Facility Medical Executive Committee.
5. Eating, drinking, smoking, applying cosmetics or lip balm and handling contact lenses is prohibited in work areas where there is a likelihood of occupational exposure to blood or other potentially infectious materials.
6. Food and drink will not be stored in any area where blood or other potentially infectious materials are present.
7. Procedures involving blood or other potentially infectious materials shall be performed in such a manner so as to prevent or minimize splash/spray/spatter and the generation of droplets of said substances.
8. All specimens of blood and body fluids will be put into a leak-proof container during collection, handling, processing, storing, transporting, or shipping.
9. When specimens of blood and/or other body fluids are transported away from the facility, they will be labeled as potentially infectious and transported according to Department of Transportation policy and procedure.
10. Only the chemical germicides that have been approved for use as hospital disinfectants will be used to decontaminate spills of blood and visible bloody body fluids and for cleaning those areas.

11. Warning labels will be prominently and firmly attached to container holding and potentially infectious materials. Labels will clearly state the contents and/or include the 'Biohazard' logo.
12. Signs will be posted at the entrance to work areas that have been determined to pose and occupational hazard for employees.
13. Each division of mental health and development disabilities hospital will provide to all employees training designed to teach the employees how to limit the risk of occupational exposure.

Surveillance, Prevention, and Control of Antibiotic Resistant Organisms (ARO)

Purpose

To prevent transmission of antibiotic resistant organisms among all persons within the health care facility; to reduce colonization among infected and non-infected persons and to reduce the possibility of transmission and subsequent infection; and to reduce morbidity and mortality associated with antibiotic-resistant organisms.

The Infection Control Nurse maintains a surveillance line listing of current and past client who are colonized and/or infected with antibiotic resistant organisms.

The ICN monitors trends in the patterns of the ARO's over time and reports these trends to the Infection Control Committee.

The ICN will immediately report outbreaks or sudden increases in the rate of ARO infection/colonization to the appropriate attending physician and clinical director as well as to the chairman of the Infection Control Committee.

The ICN will conduct an epidemic analysis of an ARO outbreak, including collection of information on all ARO- infected clients such as:

1. Client's location in the institution (before and after cohorting)
2. Date of admission and recent previous admissions
3. The names of care givers who have had directed contact with the client
4. Body site of infection or colonization
5. Age, gender, and race
6. Diagnosis, and
7. Treatment given.

These factors are evaluated for the group of ARO infected clients to aid the identification of common features that may lead to specific control strategies.

Indiscriminate use of antibiotics will be avoided at all times.

Individuals with a history of ARO infection or colonization will be identified by a label placed in the medical record. This label will remain in the chart for the duration of the hospitalization.

Staff will notify the staff of other hospital services and other facilities of the individual's history ARO colonization/infection prior to transfer/travel to those departments/facilities.

The presence of an antibiotic resistant organism does not automatically warrant admission to an acute care facility. Admission to an acute care facility for treatment is based upon the presence of clinical signs and symptoms that warrant treatment and the clinical judgment of the physician.

The decision to provide treatment for a positive culture for ARO is based on the clinical signs and symptoms of infection, not on the positive culture.

During an outbreak, all ARO infected clients will be physically separated from non-infected clients with no staff crossover between the two groups (cohorting), if possible. Should strict cohorting not be achievable, every effort to dedicate staff to those identified infected clients should be made.

Two consecutive negative cultures 24 hours apart obtained 48 hours after the completion of antibiotics is the criterion for the release from cohorting for MRSA infections.

Three negative stool cultures one week apart and two consecutive negative cultures from the site is the criterion for release from cohorting in VRE infections.

Upon discharge to home or a community agency, discharge instructions, both verbal and written, will be given to the client/family and facility or agency. These instructions will address the prevention of the spread of the antibiotic resistant organism and the risk to the individuals in the environment.

NEEDLE STICK INJURIES

What is the Risk?

The main risk of needle stick injuries is exposure of the health care worker to blood-borne virus infections like:

Hepatitis B

Hepatitis C

Human immunodeficiency virus (HIV).

In case of HBV protective vaccine is available. But for other viruses there is no such protection as on to day and these conditions are difficult to treat. Hence, it is always better to take precautions to prevent the needle stick injuries.

Who are at Risk?

Category I

Employees whose duties include routine or reasonably anticipated exposure to blood or body fluids or other potentially infectious materials. These staff include, but are not limited to:

a. Physicians, advanced practice nurses, physicians assistants
b. Nursing staff (RN, LPN, CNA)
c. Dentists
d. Dental hygienists, dental assistants
e. Direct care staff
f. Clinical laboratory personnel
g. Phlebotomists
h. Radiology technologist/technicians.

Category II

Employees whose duties include infrequently anticipated exposure to blood or body fluids or other potentially infectious materials. These staff include, but are not limited to:

a. Laundry personnel
b. Environmental service personnel
c. EEG/EKG technicians
d. PT/OT/RT personnel
e. Teachers/Instructors
f. Behavior specialists
g. Psychologists
h. Police
i. Volunteers
j. Foster grandparents.

Category III

Employees whose duties do not include routine or reasonably anticipated exposure to blood or body fluids or other potentially infectious materials. These staff include, but are not limited to:

a. Clerical staff
b. Medical records personnel
c. Plant operations personnel
d. Plant operations personnel
e. Warehouse personnel
f. Dietary staff
g. Business/administrative personnel
h. Nonnursing departments heads
i. Pharmacy staff
j. Human resources personnel.

Prevention of Needle Stick Injuries

1. Hand washing thoroughly with a disinfectant soap and running water
2. Obtain the history of vaccination
3. If vaccinated check for the antibody titers and if they are adequate no treatment is necessary
4. If not vaccinated and the source is either positive for hepatitis B or HIV or hepatitis C refer to the physician who will further follow the case with appropriate treatment such as IV human immunoglobulin G or vaccination against HBV and tetanus.
5. Use appropriate personal protection equipment such as gloves, eye-wear, aprons, etc.
6. Safe disposal of needles, sharps and broken glass pieces into appropriate puncture proof containers filled with a suitable disinfectant such as one percent sodium hypochlorite solution.

7. Do not over fill the sharp containers.
8. Follow universal precautions meticulously.
9. Never recap the needles. If it is unavoidable, place the syringe horizontally and the cap as well and carefully insert the needle into the cap.
10. Do not hand over the syringes or needles directly. Place them in a container.
11. Report all needle stick injuries and injuries due to sharps.
12. Take vaccine for hepatitis B and if needed for tetanus as well.
13. In case of any needle stick or sharp injury, please refer to procedure for HIV testing.

PROTOCOL FOR THE MANAGEMENT OF EXPOSURE TO BLOOD-BORNE PATHOGENS-EMPLOYEES

1. Determine if a true exposure has occurred. If no true exposure has occurred, there is no need to proceed. If there has been a true exposure, proceed with the following protocol.
2. Complete the employee-exposure to blood-borne pathogens report form and forward this form to occupational health.
3. Refer the employee to the identified local resource to evaluate the need for and provide HIV prophylaxis if indicated. This medication must be started within 2 hours of exposure.
4. Refer the employee to occupational health for follow-up.
   The Office of Occupational Health will maintain and make available:
   I. To the health care professional(s) responsible for the hepatitis B vaccination program, a copy of the OSHA regulation, blood-borne pathogens, and
   II. To the health care professional(s) responsible for evaluating an individual after an exposure incident.
      - A copy of the OSHA regulation, bloodborne pathogens # 1910.1030
      - A description of the exposed employee's duties as they relate to the exposure incident
      - Documentation of the route(s) of exposure and circumstances under which the exposure occurred
      - Results of the source individual's blood testing, if available; and
      - All medical records that are contained in the employee's health file and that are relevant to the appropriate treatment of the employee, including immunization status.
5. The Office of Occupational Health will establish and maintain an accurate record for the each employee who has had an occupational exposure. This record will include:
   a. The name and identification number of the employee;
   b. A copy of the employee's hepatitis B immunization status, including the dates of all the hepatitis vaccinations and any medical records related to the employee's ability to receive the vaccination;
   c. A copy of the results of the examinations, medical testing and follow-up procedures performed in the post-exposure evaluation and follow-up.

EMPLOYEE EXPOSURE TO BLOOD-BORNE PATHOGENS

Occupational Health

DateReportPrepared:____________________TimeReportPrepared:____________________

Name of Employee: ____________________ SS#: ____________________

Source of Exposure: Client Other Source ID#

HBV Status of Source: Date __________ Result ____________________

HCV Status of Source: Date __________ Result ____________________

RPR Status of Source: Date __________ Result ____________________

HIV Status of Source: Date __________ Result ____________________

If status is not known and is determined to be needed, send source individual's blood for testing HBV, HCV, RPR. And HIV after consent is obtained.

Time/Date Exposure Occurred: ____________________

Place Where Exposure Occurred: ____________________

Exposure Type (Check One)

Parenteral contact, e.g. needle stick/other sharps with blood/body fluids.

Mucous membrane exposure, e.g. eye, nose, mouth.

Blood/body fluids to non-intact skin, e.g. dermatitis, lacerations, bites, deep scratches, abrasion, cuts soiled dressing, catheters, etc.

Alleged sexual contact (oral, vaginal, rectal).

Date Referred to Health Care Provider for Evaluation: ____________________

Complete Summary of Incident:

Reporting Individual: ____________________

Date: ____________________

CONSENT FOR HIV TESTING

Please initial your choice and sign below.

I authorize the hospital to test me for HIV, the virus that causes acquired immunodeficiency syndrome (AIDS) and related syndromes.

In signing this consent form, I acknowledge that I have been provided with information about this test, about the HIV virus and about AIDS. I have been given the opportunity to ask questions regarding this information and my questions have been answered.

I have been informed that both my request for HIV test and test results are considered confidential and will be released only to me except as required or permitted by law.

If the test results are positive, I will be provided information about the consequences for my own health care so that I might take precautions to prevent transmission of the virus to others.

I understand that Georgia law requires the reporting of confirmed positive test results to the Public Health Department.

I understand that, unless otherwise limited by state and federal regulations, and except to the extent that action has been taken which was based on my consent, I may withdraw this consent at any time.

I do not authorize blood collection for HIV antibody testing.

_________________________ _________________________

Signature of Employee Signature of Witness

SSN _________________________ Date _________________________

I have consulted with the above-mentioned person about testing him or her for HIV, about availability and necessity of post-testing counseling, and that test results will be handled confidentially as prescribed by law.

_________________________ _________________________

Date Signature of Physician

(EMPLOYEES ONLY)

Glossary

BODY FLUIDS

- **Amniotic fluid**—fluid produced by the innermost layer of the placenta early in gestation and contained within the amniotic sac surrounding the embryo *in utero*.
- **Ascitic fluid**—serous fluid aspirated from the abdominal cavity (the peritoneum).
- **Bile**—a brown-green fluid secreted by the liver and either poured into the intestine or concentrated in the gallbladder.
- **Bone marrow**—the soft, highly cellular, blood-forming tissue that fills bone cavities.
- **Joint (synovial) fluid**—alkaline, thick fluid contained in joint cavities, bursae, and tendon sheaths serving as a lubricant.
- **Pericardial fluid**—fluid contained within the membranous sac that encases the heart.
- **Peritoneal fluid**—same as ascitic fluid.
- **Pleural fluid**—fluid within the thoracic cavity which encases the lungs.
- **Spinal fluid**—fluid contained within the membranous coverings of the spinal cord and brain within the space known as the subarachnoid space.
- **Transudate**—fluid which has passed through a membrane or extruded from a tissue and characterized by its low viscosity, lack of protein, and cells or cellular debris, and by having a specific gravity under 1.013.

EYE

- **Conjunctiva**—the mucous membrane covering the anterior surface of the eyeball and the under surfaces of the eyelids.
- **Inner canthus**—the inner (nasal) angle formed by the union of the upper and lower eyelids.
- **Lid**—folds of skin that protect the anterior eyeball surface.

GENITAL (FEMALE)

- **Bartholin's gland**—one of two, small, mucus-secreting glands on either side of the vaginal orifice.

- **Cervical aspirate**—mechanical withdrawal of material from the cervix.
- **Culdocentesis**—aspiration of fluid from rectouterine excavation by puncture of the vaginal wall.
- **Endocervical**—from the interior of the cervix.
- **Endometrium**—the mucous membrane comprising the inner lining of the uterine cavity.
- **Fallopian tube**—tube from uterus to ovary.
- **Female genital**—nondescript term generally taken to mean a vaginal/cervical specimen.
- **Lochia**—the final vaginal discharge occurring 1 to 2 weeks after childbirth.
- **Ovary**—reproductive egg-forming gland within the pelvis in the female, lying lateral to the uterus.
- **Perineum**—the space between the anus and the scrotum of the male and the anus and vulva of the female.
- **Placenta**—highly vascularized organ of pregnancy, composed of multiple layers within the gravid uterus, supplying nutrients and gas exchange to the fetus.
- **Placenta (C-section)**—(see placenta) a result of a cesarean section.
- **Urethra**—from the membraneous canal conveying urine from the bladder to the exterior of the body.
- **Uterus**—hollow, muscular organ in the female in which the fetus develops.
- **Vaginal**—from the canal that extends from the vulva to the cervix.
- **Vulva**—the region of the external female genitals.

GENITAL (MALE)

- **Lesion**—a more or less circumscribed pathologic or traumatic injury to tissue.
- **Penile exudate**—exudate expressed through the urethra.
- **Prostate**—a gland which, in the male, surrounds the neck of the bladder and the urethra.
- **Urethral**—see above.

LOWER RESPIRATORY TRACT

- **Bronchial**—referring to the large air passages which dichotomously branch within the lungs.
- **Bronchial aspirate**—material collected from the bronchi by means of instrumentation.
- **Fiberoptic**—collection of material with an instrument designed for visualization of the lower respiratory area and for specimen collection.
- **Sputum**—matter ejected from the lungs, bronchi, and trachea through the mouth.
- **Tracheal**—the tube from the larynx to the bronchi.
- **Transtracheal aspirate**—material obtained by surgical passage of a catheter through the tracheal wall and into the lower respiratory area.

UPPER RESPIRATORY TRACT

- **Ear**—unless specified, refers to the external ear.
- **Mouth and dental**—gums, gingivae, teeth, root canals, tongue, etc.
- **Nasopharynx**—that part of the pharynx above the soft palate.
- **Nose (nasal)**—in microbiology the term usually refers to culture obtained from about 1 to 2 cm deep within the nostril.
- **Sinus**—anybody cavity, hollow space, or open channel.
- **Throat**—that area within the deep oral cavity between and including the tonsillar pillars from where cultures are obtained.
- **Stool/rectal**—a term referring to the fecal discharge from the bowels.

SURFACE SPECIMENS

- **Burn**—traumatic lesion caused by contact of tissue with heat.
- **Cyst**—any liquid- or exudate-containing sac.
- **Decubitus**—ulceration due to prolonged pressure of lying down or sitting.
- **Exudate**—fluid containing protein, cells or solid material, which has escaped from blood vessels as a result of injury or inflammation.
- **Laceration**—a cut.
- **Lesion**—see genital (male).
- **Paronychia**—inflammation involving the folds of skin around the fingernails.
- **Skin**—external body covering.
- **Stoma**—any small opening or orifice on a free surface, i.e. the opening from a colostomy or ileostomy site.
- **Suture**—a surgical "stitch".
- **Ulcer**—a loss of integrity of a cutaneous or mucous surface lining resulting from the sudden or gradual sloughing of necrotic tissue.
- **Vesicle**—a small blister containing a serous liquid.

SURGICAL SPECIMENS

- **Abscess**—localized collection of pus in a cavity formed by disintegration of tissue.
- **Aspirate**—removal of fluids from a cavity by suction.
- **Biopsy**—surgical removal of small portions of tissue from a living body for the purpose of establishing a precise diagnosis.
- **Bone**—mineralized connective tissue that makes up the skeleton of vertebrates.
- **Clot**—a semisolid mass, usually of blood or lymph.
- **Drain**—an artifically placed device used to create a channel by which fluid or pus can be exited from a cystic space or body cavity.
- **Exudate**—see surface specimens.
- **Fistula**—an abnormal passage or communication between two organs or to the outside.

- **Hematoma**—a tumor of effused blood—a bruise.
- **IV catheter**—tubing used to infuse sterile material into the veins.
- **Prosthesis**—an artificial body part.
- **Pus**—a liquid inflammatory product of leukocytes and fluid.
- **Stone**—a very hard mass or calculus usually composed of mineral salts.
- **Tissue**—a surgically removed mass of body cells.
- **Wound**—see lesion, genital (male).

URINE

- **Catheterized**—urine aspirated from a urinary catheter.
- **Midstream**—urine collected in a container after the first few milliliters of urine has been passed.
- **Suprapubic**—urine surgically aspirated with syringe and needle by direct puncture into the bladder.

Index

Page numbers followed by *f* refer to figure and *t* refer to table, respectively.

B

C

Q

R

U

V

W

X

Y

Z